Neurological and Mental Disorders

Edited by Kaneez Fatima Shad and Kamil Hakan Dogan

Published in London, United Kingdom

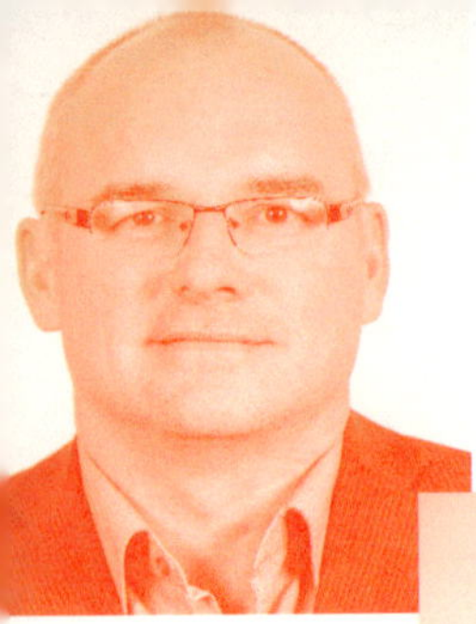
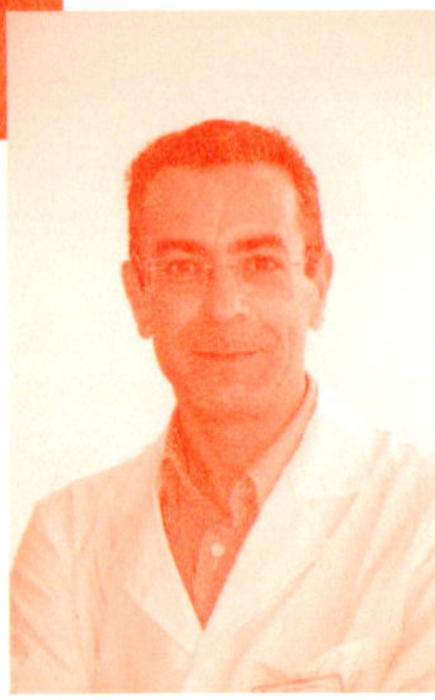
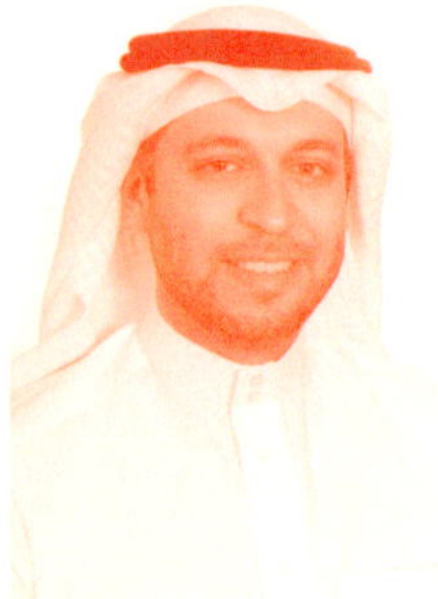
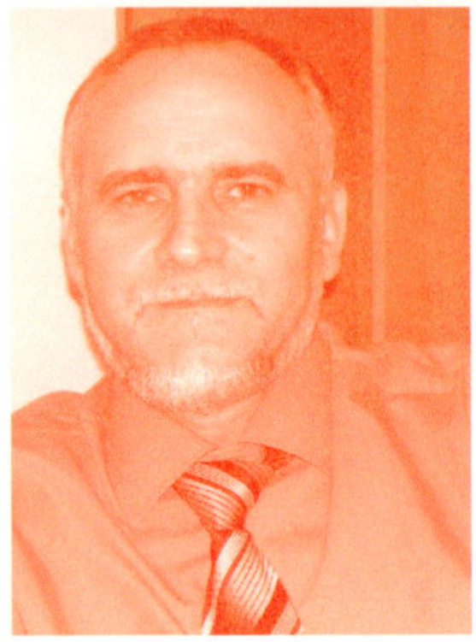
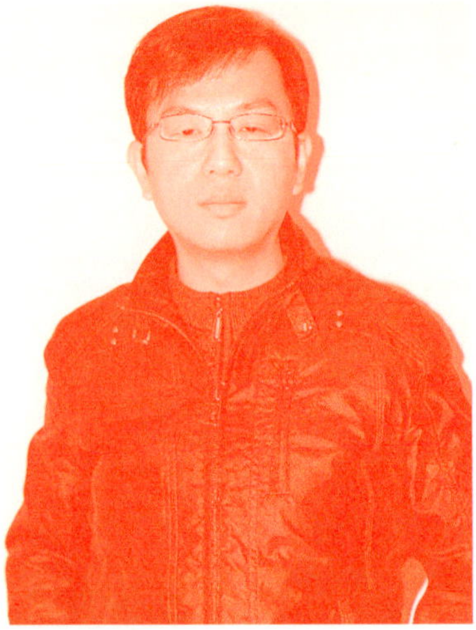
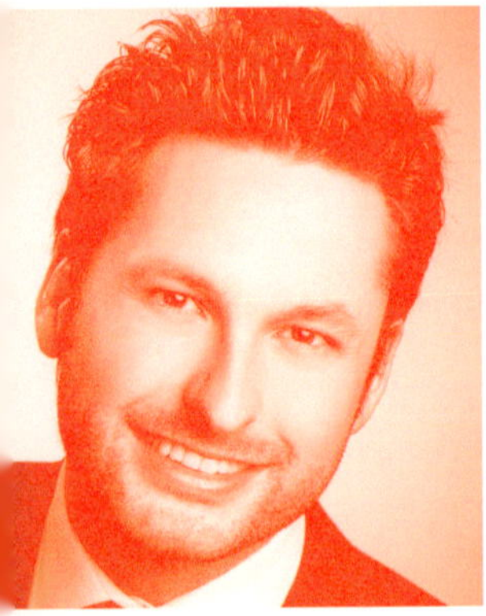
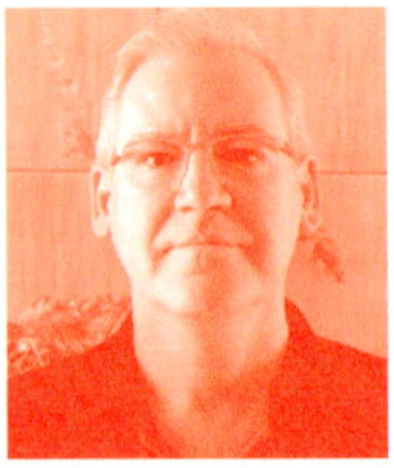

IntechOpen

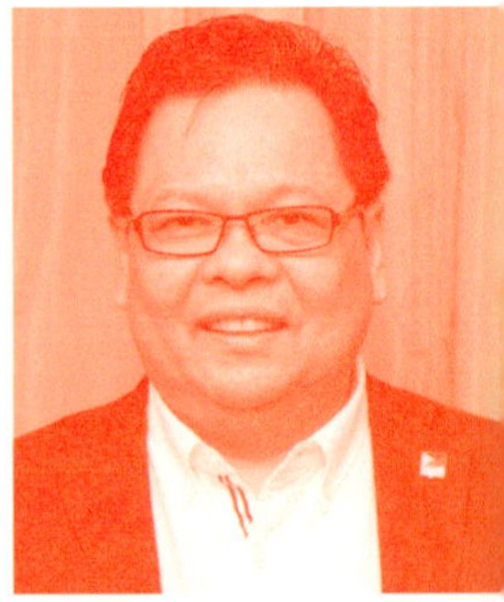
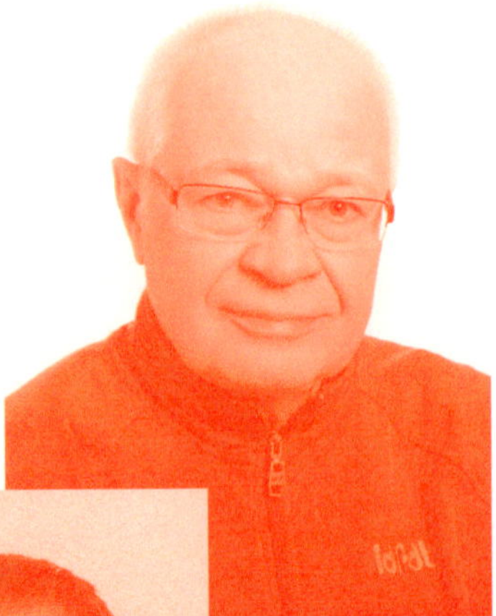
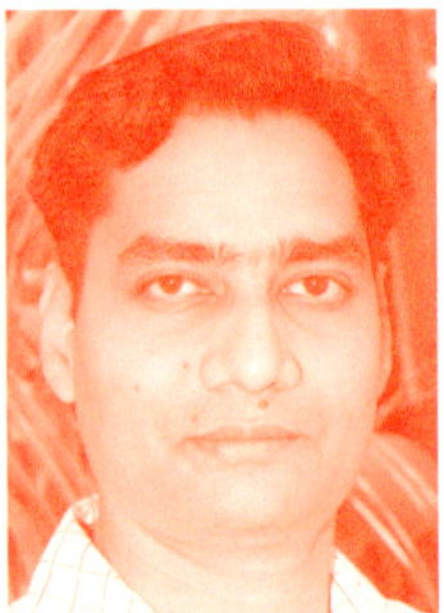
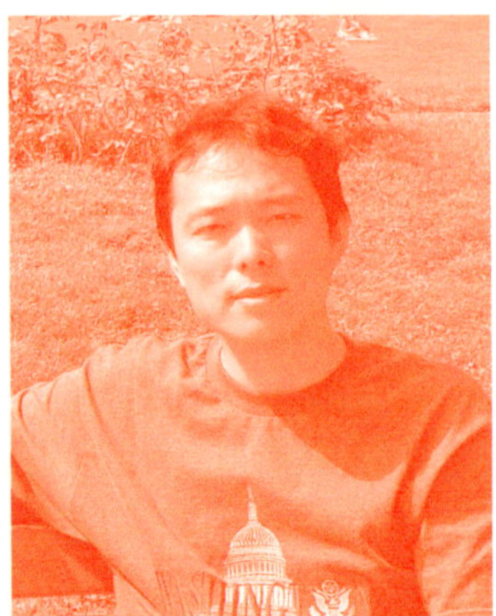
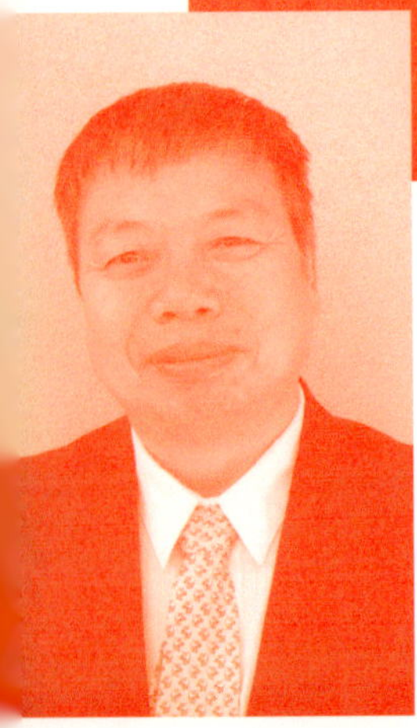
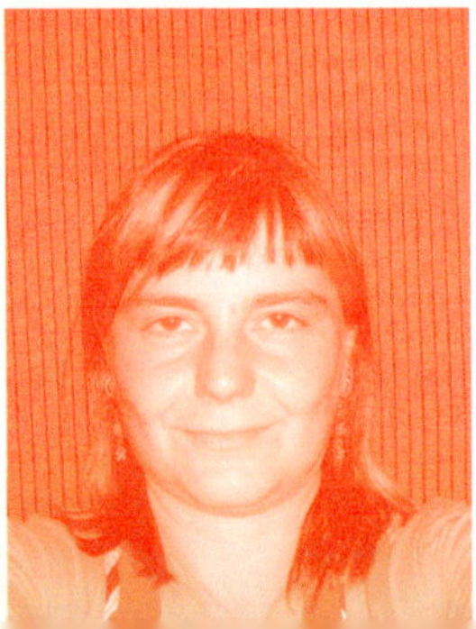

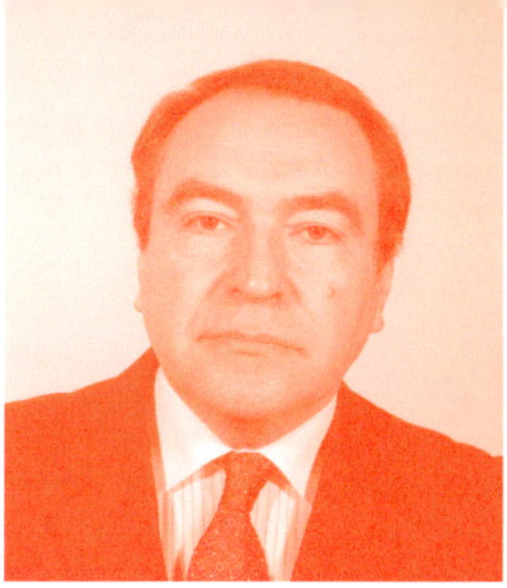
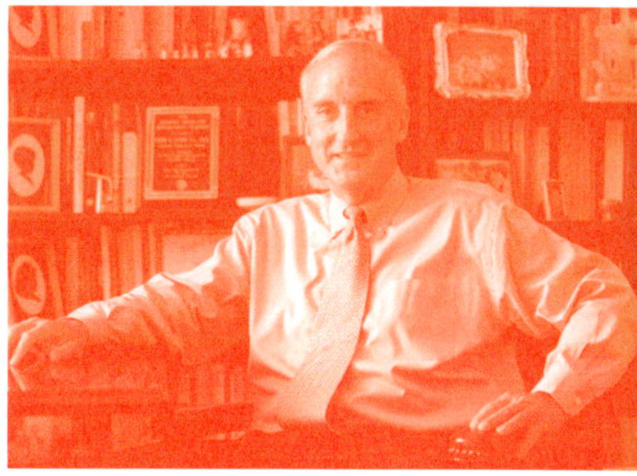
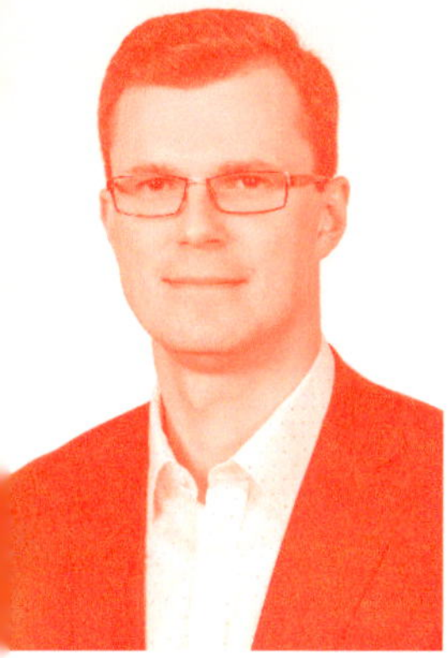
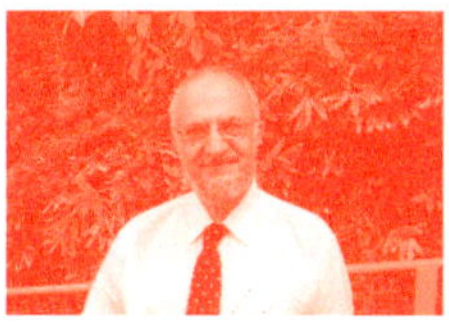
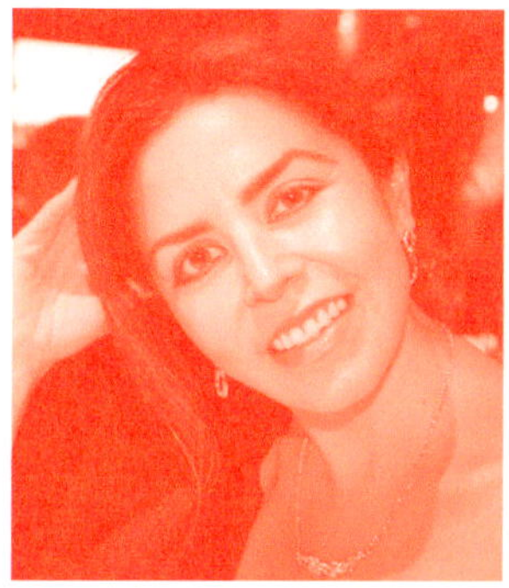

Supporting open minds since 2005

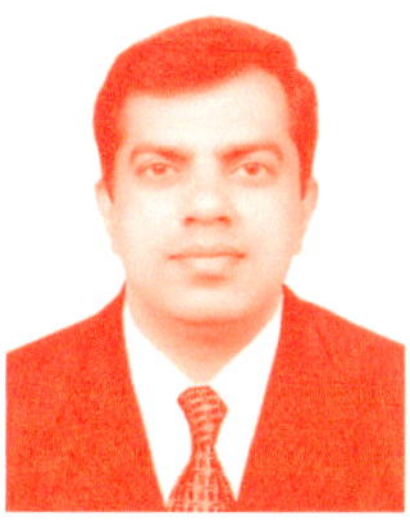
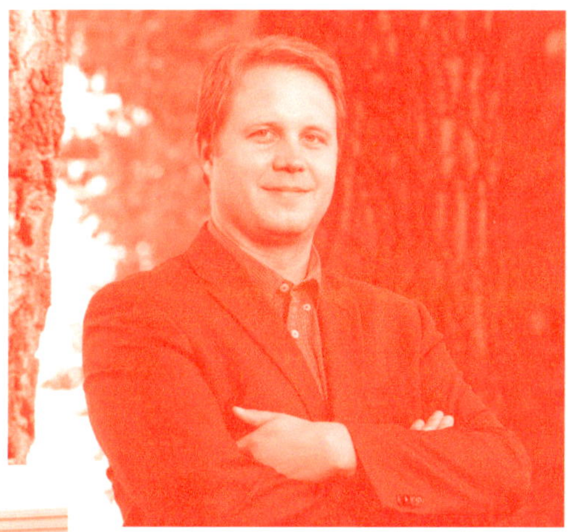
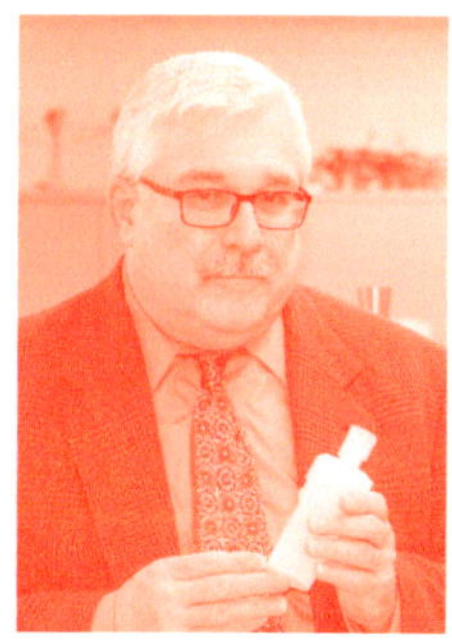
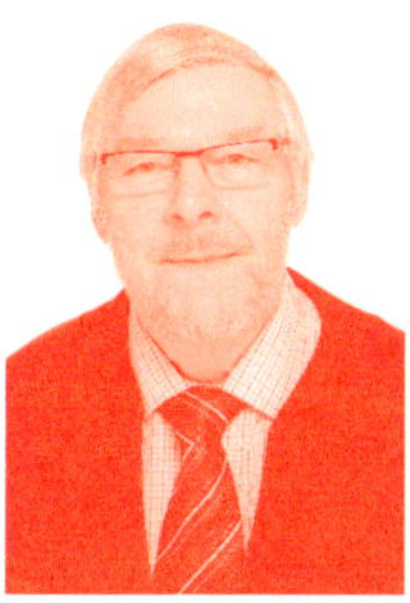
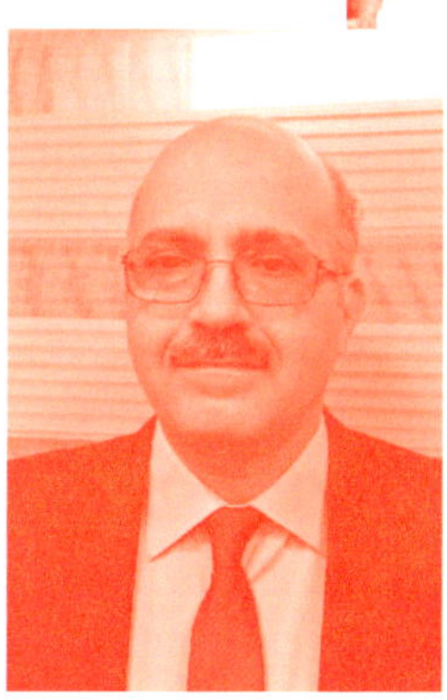
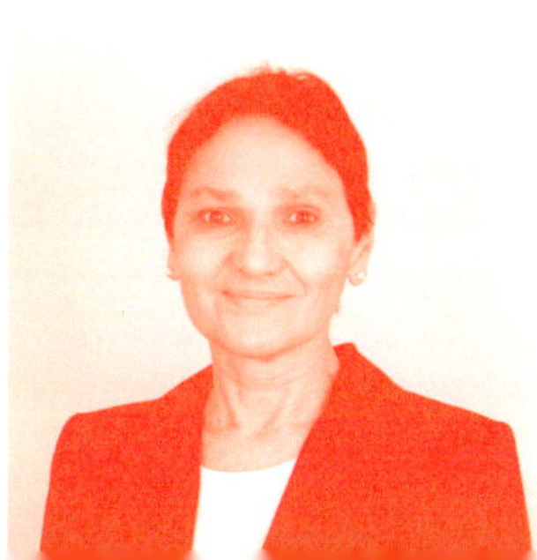
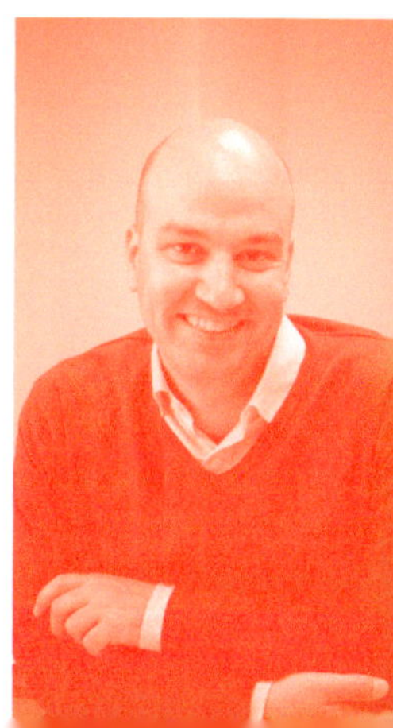

Neurological and Mental Disorders
http://dx.doi.org/10.5772/intechopen.87273
Edited by Kaneez Fatima Shad and Kamil Hakan Dogan

Contributors
Eugenia Marin-Garcia, Stamatios Papadakis, Dimitrios Pallis, Spyridon Galanakos, Konstantinos Kateros, Grigorios Leon, George Macheras, George Sapkas, Nishi Misra, Harshita Jha, Komal Tiwari, Alison Husain, Valeska Kouzak Campos Da Paz, Carlos Alberto Bezerra Tomaz, Silvia Fernanda Lima De Cal, Tatiana Farias, Rebeca Cerqueira, Danton Ferraz, João Freira, Ana Lopes, Sophia Bakhtadze, Tinatin Tkemaladze, Tinatin Kutubidze, Xiaoxia Wang, Kaneez Fatima Shad, Saima Khan, Dominik Havsteen-Franklin, Jorge Camarena Altamirano, Greta Somaini, Maria Patsou, Catalina Crisan, Bianca Suciu, Hojka Gregoric Kumperscak

First published in London, United Kingdom, 2020 by IntechOpen
IntechOpen is the global imprint of INTECHOPEN LIMITED, registered in England and Wales, registration number: 11086078, 5 Princes Gate Court, London, SW7 2QJ, United Kingdom
Printed in Croatia

British Library Cataloguing-in-Publication Data
A catalogue record for this book is available from the British Library

Additional hard and PDF copies can be obtained from orders@intechopen.com

Neurological and Mental Disorders
Edited by Kaneez Fatima Shad and Kamil Hakan Dogan
p. cm.
Print ISBN 978-1-83962-973-0
Online ISBN 978-1-83962-974-7
eBook (PDF) ISBN 978-1-83962-975-4

For EU product safety concerns:
IN TECH d.o.o., Prolaz Marije Krucifikse Kozulić 3, 51000 Rijeka, Croatia, info@intechopen.com or visit our website at intechopen.com.

Meet the editors

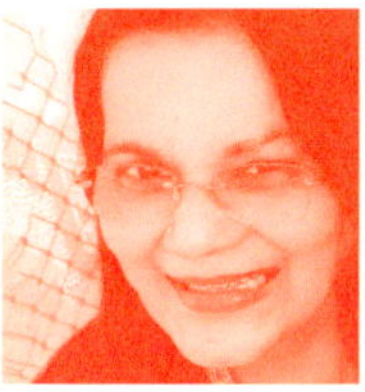

Professor Kaneez Fatima Shad, a Pakistani born Australian Neuroscientist with a medical background, received her PhD in 1994 from the Faculty of Medicine, UNSW, Australia, followed by a post doctorate degree at the Allegheny University of Health Sciences, Philadelphia, USA. She has taught Medical and Biological Sciences in various universities in Australia, USA, UAE, Bahrain, Pakistan and Brunei. During this period, she was also engaged in research by obtaining local and international grants (total of over 2.4 million USD) and translating this into products such as a rapid diagnostic test for stroke and other vascular disorders such as schizophrenia. She has published over 65 articles in refereed journals, edited five books, written 8 book chapters, presented at over 80 international conferences and mentored thirty-four postgraduate students.

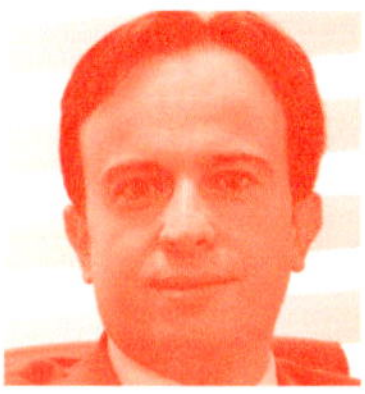

Kamil Hakan Dogan MD, PhD is a Full Professor and Chair in the Department of Forensic Medicine at Selcuk University, Faculty of Medicine in Turkey. Dr. Dogan received his MD from Gazi University, Faculty of Medicine in 2000. After his extensive research in the forensic medicine field, he received his PhD in Biochemistry in 2012. He gives lectures on Forensic Medicine and Medical Ethics to medical students as well as students of the dentistry and law faculties. He is a reviewer for several international journals and he has published over 200 articles in refereed journals, chapters in textbooks and abstracts in scientific meetings. His publications have been cited more than 700 times.

Contents

Preface

Neurological and mental disorders affect an extensive network of neurons spread throughout the brain and body. An intact neuronal system is essential for synaptic interactions and for the normal functioning of the brain.

Mental disorders can result from disruption of neuronal circuitry, damage to the neuronal and non-neuronal cells, altered circuitry in the different regions of the brain and any changes in the permeability of the blood brain barrier. Early identification of these impairments through investigative means could help to improve the outcome for many brain and behaviour disease states.

This book rightly entitled "Neurological and Mental Disorders" effectively describes the basic biochemical concepts of the neurological circuitry and their role in the mental state of a person. The role of the BDNF protein in anxiety disorders is very well described in the first chapter.

The following chapters describe how different therapeutic management techniques can stabilize diseases such as personality disorders and feeding and eating disorders. Later in this segment, the role of neurofeedback training was analysed in maintaining cognitive reserve in aging adults.

The medical section of the book begins with describing the neuroprotective role of non-allopathic medicine curcumin and supplement vitamin D3 in the animal model of Alzheimer's disease, followed by revealing the aetiology and characteristics of ADHD and the effect of stimulants in alleviating its symptoms. The next chapter in this section explains the demographic traits, symptoms and outcomes of "falls from height" patients, followed by another interesting chapter on using computational modelling and machine learning for the detection of depressive disorders. Similarly, art-based practices and psychological interventions were clearly shown to be effective in the treatment of Borderline Personality Disorder.

The social aspects section commences with a remarkably interesting chapter illustrating the effect of intergenerational and psychosocial traumas on the degree of amnesia in indigenous and non-indigenous Australians. In another chapter, the author thoroughly describes the changes in the pattern of mass suicide with the advent of computers and social media. Last but not the least, the readers will be captivated by how transient global amnesia is associated with hippocampal perturbation and memory loss paradigm.

I hope those who read this book gain a better understanding of the various facets of neurocircuitry and behavioural patterns under the influence of social aspects around the globe.

I would like to thank my co-editor Dr Kamil Hakan Dogan (Forensic Medicine Specialist at Selcuk University Faculty of Medicine, Konya, Turkey) for his contribution towards compiling this book, editing the chapters and writing the preface.

Production of this book would not have been possible without the contribution from the experts in the field and the continuous hard work of Ms Dolores Kuzelj, Author Service Manager from IntechOpen Publication.

In the end I would like to emphasise that this book is meant for a broad range of readers including undergraduates, graduates, researchers, teachers, medical professionals and specialists such as neurologists, psychiatrists, psychologists, forensic pathologists and social scientists.

Kaneez Fatima Shad
Professor,
School of Life Sciences,
Faculty of Science,
Centre for Health Technologies,
University of Technology Sydney,
Sydney, Australia

Kamil Hakan Dogan
Selçuk University,
Konya, Turkey

Section 1

Behavioral Aspects

Chapter 1

BDNF Protein and Anxiety Disorders

Tatiana Marins Farias, Rebeca Ataíde Cerqueira, Danton Ferraz Sousa, João Vitor Costa Freire, Ana Carolina Tavares Lopes and Silvia Fernanda Lima De Moura Cal

Abstract

An increase in the prevalence of anxiety disorders (ADs), in individual, social, and economic losses, due to the high prevalence, chronicity, and disability of the individual besides the growth of multiple environmental stressors that are related to lifestyles, has been observed, which are all more harmful to one's health, and associated with genetic inheritances, among other factors. This reality may contribute to the risk of losing neurological functions, for example, cognition and memory, as well as to the development of more severe psychiatric disorders, with high levels of heritability and risk of suicide. Brain-derived neurotrophic factor (BDNF) is one of the most abundant neurotrophins in the human brain. Studies with neurotrophins allowed the introduction of one more hypothesis, called neurotrophic hypothesis, that would explain the physiopathology of mental disorders (MD), where deficits of neuroplasticity would occur and cause atrophy of certain regions of the brain (mainly cortical and the hippocampus), contributing to the development of mental disorders. Knowing the neurobiology of the ADs, as well as its relation to BDNF levels, may contribute to preventive actions regarding the said disorder in the general population. The objective of this chapter is to analyze the relation between levels of BDNF and AD.

Keywords: anxiety disorders, BDNF, mental disorders, neurobiology, neurotrophic theory

1. Introduction

Anxiety disorders (ADs) have become a significant public health issue worldwide, with individual, social, and economic losses, due to their high prevalence, chronic condition, and the individual's disability [1].

This reality may contribute to the risk of losing neurological functions, for example, cognition and memory, as well as to the development of more severe psychiatric disorders, with high levels of heritability and risk of suicide.

Anxious disorders like panic disorder (PD) with or without agoraphobia, generalized anxiety disorder (GAD), social anxiety disorder (SAD), specific phobias (SPs), and separation anxiety disorder are the most prevalent mental disorders (MD) and are associated with immense healthcare costs and a high burden of disease [1].

The word anxiety is derived from Latin *anxietatis* (desire, worry); *anxi* (contract, narrow); *anxietas* (narrowing); and *anxia* (craving, vulgar Latin) and is considered a physiological manifestation when facing some type of danger (real or imaginary), with adaptability in forming responses to threatening stimuli, in order to foment the individual's safety and survival, leading to an unpleasant somatic and psychological experience [2].

When the severity, frequency, and persistence of the anxious symptoms become inconsistent with the presented circumstances, and the anxious reaction causes the behavior to be dysfunctional, then these are characterized as the anxiety disorders, which present high levels of morbidity, with a possible increase in mortality [1], since 6.1% of suicide cases are associated with AD [3].

Mental disorders were only recognized as a serious public health problem in 1996, in a study conducted by researchers from Harvard University and the World Health Organization (WHO), when out of the 10 main causes of disability worldwide, 5 were associated with mental disorders [4]. In the metropolitan region of São Paulo, 29.6% of individuals presented mental disorders with anxiety disorders being the most common, affecting 19.9% of the population, occurring twice as much in females [5]. Among the types of anxiety disorders, it is estimated that up to 5% of the population suffers from generalized anxiety disorder [1].

Generalized anxiety disorder, a type of AD, has high rates of comorbidity and stands out from mood disorders and other types of anxiety disorders. A recent study indicates that in 67% of the cases, GAD precedes (or is concomitant) depressive disorders (unipolar), 17% have bipolar disorder, and only 16% have no lifetime mood disorder and can be considered a risk factor. Furthermore, it is also associated with renal and cardiovascular diseases, rendering a more reserved prognosis in either situation [5, 6].

According to Bandelow and Michaelis, 33.7% of the world population suffers from anxiety disorders; however, it is difficult to find reliable evidence to demonstrate the evolution of this prevalence. Because the patients with anxiety disorders are mostly treated as outpatients, they probably receive less attention from clinical psychiatrists [1].

Epidemiological data from the National Comorbidity Survey suggest that 67% of the individual with GAD have depressive disorder (unipolar), 17% have bipolar disorder, and only 16% have no lifetime mood disorder [6].

ADs are highly comorbid with other mental problems like additive psychiatric disorders, leading to disability and impairment in quality of life [6].

Brain-derived neurotrophic factor (BDNF) is one of the most abundant neurotrophins in the human brain. Studies with neurotrophins allowed the introduction of one more hypothesis, called neurotrophic hypothesis, that would explain the physiopathology of mental disorders, where deficits of neuroplasticity would occur and cause atrophy of certain regions of the brain (mainly cortical and the hippocampus), contributing to the development of mental disorders [7]. Knowing the neurobiology of the AD, as well as its relation to BDNF levels, may contribute to preventative actions regarding the said disorder in the general population. The objective of this chapter is to analyze the relation between levels of BDNF and AD.

2. Methods

The two main types of review articles are commonly found in the scientific literature: systematic and narrative review of the literature. These two types of review articles have distinct characteristics and goals. The review of narrative or traditional literature, when compared to systematic review, presents a more open theme. This makes part of a specific and well-defined problem difficult and does not require a strict protocol for its preparation. The search for sources is not predetermined and specific and is generally less comprehensive. Studies on BDNF protein and anxiety disorders are the focus of this narrative review of the literature [8].

3. Clinical picture

For the individual, anxiety is a form of protection, a defense mechanism, with an important role in the preservation of life, with symptoms that are somatic (breathing discomfort, tachycardia and precordial chest pain, excessive perspiration, increased peristalsis, epigastric pain, nausea, pallor or skin redness and flushing, paresthesia, chills, muscular changes, headache, dizziness, dry mouth, inability to remain seated or immobile for very long, etc.) and psychic (feeling of internal unrest, insomnia, feeling of oppression and discomfort, exaggerated worry, insecurity, irritability, undefined uneasiness, difficulty concentrating, depersonalization and derealization, among others). The effects of anxiety on thought, perception, and the learning process may be quite intense.

Anxiety tends to produce confusion and perspective distortions, not only in terms of time and space but also of people and the significance of events. These distortions may cause interference in learning, lowering concentration, reducing memory, and impairing the capability of association.

Pathological anxiety constitutes an inadequate response to a certain stimulus, as a result of its greater intensity and duration. Pathological anxiety paralyzes the individual, not allowing him/her to be prepared and to face threatening situations, differentiating itself from normal anxiety by the assessment of the intensity from the patient, his/her family, as well as from the physician [1]. The state of anxiety, its traits, and the ADs are differentiated by the degree of impairment and the duration of the anxiety symptoms on the individual. The state of anxiety is normally defined as a measure of acute or intermediate level of anxiety. Now, the anxiety trait is considered a tendency of the individual to produce an anxious response to environmental events. And, lastly, the anxiety disorders are the most severe, due to the excessive worry and fear and the greater duration and complexity of the anxious symptoms, which are dysfunctional and accompanied by impairment [8].

4. Classification

There are two types of international classification for anxiety disorders. According to the International Classification of Diseases, 10th edition, and more utilized in clinical psychiatry, there are seven main anxiety disorders: specific phobias, social phobia, panic disorder, generalized anxiety, obsessive-compulsive disorder, reaction to severe stress, and mixed anxiety-depressive disorder [9].

On the other hand, with the main goal of research purposes, the *Diagnostic and Statistical Manual of Mental Disorders, 5th edition* (DSM-V), classifies the most important ADs as (1) generalized anxiety disorder, (2) panic disorder, (3) agoraphobia, (4) separation anxiety disorder, (5) social anxiety disorder or social phobia, (6) specific phobias, and (7) selective mutism [10].

5. Etiology

Biologically, the etiology of anxiety, with complex neurobiological mechanisms, according to the literature in neuroscience [2] seems to be related to the noradrenergic, GABAergic, and serotoninergic systems and the frontal lobe and limbic systems. The anxious patients tend to have increased sympathetic tone, causing delays in adapting to changes in the autonomic nervous system [1].

However, studies with neurotrophins gave rise to one more hypothesis that would explain the physiopathology of mental disorders in general, called the neurotrophic hypothesis, where deficits in the neuroplasticity would occur as well as cause atrophy of certain brain regions, mainly the cortex and hippocampus [7]. Nevertheless, there are gaps in the literature on whether the ADs take this explanation into consideration.

Increased activity in emotion-processing brain regions in patients who have an anxiety disorder could result from decreased inhibitory signaling by g-aminobutyric-acid (GABA) or increased excitatory neurotransmission by glutamate [11].

The connection between the sympathetic nervous system and the psyche is best seen in anxiety and especially in social phobia. The hippocampus may predominantly control the avoidance components of phobic anxiety by the serotonergic system, with other regions, such as the dorsomedial hypothalamus, controlling the escape components with the cholinergic system. Furthermore, the autonomic dysfunction and the overactivity of the sympathetic nervous system appear to induce many of the symptoms of anxiety, such as sweating, trembling, and heart racing [12].

There is increasing evidence that development and maturation of neuronal connectivity are critical components in the pathophysiology of essentially all neuropsychiatric disorders. As neurotrophins have been implicated in brain development and in particular in the plasticity and maturation of neuronal circuits, it is understandable that neurotrophins have been popular candidate genes for psychiatric diseases [13]. However, there are gaps in the literature on whether anxiety disorders include this explanation.

6. Genetic predisposition and precursor factors

More well-defined classifications tend to standardize the studies on ADs, contributing toward the biological evidence associated with these disorders, as well as making the "phenotypic complexity" a challenge to genetic psychiatry [14].

Upon including twins and their biological families, a meta-analysis indicated a heritability between 30 and 40% for anxiety disorders [15]. Now, a longitudinal study estimated a heritability ranging from 72 to 89%. The results of this study also showed a "developmental dynamic" pattern, for, over time, there is a mitigation of the genetic influence as a risk factor for anxious and depressive symptoms [16], leading one to ponder over the influence of protective factors in the prognosis of ADs.

7. Environmental factors

Individuals with AD present attentional bias to the threatening stimulus, which increases the vulnerability to stress, considering these "complex disorders," due to being influenced by multiple factors that flee from what are called "deterministic effects" of the genes, therefore making them liable to modulation by interference [2].

According to an experimental study with laboratory animals, stress by social subjugation is able to foster hyperalgesia with a decrease in the BDNF levels; this condition is more evident in "susceptible" subjects rather than in "resilient" ones [17], reinforcing the complex multifactorial theory that the neurobiological response to stress is not only genetic but also environmental.

BDNF exons decrease markedly after high corticosterone levels. BDNF levels are controlled by epigenetic mechanisms with extinction assisted by partial NMDA receptor agonists (e.g., D-cycloserine) and histone deacetylase inhibitors [18].

Environmental factors, via epigenetic factors, control the alterations of BDNF gene expression, especially when young. Harmful environmental influences while growing can cause a decrease in BDNF expression in adulthood, in addition to the serotonin transporter and FKBP5, leading to problems in patient response to drug and behavior therapies [19, 20].

Problems during youth lead to DNA methylation of BDNF promoter IV and a decrease in prefrontal cortex total BDNF mRNA [21]. However, after exercise and a healthy environment, total BDNF mRNA in the hippocampus increases due to increases in histone acetylation at promoter IV or decreases in its methylation [19].

In response to fear conditioning, the levels of BDNF exon mRNAs change markedly. As an example, after fear conditioning using light shock, exon I and III mRNA levels increase markedly, different from the exons II and IV which remain constant [18].

Several psychological factors have been associated with increased risk for anxiety disorders. Among the most intensively researched has been the concept of anxiety sensitivity (AS). AS has been defined as the individual response to physiological alterations associated with anxiety and fear. Patients with anxiety disorders have exaggerated psychological reactions that are reflective of misinterpretation of bodily cues such that the patient misperceives these sensations inappropriately as being harmful and dangerous, leading in a circular fashion to increased anxiety and fear. AS is associated with a selective cognitive bias toward threat. AS predicts the frequency and intensity of panic attacks [21].

The above section identifies several possible mediators of the psychobiological response to extreme stress and how each may contribute, alone or through functional interactions, to resilience or vulnerability to anxiety disorders. One prediction is that individuals in the highest quartile for measures of HPA axis, CRH, LC-NE, and estrogen activity and the lowest quartile for DHEA, NPY, galanin, testosterone, and 5-HT1A receptor and benzodiazepine receptor function will have an increased risk for anxiety disorders. Other mediators that can be included for the characterization of the vulnerable or resilient profile are glutamate and neurotrophic factors, such as brain-derived neurotrophic factor, and neuropeptides, such as substance P and cholecystokinin [21].

8. Pharmacologic and non-pharmacologic treatments

Patients should receive "psychoeducation" about their diagnosis, the possible etiology, and the mechanisms of action of the available treatment approaches. The treatment plan should include psychotherapy, pharmacotherapy, and other interventions, which should be chosen after careful consideration of individual factors, e.g., the patient's preference, the patient's history with previous treatment attempts, illness severity, comorbidities such as personality disorders, suicidality, local availability of treatment methods, wait time for psychotherapy appointments, costs, and other factors [22].

For all types of anxiety disorder, cognitive-behavioral therapy is the type of psychotherapy for which there is the strongest evidence and which receives the highest-level recommendation [23].

Cognitive-behavioral therapy has been found to have a moderately strong beneficial effect against all types of anxiety disorder compared to a placebo drug

(Cohen's d = 0.57); the same is true of pharmacotherapy (e.g., sertraline, d = 0.54; venlafaxine, d = 0.50) [24, 25].

It is important to highlight that no articles were found that evaluated the effectiveness of Jungian and integrative psychotherapy.

Pharmacological treatments for anxiety disorders have become more tolerable, available, and numerous over the past half century. At the same time, research has yielded a vastly improved understanding of the neurobiological and physiological mechanisms involved in chronic anxiety and stress responses, suggesting new approaches to the treatment of anxiety disorders [26].

Numerous neurotransmitters play a role in normal states and in pathological anxiety states. Each of these systems is a potential target for pharmacological intervention, but relatively few classes of medications are used in clinical practice for the treatment of anxiety [27].

Due to their positive benefit/risk balance, selective serotonin reuptake inhibitors (SSRIs) and selective serotonin norepinephrine reuptake inhibitors (SNRIs) are recommended as first-line drugs. Patients should be informed that the onset of the anxiolytic effect of these antidepressants has a latency of 2–4 weeks (in some cases up to 6 weeks) [22].

We should continue to test alternative therapies for treating and preventing anxiety disorders and to help patients whose anxiety is resistant to conventional treatments; also, we need to consider the patient's feelings about mental illness and address their responses early in treatment. All of these measures will enhance the care of patients with anxiety [27].

9. Brain-derived neurotrophic factor

BDNF is one of the most abundant neurotrophins in the human brain, identified in 1982 by Yves Barde and Hans [17]. It is found in two distinct forms, pro-BDNF and the mature BDNF, which have antagonistic functions. The pro-BDNF is the precursor protein that is synthesized and undergoes cleavage to produce its mature form, BDNF, presenting greater physiological activity in the central nervous system [28, 29].

The pro-BDNF has high affinity to the p75 neurotrophin receptor, triggering pro-apoptotic effects and anti-plasticity [17]. On the other hand, the main receptor where the binding of the mature BDNF occurs is the tropomyosin-related kinase receptor type B (TrkB), distributed in the cortex, hippocampus, multiple bridged nuclei, and the spinal cord. When activated, this receptor causes a series of intracellular cascades that are responsible for growth, survival, and neural differentiation [15, 18].

Studies on neurotrophins allowed the release of one more hypothesis that would explain the physiopathology of mental disorders, called neurotrophic hypothesis, where deficits of neuroplasticity would occur and cause atrophy of certain regions of the brain (mainly cortical and the hippocampus), contributing to the development of mental disorders [7].

The main origin of these alterations is a decrease in the BDNF expression, caused by stress [19]. However, the association between the BDNF serum levels and mental disorders has yet to be completely clarified. There is evidence that the BDNF serum levels are reduced in patients with mental disorders, regardless of the diagnosis [7].

A meta-analysis that studied the peripheral values of BDNF in different mental disorders with the hypothesis of proving its nonspecificity obtained results pointing to a valid reduction of BDNF levels in acute cases as well as in other periods of treatment (i.e., with symptom remission and in the presence of residual symptoms), in comparing groups of patients with healthy controls [30].

It is known that in a severe and prolonged state of stress, with sustained increase of glucocorticoid (GC) hormone levels due to the activation of the HPA axis, neuroplastic changes occur, as well as a decrease in the BDNF hippocampal levels. Thus, a persistence and intensity of stressors may produce hippocampal dysfunction, causing a decline in the inhibitory control that the hippocampus exerts over the HPA axis [31].

The BDNF has become an important tool in understanding cognitive deficits, especially those related to memory loss. One of the reasons to use this neurotrophin in these studies is its participation not only in processes of differentiation, neuronal survival, and synaptic plasticity but also in processes involving learning and memory [32].

The BDNF also enables the strengthening of connections between neurons (synapsis), mainly in the hippocampus, cortex, and basal forebrain—important regions for learning, maintaining memory, and higher thinking.

10. Changes in BDNF levels in psychiatric illnesses

The BDNF may cause neurogenesis mainly in the hippocampal region of adult brains. At the same time, in patients who suffer from psychiatric illnesses, a smaller hippocampus has been identified, associated with a decrease in BDNF plasma levels, than healthy individuals. Clarifying the exact mechanism of the action of BDNF will permit a better understanding of the cognitive deficits.

BDNF crosses the blood-brain barrier, possibly through its dosage in peripheral blood, whose serum levels correlate with the levels in the central nervous system [7]. However, this has not become a clinical reality, despite the biological plausibility, due to great heterogeneity between the studies, which presented low power of detection of differences and biases of publication, and influence of confounding variables (physical exercise, smoking, body mass index, laboratory techniques that lack standardization, kits that do not distinguish between pro-BDNF and mature BDNF). The high number of variations limits comparisons between the studies [7].

The regular practice of physical activity has been shown to be a prophylactic and therapeutic intervention for several dysfunctions, such as stress, by way of the increase in adaptive responses of the HPA axis, improvement of adaptive response to stress, and a decrease in anxiety.

It is believed that identifying variations of the epigenetic pattern of DNA and of the gene expression of rats exposed to stress, as well as rat practitioners and non-practitioners of physical activity, may reveal additional data that could be extrapolated to the human population, regarding the importance of physical activity in illness prevention [24].

The interest in knowing the molecular aspects of the effect of physical activity and/or exercise is evident; however, little is known yet regarding the epigenetic changes resulting from physical exercise [24].

Thus, several studies have been conducted to clarify the connection between the regular practice of physical exercise and the increased concentration of BDNF, making it necessary to shed light on the role of this gene in suppressing the harmful effects resulting from stressful situations [24].

11. Conclusion

There is evidence that it is important to study aspects in common of the neurobiology of anxiety disorders, and its relation to the BNDF protein, to obtain preventive measures in mental health.

Recent clinical trials, in animals and humans, increasingly seek an association between different spectra of mental disorders and BDNF levels and their subforms, in different collection sites, leading to the question of the possibility of using it as a biomarker of susceptibility to anxious disorders. The early titration and serialization of BDNF and subforms in families with a high probability of ED heritability are shown as a future perspective for primary and integrated actions in mental health, with modulation of gene expression, using the "dynamic developmental" pattern for a reduction of future medication for susceptible individuals, as well as the possibility of discovering acute illnesses early, with a positive change in the history of the disease and a reduction in social economic losses. From this perspective, we highlight the importance of further studies on the neurobiology of anxiety disorders, on BDNF protein and its physiology, and the association between both for preventive measures in mental health.

Author details

Tatiana Marins Farias[1,2,3], Rebeca Ataíde Cerqueira[1], Danton Ferraz Sousa[1], João Vitor Costa Freire[1], Ana Carolina Tavares Lopes[1] and Silvia Fernanda Lima De Moura Cal[1*]

1 UNIME - Metropolitan Union for the Development of Education and Culture, Brazil

2 Federal University of Bahia (UFBa), Brazil

3 Federal Government Economy Ministry, Brazil

*Address all correspondence to: silviacal@uol.com.br

References

[1] Bandelow B, Michaelis S. Epidemiology of anxiety disorders in the 21st century. Dialogues in Clinical Neuroscience. 2015;**17**(3):327-335. Available from: http://www.ncbi.nlm.nih.gov/pubmed/26487813

[2] Crocq M-A. A history of anxiety: From Hippocrates to DSM. Dialogues in Clinical Neuroscience. 2015;**17**(3):319-325. Available from: http://www.ncbi.nlm.nih.gov/pubmed/26487812

[3] Bertolote JM, Fleischmann A. Suicide and psychiatric diagnosis: A worldwide perspective. World Psychiatry. 2002;**1**(3):181-185. Available from: http://www.ncbi.nlm.nih.gov/pubmed/16946849

[4] Lopez AD, Murray CC. The global burden of disease, 1990-2020. Nature Medicine. 1998;**4**(11):1241-1243. Available from: http://www.ncbi.nlm.nih.gov/pubmed/9809543

[5] Andrade LH, Wang YP, Andreoni S, Silveira CM, Alexandrino-Silva C, Siu ER, et al. Mental disorders in megacities: Findings from the São Paulo megacity mental health survey, Brazil. PLoS One. 2012;7(2):1-11

[6] Simon NM. Generalized anxiety disorder and psychiatric comorbidities such as depression, bipolar disorder, and substance abuse. The Journal of Clinical Psychiatry. 2009;**70**(Suppl 2):10-14

[7] Nagahara AH, Tuszynski MH. Potential therapeutic uses of BDNF in neurological and psychiatric disorders. Nat Rev Drug Discov [Internet]. 2011;**10**(3):209-219. Available from: https://www.nature.com/articles/nrd3366

[8] Cordeiro AOG. Revisão sistemática: uma revisão narrativa. Rev do Colégio Bras Cir. 2007;**6**(34):428-431. Available from: http://www.scielo.br/scielo.php?script=sci_arttext&pid=S0100-69912007000600012&lng=pt&tlng=pt

[9] Publication AP. Diagnostic and Statistical Manual of Mental Disorders. DSM-5 [Internet]. Washington DC: American Psychiatric Publication; 2013. Available from: https://books.google.com.br/books?hl=pt-BR&lr=&id=-JivBAAAQBAJ&oi=fnd&pg=PT18&dq=diagnostic+and+statistical+mental+disorders&ots=ceSN16OHyc&sig=VBVXcQ2KuBON36zYhC84Nflx_-o#v=onepage&q=diagnostic and statistical mental disorders&f=false

[10] Martin E, Ressler K, Binder E, Nemeroff C. The neurobiology of anxiety disorders: Brain imaging, genetics, and Psychoneuroendocrinology. The Psychiatric Clinics of North America. 2013;**32**(3):549-575

[11] Pohjavaara P, Telaranta T, Väisänen E. The role of the sympathetic nervous system in anxiety: Is it possible to relieve anxiety with endoscopic sympathetic block? Nordic Journal of Psychiatry. 2003;**57**(1):55-60. Available from: https://www.tandfonline.com/doi/abs/10.1080/08039480310000266

[12] Castrén E. Neurotrophins and psychiatric disorders. Handb Exp Pharmacol [Internet]. 2014;**220**:461-479. Available from: http://www.ncbi.nlm.nih.gov/pubmed/24668483

[13] Kupfer DJ. Anxiety and DSM-5. Dialogues in Clinical Neuroscience. 2015;**17**(3):245-246

[14] Hettema JM, Neale MC, Kendler KS. A review and meta-analysis of the genetic epidemiology of anxiety disorders. Am J Psychiatry [Internet]. 2001;**158**(10):1568-1578. Available from: http://www.ncbi.nlm.nih.gov/pubmed/11578982

[15] Kendler KS, Gardner CO, Lichtenstein P. A developmental twin study of symptoms of anxiety and depression: Evidence for genetic innovation and attenuation. Psychological Medicine. 2008;**38**(11):1567-1575. Available from: https://www.cambridge.org/core/product/identifier/S003329170800384X/type/journal_article

[16] Lu B, Pang PT, Woo NH. The yin and yang of neurotrophin action. Nature Reviews. Neuroscience. 2005;**6**(8):603-614. Available from: http://www.ncbi.nlm.nih.gov/pubmed/16062169

[17] Farach FJ, Pruitt LD, Jun JJ, Jerud AB, Zoellner LA, Roy-Byrne PP. Pharmacological treatment of anxiety disorders: Current treatments and future directions. Journal of Anxiety Disorders. 2012;**26**(8):833-843. Available from: http://www.ncbi.nlm.nih.gov/pubmed/23023162

[18] Boulle F, van den Hove DLA, Jakob SB, Rutten BP, Hamon M, van Os J, et al. Epigenetic regulation of the BDNF gene: Implications for psychiatric disorders. Molecular Psychiatry. 2012;**17**(6):584-596. Available from: http://www.ncbi.nlm.nih.gov/pubmed/21894152

[19] van Winkel R, van Nierop M, Myin-Germeys I, van Os J. Childhood trauma as a cause of psychosis: Linking genes, psychology, and biology. Canadian Journal of Psychiatry. 2013;**58**(1):44-51. Available from: http://journals.sagepub.com/doi/10.1177/070674371305800109

[20] Bennett M, Lagopoulos J. Stress, Trauma and Synaptic Plasticity [Internet]. Cham: Springer International Publishing; 2018. Available from: https://link.springer.com/book/10.1007/978-3-319-91116-8

[21] Charney DS. The psychobiology of resilience and vulnerability to anxiety disorders: Implications for prevention and treatment. Dialogues in Clinical Neuroscience. 2003;**5**(3):207-221. Available from: http://www.ncbi.nlm.nih.gov/pubmed/22034473

[22] Bandelow B, Michaelis S, Wedekind D. Treatment of anxiety disorders. Dialogues in Clinical Neuroscience. 2017;**19**(2):93-107. Available from: http://www.ncbi.nlm.nih.gov/pubmed/28867934

[23] Ströhle A, Gensichen J, Domschke K. The diagnosis and treatment of anxiety disorders. Deutsches Ärzteblatt International. 2018;**155**(37):611-620. Available from: http://www.ncbi.nlm.nih.gov/pubmed/30282583

[24] Bandelow B, Reitt M, Röver C, Michaelis S, Görlich Y, Wedekind D. Efficacy of treatments for anxiety disorders. International Clinical Psychopharmacology. 2015;**30**(4):183-192. Available from: http://content.wkhealth.com/linkback/openurl?sid=WKPTLP:landingpage&an=00004850-201507000-00002

[25] Bystritsky A, Khalsa SS, Cameron ME, Schiffman J. Current diagnosis and treatment of anxiety disorders. PT. 2013;**38**(1):30-57. Available from: http://www.ncbi.nlm.nih.gov/pubmed/23599668

[26] Teche SP, Nuernberg GL, Sordi AO, De Souza LH, Remy L, Cereser KMM, et al. Measurement methods of bdnf levels in major depression: A qualitative systematic review of clinical trials. The Psychiatric Quarterly. 2013;**84**(4):485-497

[27] Farooqui T, Farooqui AA, editors. Diet and Exercise in Cognitive Function and Neurological Diseases. John Wiley & Sons, Inc: Hoboken, NJ; 2015. Available from: https://onlinelibrary.wiley.com/doi/book/10.1002/9781118840634

[28] Fernandes BS, Steiner J, Berk M, Molendijk ML, Gonzalez-Pinto A, Turck CW, et al. Peripheral brain-derived neurotrophic factor in schizophrenia and the role of antipsychotics: Meta-analysis and implications. Molecular Psychiatry. 2015;**20**(9):1108-1119

[29] Nooshinfar E, Akbarzadeh-Baghban A, Meisami E. Effects of increasing durations of immobilization stress on plasma corticosterone level, learning and memory and hippocampal BDNF gene expression in rats. Neuroscience Letters. 2011;**500**(1):63-66. Available from: http://www.ncbi.nlm.nih.gov/pubmed/21683767

[30] Li G, Peskind ER, Millard SP, Chi P, Sokal I, Yu C-E, et al. Cerebrospinal fluid concentration of brain-derived neurotrophic factor and cognitive function in non-demented subjects. PLOS One [Internet]. 2009;**4**(5):e5424. Available from: http://www.ncbi.nlm.nih.gov/pubmed/19412541

[31] Lee E, Son H. Adult hippocampal neurogenesis and related neurotrophic factors. BMB Rep [Internet]. 2009;**42**(5):239-244. Available from: http://www.ncbi.nlm.nih.gov/pubmed/19470236

[32] Zoladz JA, Pilc A. The effect of physical activity on the brain derived neurotrophic factor: From animal to human studies. Journal of Physiology and Pharmacology. 2010;**61**(5):533-541. Available from: http://www.ncbi.nlm.nih.gov/pubmed/21081796

Chapter 2

Personality Disorders in Adolescents and Different Therapeutic Approaches

Hojka Gregoric Kumperscak

Abstract

A personality disorder can be diagnosed at any age if the diagnostic criteria are met, which means also in adolescence. Diagnosing personality disorders is important since only with clear diagnosis specialized treatment can be applied. Several specialized (psycho)therapies have been developed for treating adolescent personality disorder with evidence-based efficiency, especially in borderline personality disorder—adolescent identity treatment (AIT), mentalization-based therapy (MBT), and dialectical behavior therapy (DBT). All are evidence-based therapies. Pharmacotherapy is not the therapy of choice and only a few studies have clearly demonstrated its efficiency; however, it is still largely utilized in clinical practice.

Keywords: personality disorders, adolescent, borderline personality disorder, adolescent identity treatment, mentalization-based therapy, dialectical behavior therapy

1. Introduction

Each person has a set of personality traits that are unique and make up one's personality. *Personality* can be defined as recognizable and permanent characteristics and attitudes that are reflected in thinking, feeling, and behaving (impulse control, the way of establishing and managing interpersonal relationships) [1]. Personality develops and evolves since childhood and shapes throughout life. *Temperament* is a biologically determined trait manifested from birth [2]. Rothbart et al. introduced three factors of temperament for the early and middle childhood that, later on in the development, shape personality dimensions, such as negative affectivity, extraversion, and effortful control [2].

Temperamental characteristics show high stability and are developmentally associated with personality traits during adulthood including extraversion or high energetic level, agreeableness, conscientiousness, neuroticism (emotional stability), and openness [2]. An important personality trait is *character*, which mainly refers to the substantive aspects of experiencing and related behavior. At the heart of the psychological understanding of character are traits that are important in terms of the individual's will, morality, and ethical and value orientation [3]. Naturally, our achievements in solving mental and life's problems depend on our abilities. The great scope of competence can be combined with various talents and the scope of skills as well [3].

Personality disorder (PD) is defined as an enduring pattern of inner experience and behavior that deviates markedly from the expectations of the individual's culture, is pervasive and inflexible, and leads to distress or impairment [4]. People with PD have disrupted behavior, cognition, and emotions when in contact with other people and society, while the individuals and the people around them suffer [1]. The ICD-10 classifies the following PD: paranoid, schizoid, dissocial, emotionally unstable (impulsive and borderline type), histrionic, anankastic, anxious (avoidant), dependent, and other (e.g., narcissistic) [5]. The DSM-5 divides PD into three clusters. Cluster A personality disorders are characterized by unusual and odd-eccentric behavior and introverted individuals including paranoid, schizoid, and schizotypal PD. Cluster B personality disorders are associated with dramatic, emotional, and erratic behavior: antisocial, borderline, histrionic, and narcissistic PD. Cluster C includes avoidant, dependent, and obsessive-compulsive PD associated with anxious and fearful disorders. The division into three groups is useful for educational and research purposes; however, it also has its limitations. Clinically, there is a lot of overlapping between various PDs. The frequency of individual PD varies from study to study, and even greater differences are present when looking at the frequency of individual PD in a given population. Borderline PD is present in 0.9–3% of the general adolescent population, in 11% of outpatient adolescents, and 49% of admitted adolescents [4].

People diagnosed with PD from one group may also meet the diagnostic criteria of PD from the other, which occurs in about 9% [4]. Individuals from group C and A most commonly have an associated PD (6.0 and 5.7%, respectively), while this occurs only in 1.5% of individuals in the group B [4]. Due to PD overlapping and for other reasons as well, the PD criteria in ICD-11, which will come into effect in January 2022, have been modified [6]. ICD-11 follows a dimensional understanding of PD and largely abandons the categorical view. The new division of PD follows the psychodynamic tradition, the scientific model of the core PD characteristics, and thus provides guidance for clinical treatment [7]. It provides an assessment of the severity of the disorder, and enables to diagnose three levels of PD and code subthreshold personality difficulty. ICD-11 specifies five domain qualifiers of personality, which include negative affectivity, detachment, dissociality, disinhibition, and anankastia. In addition to these five markers, a borderline pattern qualifier can also be specified. The latter may be applied if at least five out of nine borderline PD criteria according to DSM-5 are present. An example of a diagnosis of borderline PD following the new features in ICD-11 is for example a moderate PD with borderline pattern, negative affectivity, disinhibition, and dissociality [7].

2. Borderline personality disorder

Borderline PD is one of the most common PDs and these individuals are also more likely to seek medical help and suffer from significantly more associated mental disorders (depression, anxiety disorders, psychoactive substances abuse, and hyperkinetic disorder) compared to the general population [8]. Vulnerability for borderline PD can be clearly recognized during the development period. The concept of borderline personality has evolved throughout history. Morel and Kraepelin used this term to describe the states between neurotic and psychotic conditions primarily based on phenomenological clinical descriptions and by ignoring the developmental and dynamic aspects of pathology [9].

Kernberg linked the classical psychoanalysis, the object relations theories, the psychology of self (immature integrative self-functions) with the psychobiological and neurobiological theories, and defined the concept of borderline personality disorder as a pathological personality organization that is intermediate between psychotic disorders and neuroses—symptomatically, structurally, and genetically-dynamically [10, 11]. This concept was further enhanced by the Linehan's biosocial model [12].

According to DSM-5, at least five of the following nine criteria must be present to code borderline personality disorder [4].

1. Frantic efforts to avoid real or imagined abandonment

2. Unstable and intense relationships

3. Identity disturbance, seen in an unstable self-image or sense of self

4. Impulsivity

5. Suicidal behavior

6. Affective instability (episodic dysphoria, irritability, anxiety: lasting a few hours to days)

7. Chronic feelings of emptiness

8. Displays of inappropriate anger (verbal/physical fights)

9. Micropsychotic episodes, transient stress-related paranoid ideation/dissociative symptoms

In addition, these patterns are enduring, inflexible, and clinically relevant to diminish social, educational, or professional functioning. The onset of this pattern is traced back at least to adolescence or early adulthood and it is not a manifestation of another mental disorder and is not due to the consumption of psychoactive substances [4].

Quite a few features of borderline PD (impulsivity, emotional instability, dysfunctional interpersonal relationships, impaired self-image, and identity diffusion) may also—to some extent—be characteristics of adolescent period. In order to diagnose a borderline PD in an individual during adolescence, the features must have been present for at least 1 year and cause severe dysfunction [4]. If the adolescent reacts highly destructive, has transient psychotic reactions and behavioral problems, uses psychoactive substances, has emotional disorders associated with the loss of a relationship with the important other or negative emotions, one can suspect a borderline PD [13].

In the clinical picture of borderline PD in adolescents, one often sees anger towards parents, depression without any existential despair, tension, loss of empathy, impulsive behavior, and brief psychotic episodes including a paranoid thoughts and depersonalization without thought disorder [14].

3. Personality disorders during adolescence

It is a legitimate question whether to diagnose or not to diagnose PD before the age of 18. That is during adolescence – the time of major developmental changes, when the personality is not yet fully formed. However, relevant classifications and guidelines, based on a number of studies, allow us to diagnose a PD before 18 years of age. According to ICD-10, a PD can be diagnosed regardless the age of person if the diagnostic criteria are met; however, this is exceptionally rare before the age 16 or 17 years [5]. This is even more clearly defined in ICD-11, where the diagnosis of PD is made whenever the diagnostic criteria are met [6].

The DSM-5 allows for a diagnosis of PD in children and adolescents, when personality traits are particularly maladapted, permanent, and not related to a specific developmental period, mental disorder, or cultural background with the exception of antisocial PD, which cannot be diagnosed before the age of 18. For a diagnosis to be made, the characteristics of PD should have been present persistently for at least 1 year [4]. One should keep in mind that the characteristics of PD identified in childhood will change and that some types of PD will become less obvious or even disappear in later developmental periods (borderline, antisocial PD). The NICE recommendations do not define a chronological age at which a PD can be diagnosed. Instead, they focus on the individual level of developmental maturity and an understandable therapeutic plan to be provided to the person diagnosed with PD [15]. However, PD should not be diagnosed in individuals under the age of 13 and is not applicable until an individual finishes puberty. Because PDs have long been considered as therapy resistant, this diagnosis is misused even today as an excuse to refuse a patient. When diagnosing a person with PD, especially if it is an adolescent, an appropriate treatment must be provided along with the diagnosis. Prevention, early detection, and timely treatment are essential [15].

4. Personality disorders treatment in a development period

The purpose of diagnosing PD is to provide the adolescent with the appropriate treatment. It is the adolescent period that has a corrective potential and by introducing a therapy in time, we can significantly influence the course of PD. Adolescents with PD should be treated by a team of highly qualified professionals with a clearly structured intervention model and therapeutic plan [8, 13, 15]. Primarily, the patient must be provided with continuity and consistency. Adolescents with PD, especially borderline patients, have a tendency to form intense relationships; therefore, it is necessary to set clear time and space framework for treatments with different therapists. It is essential to organize treatments adequately—not too much and too little. Team members often have different views on the adolescent's problems and symptoms, which often lead to conflicts within the team; therefore, supervision is necessary. Often, many services (social services, school, general physician, previous therapist) are involved in the treatment; therefore, roles and tasks need to be clearly identified and coordinated. One of the main treatment goals of all team members is to support the adolescent in his separation and individualization and to actively involve him in the decision-making process. Many adolescents with borderline PD have experienced traumatic events; however, trauma processing is often not the primary intervention. Primarily, it is necessary to reduce suicidality and increase emotional stability [15, 16].

There are many different psychotherapeutic approaches to treat PD. Mentalization-based therapy (MBT), dialectical-behavioral therapy (DBT), and adolescent identity treatment (AIT) are among the most common. It is not so important which specific psychotherapeutic approach is used in the therapy but that certain changes outside the therapeutic relationship are triggered [13, 16]. According to Lambert, these changes are to be accountable for 40% of success in psychotherapy [17]. It is important to include the rest of the family in the therapy, to generate changes in the school, and that all significant others receive appropriate psychoeducation. Psychotherapeutic factors such as therapeutic posture, curiosity, optimism, consistency, empathy, and warmth contribute 30% to the success of a therapy. The adolescent's expectations of how successful the therapy will be contributing a further 15%. In addition, 15% is contributed by the specific psychotherapeutic techniques [17].

To achieve an optimal therapeutic process, regardless of the type of therapy, the therapist needs to be open, accepting, and optimistic and maintain a positive mental representation of the adolescent as well as curiosity and interest in getting to know the adolescent as a holistic personality, not only in the context of his or her disorder [16]. Since AIT is a younger and not so known therapy as MBT and DBT, it will be explained in more detail than the last two therapies below.

5. Adolescent identity treatment

Adolescent identity treatment (AIT) is an integrative therapeutic approach based on the principles of Paulina Kernberg, which includes modified elements of transference- focused psychotherapy, psychoeducation, behavior-oriented home plans, therapeutic contract, and intensive family work with adolescents and parents (adapted from [16]). Identity diffusion and interpersonal misfunctioning are regarded as the core of the borderline PD in adolescents and, as such, forming a base for the essential principles of AIT. The AIT focuses on identity stabilizing and integration of the concepts of the self and significant others, which gradually affects interpersonal relationships and leads to resolving interpersonal conflicts. The AIT applies verbal and nonverbal communication as well as countertransference. The basic principle of the AIT is to work on the dominant affect. The therapist focuses on the dominant affect the adolescent is affected by—here and now. Clarification, confrontation, and interpretation are applied as therapeutic techniques.

Clarification is the most common AIT therapeutic technique. It is used to explore and understand what the patient is saying. The adolescent's subjective feelings and perceptions are explored in detail until the therapist is able to understand exactly what the patient has in mind. Clarification is the therapist's invitation to the adolescent to explain information that is vague, not clear, confusing, chaotic, and contradictory. It allows the adolescent to fully access the internalized, unconscious meaning of his/her actions and encourages self-reflection. This method is of essential importance for borderline PD, as identity diffusion is strongly pronounced in borderline patients. Examples of clarification:

- I did not understand...
- Did I get this right? You said...
- What did you mean by saying...?
- Please, could you explain that to me in detail?
- Is it because you do not have words to describe it, or because you have not thought about it?

Confrontation is not a common therapeutic technique, especially not at the beginning of a therapy, as adolescents may feel attacked when it is used too soon. Confrontation is supposed to be an invitation to the adolescent to look at the inconsistencies and contradictions and to bring to attention information (verbal or nonverbal) he or she is not aware of or regards as completely normal. It is important to use it as an encouragement to talk about auto- and hetero-aggressive thoughts and behaviors that interfere with therapy. Examples of confrontation are:

- You are telling me about a rather excruciating pain, but you are laughing at the same time. This does not fit. Do you have any idea what could this mean?
- You are saying that you are fine, but I see fresh cuts. How do these things fit?
- You are telling me you are not disappointed, yet you are struggling with tears. Can you explain this?

Interpretation helps the adolescent to self-reflect and explain the meaning of his/her thoughts and actions. The interpretation does not reflect the therapist's point of view, who knows everything, but as a hypothesis offered to the adolescents for their consideration. It is applied when clarification and confrontation have not had the desired effect and when the therapist thinks it is unrealistic to expect the adolescent will reach a certain insight on his or her own. Interpretation must follow the emotions (anger, hatred, anxiety, envy). Examples of interpretation are:

- This is how I see it, but correct me, if I am wrong.
- On the one hand, you are telling me that you are fine, but I see many fresh wounds on your arm.
- Then you tell me that no one would be sad if you killed yourself.
- Could it be that all these contradictory images are within you and that you do not know exactly whether you are feeling well or maybe you are still sad?

Regardless of the psychotherapeutic approach, sincerity, empathy, and warmth are the key characteristics of a therapist. AIT, however, added playful flexibility to the list, with the therapist explaining his/her thoughts, offering possible explanations as a hypothesis (interpretation) and adjusting to the adolescent. The therapist maintains a sound and meaningful stance, knows right from wrong, and maintains his or her position. Optimism is a necessary condition for the therapist to develop an idea of the adolescent as a healthy and stable person, including therapist's attitude that the adolescent is able to cooperate in sessions and that he or she can develop. The therapist maintains hope for change during therapy stagnation and when the risk of discontinuation of therapy occurs. The absolute presence of the therapist is crucial for the therapy. It can be manifested as curiosity and a genuine interest in the adolescent's experiences. The therapist is absolutely present when his or her nonverbal/body language and tone of speech reflect the adolescent's experience of the here and now. The therapist is a role model. For an adolescent, therapist may be the first person to ever really take a truly interest in him or her. By doing so, the therapist engages the adolescent to be curious, motivated, and interested in himself/herself.

Body language is an important factor in AIT. Therapists must be fully aware of their tone, facial expressions, thinking, and interest, paying attention to the adolescent in the treatment, and how all of this is being acknowledged by the adolescent. Nonverbal information is vital in therapy with PD adolescents, who are overly sensitive to possible rejection, split, and are not able to recognize contradictions in verbal and nonverbal communication or are prone to misjudging it. It does matter how the therapist dresses and whether he/she has a piercing or a tattoo. The latter, in particular, can be an important message of how a therapist treats his/her body or allows for various manipulations.

Intensive parental involvement in therapy is especially important in adolescents with PD and is therefore a crucial element of AIT. Working with parents can only be successful if there is no attribution of blame to the parents for the development of PD in their adolescent. If the parents are viewed as the "bad guys," then the therapist may cause the adolescent to see him/her as a "better parent" and a "savior," which brings many risks to the therapy. At the beginning of therapy, even very competent and functional parents can appear to be "pathological" due to psychological burden when living with an adolescent with PD.

It is important that the parents are not viewed as bad and invalidating by the therapist. If parents are not included in the therapy, the power of family dynamics and interactions significantly shaping the adolescent is being underestimated. It is essential to educate parents on the adolescent's heightened sensitivity to emotional stressors, such as criticism, rejection, and separation, and how stressors can be avoided or reduced. Parents need an explanation that the therapy will not change the adolescent's temperament; however, it will help him to control it more easily. Their job is to encourage the adolescent to go to therapy.

Therefore, *a contract with the parents* is delineated as well, which covers all issues described above. The goal of the contract is to optimize the family's potential in therapy and to record the expectations and limitations of therapy. Possible factors that could lead to discontinuation of therapy are also included in the contract. The contract contains previously agreed and expected changes in the family (and not just in the adolescent) and clear rules regarding suicidal and self-harming behavior.

At the beginning of therapy, a *treatment contract with the adolescent* is drawn up with the adolescent and therapist responsibilities. The adolescent undertakes to attend therapy regularly, that is, 25 weekly sessions, to arrive "clean" and not to use any psychoactive substances before therapy, to talk about important issues (e.g., self-harming) at the very beginning of each therapy and not at the end of therapy. The contract also includes the duties of the therapist and exceptions to confidentiality (such as severe abuse of psychoactive substances, suicide, pregnancy), support for the patient not to discontinue therapy (external superego; e.g., the therapist calls the adolescent 2 hours prior to the therapy and reminds him or her of the appointment), and clear rules of a therapist conduct in case of suicidal and/or self-harming behavior (to call parents, hospitalization).

A home plan involves clearly agreed responsibilities of both the adolescent and parents. This includes clear measures for self-injurious behavior such as addressing the wound without any additional comments, threats, rewards, or conversation; the adolescent will discuss this with his/her therapist at the next regular session. If the wounds are deep, the adolescent should be taken to see a surgeon. Behaviors that violate the home plan resulting in the revocation of privileges are agreed upon and set out in the contract, including a reward system for behavior if the adolescent sticks to the home plan.

6. Mentalization-based therapy

Mentalization-based therapy is a psychosocial therapy to treat borderline PD (adapted from [18]). It derives from psychoanalysis, attachment theory, and developmental psychopathology and is based on mentalization. It was first intended for the treatment of adults with borderline PD, later on a version for adolescents (MBT-A) was developed. Mentalization is the ability to understand our own mental states and the mental states of other people and represents the capacity that makes us human. We mentalize when we are aware of the mental states of others and ourselves. MBT is based on the assumption that instability in mentalization is a key problem of borderline PD. Similar to AIT, the therapist takes the position of a curious listener, who does not know what is going on and therefore encourages the adolescent to explain. The therapist observes the capacity for attachment and mentalization and applies various interventions to improve or at least maintain the adolescent's capacity to mentalize.

7. Dialectical behavioral therapy

Dialectical behavioral therapy was developed by the psychologist Marsha M. Linehan and colleagues in the late 1980s to treat borderline PD [19]. Later on, Rathus and Miller developed a version of DBT for adolescents (DBT-A) [20].

The DBT is based on cognitive-behavioral therapy, dialectical philosophy, and on the findings of M. Linehan that people with borderline PD are prone to more intense and dramatic responses when facing specific emotional situations (e.g., romantic, friendly, and family relationships) compared to people without PD. People with borderline PD have quick and strong emotional reactions in the situations described above, remain emotionally aroused, and require more time to calm down than people without borderline PD [19]. As a result, DBT does not focus on the core unconscious conflict, such as in MBT. Instead, it focuses on how to change problematic responses with a range of different behavioral strategies [21].

DBT-A is a 16-week treatment that includes individual adolescent therapy once a week, family therapy as required, and a skills training group for families of adolescents with borderline PD [22]. It is aimed at reducing life-threatening and undesirable behaviors in therapy and behaviors that impair the quality of life. It empowers the adolescents to regulate their emotions, to appropriately deal with interpersonal relationships and cope with stress, and encourages mindfulness [20].

8. Pharmacotherapy

The 2001 American Psychiatric Association recommendations [23], the 2009 NICE guidelines [15], which were reaffirmed in 2018 [24], and the Australian NHMRC guidelines for the treatment of borderline PD [25] do not recommend the use of pharmacotherapy as the first-line therapy. The World Federation of Societies of Biological Psychiatry recommendations mentions several studies reporting the efficacy of serotonin reuptake inhibitors (SSRIs), such as fluoxetine and fluvoxamine and second-generation antipsychotics in the treatment of PD [26].

The 2019 Timaus et al. study confirms clinical observations that most patients with PD are also treated pharmacotherapeutically [27]. Polypharmacy is high, which can also be attributed to the great comorbidity of PD with at least one additional mental disorder. For the most part, tricyclics, first-generation antipsychotics, and mood stabilizers are being omitted in the pharmacotherapy of PD. The mood stabilizer lamotrigine did not prove to be successful in the treatment of PD in a 2018 study [28]. The use of the atypical antipsychotic quetiapine and the opioid antagonist naltrexone has been increasing [27]. However, more studies are required to support the justification for using these medicines.

9. Conclusions

Prevention and early detection of PD are essential in order to prevent long-lasting effect of PD on adolescent's overall functioning and interpersonal relationships.

When diagnosing a PD in adolescence, we are obliged to provide an appropriate and a PD specialized treatment (AIT, DBT-A, MBT-A). By introducing a therapy in time and by a licensed therapist PD treatment is very effective especially in the adolescent period which has a strong corrective potential.

Acknowledgements

This work was part of a Slovenian Research Agency project J4-9434.

Author details

Hojka Gregoric Kumperscak[1,2]

1 Child and Adolescent Psychiatry Unit, University Medical Centre, Maribor, Slovenia

2 Faculty of Medicine, University of Maribor, Maribor, Slovenia

*Address all correspondence to: hojka.gregoric@guest.arnes.si

References

[1] Pregelj P, Kores-Plesnicar B, Tomori M, Zalar B, Ziherl S, editors. Psychiatry. Ljubljana: Psihiatricna klinika; 2013

[2] Rothbart M, Ahadi SA, Hershley KL, Fisher P. Investigations of temperament at three to seven years: The children's behaviour questionnaire. Child Development. 2001;**72**:1394-1408

[3] Musek J, editor. Personality, Values and Psychological Well-Being. Ljubljana: University of Ljubljana, Philosophic Faculty; 2015

[4] American psychiatric association. Diagnostic and Statistical Manual of Mental Disorders 5 (DSM – 5) [Internet]. 2013. Available from: https://www.psychiatry.org/psychiatrists/practice/dsm [Accessed: 08 March 2020]

[5] World health organization. Classification of mental and behavioural disorders (ICD-10) [Internet]. 1993. Available from: https://www.who.int/classifications/icd/en/GRNBOOK.pdf?ua=1 [Accessed: 08 March 2020]

[6] World health organization. International classification of diseases for mortality and morbidity statistics (11th Revision) [Internet]. 2018. Available from: https://icd.who.int/browse11/l-m/en [Accessed: 08 March 2020]

[7] Bach B, First MB. Application of the ICD-11 classification of personality disorders. BMC Psychiatry. 2018;**18**(351):1-14. DOI: 10.1186/s12888-018-1908-3

[8] Friedel RO. Borderline personality disorder demystified [Internet]. 2018. Available from: http://www.bpddemystified.com/overview/ [Accessed: 08 March 2020]

[9] Steinert T, Schmidt-Michel PO. Borderlinestorungen und schizophrenie. Der Nervenarzt. 1995;**66**:858-863

[10] Volkan VD, Ast G, editors. Eine Borderline-therapie. Gottingen: Vandenbboeck & Ruprecht; 1996

[11] Caran N. Borderline Case. Naučna knjiga: Beograd; 1983

[12] Linehan MM, Tutek DA, Heard HL, Armstrong HE. Interpersonal outcome of cognitive behavioral treatment for chronically suicidal borderline patients. The American Journal of Psychiatry. 1994;**151**:1771-1776

[13] Nagy Zunter AM, Stamos V, Jogan H, editors. Borderline Personality Disorder. Pozeg: Tiskarna Grafis; 1999

[14] Bennett Roth E. Six types of borderline and narcissistic patients: An initial typology. International Journal of Group Psychotherapy. 1982;**32**(1):9-27

[15] National collaborating centre for mental health, British psychological society. Borderline personality disorder: treatment and management. National clinical practice guidelines Number 78 [Internet]. 2009. Available from: https://www.nice.org.uk/guidance/cg78/evidence/bpd-full-guideline-242147197 [Accessed: 08 March 2020]

[16] Foelsch PA, Schlüter-Müller S, Odom AE, Arena HT, Borzutzky HA, Schmeck K, editors. Adolescent Identity Treatment. Cham, Heidelberg, New York, Dordrecht, London: Springer; 2014

[17] Lambert MJ. Psychotherapy outcome research: Implications for integrative and eclectic therapists. In: Norcross JC, Goldfried MR, editors. Handbook of Psychotherapy

Integration. New York: Basic Books; 1992. pp. 94-129

[18] Fonagy P, Gergeley G, Jurist E, Target M, editors. Affect Regulation, Mentalization, and the Development of the Self. New York: Other Press; 2002

[19] Linehan MM, Armstrong HE, Suarez A, Allmon D, Heard HL. Cognitive-behavioral treatment of chronically parasuicidal borderline patients. Archives of General Psychiatry. 1991;**48**:1060-1064

[20] Rathus JH, Miller AL. Dialectical behavior therapy adapted for suicidal adolescents. Suicide & Life-Threatening Behavior. 2002;**32**:146-157. DOI: 10.1521/suli.32.2.146.24399

[21] Swenson CR, Choi-Kain LW. Mentalization and dialectical behavior therapy. American Journal of Psychotherapy. 2015;**69**(2):199-217

[22] Fleischhaker C, Böhme R, Sixt B, Brück C, Schneider C, Schulz E. Dialectical behavioral therapy for adolescents (DBT-A): A clinical trial for patients with suicidal and self-injurious behavior and borderline symptoms with a one-year follow-up. Child and Adolescent Psychiatry and Mental Health. 2011;**5**(1):3

[23] American Psychiatric Association. Practice guideline for the treatment of patients with borderline personality disorder. The American Journal of Psychiatry. 2001;**158**:1-52

[24] National institute for health and care excellence. Surveillance of personality disorders (NICE guidelines CG77 and CG78) [Internet]. 2018. Available from: https://www.nice.org.uk/guidance/cg78/resources/2018-surveillance-of personality-disorders-nice-guidelines-cg77-and-cg78-pdf-6358811143669 [Accessed: 08 March 2020]

[25] National Health and Medical Research Council. Clinical practice guideline for the management of borderline personality disorder – Appendix H [Internet]. 2012. Available from: https://www.nhmrc.gov.au/sites/default/files/documents/reports/clinical%20guidelines/mh25c-bpd-appendix-h.pdf [Accessed: 08 March 2020]

[26] Herpertz SC, Zanarini M, Schulz CS, Siever L, Lieb K, Möller HJ. WFSBP task force on personality disorders; world Federation of Societies of biological psychiatry (WFSBP). WFSBP guidelines for biological treatment of personality disorders. The World Journal of Biological Psychiatry. 2007;**8**:212-244

[27] Timäus C, Meiser M, Bandelow B, et al. Pharmacotherapy of borderline personality disorder: What has changed over two decades? A retrospective evaluation of clinical practice. BMC Psychiatry. 2019;**19**:393. DOI: 10.1186/s12888-019-2377-z

[28] Crawford MJ, Sanatinia R, Barrett B, Cunningham G, Dale O, Ganguli P, et al. The clinical effectiveness and cost-effectiveness of Lamotrigine in borderline personality disorder: A randomized placebo-controlled trial. The American Journal of Psychiatry. 2018;**175**(8):756-764

Chapter 3

Neurofeedback Training on Aging: Prospects on Maintaining Cognitive Reserve

Valeska Kouzak Campos da Paz and Carlos Tomaz

Abstract

Neurofeedback is a neuromodulation technique based on a brain-computer interface. An individual receives feedback from a computer about their brain activity and is conditioned to improve performance according to a training target. Therefore, it may be used to help individuals who suffer from cognitive decline, which is predicted to occur during aging. Cognitive decline affects working memory, which involves the medial temporal lobe—an important area for temporarily storing information—and recruits the prefrontal cortex, an area associated with higher cognitive functions, such as executive function. Since memory and executive function are fundamental components for every healthy and independent human life, cognitive decline fundamentally impairs a person's well-being. As such, since the aging population has been increasing at higher rates, methods to enhance their cognitive performance have become increasingly important. These methods may be used to increase brain reserve and help the elderly maintain a socially active life. The purpose of this chapter is to add neurofeedback to the box of promising tools that maintain cognitive reserve and as such promote a healthy and active life.

Keywords: neurofeedback, memory storage, executive function, brain reserve, SMR protocol, prefrontal cortex

1. Introduction

Across a life span, changes in cognition are expected to occur as individuals grow older. Most of the changes experienced in aging are related to a decline in fluid intelligence, defined as the capacity to solve problems and articulate ideas, to navigate new situations, and to acquire knowledge. On the other hand, crystallized intelligence, defined as acquired general knowledge (e.g., vocabulary and procedures), is preserved for longer periods [1]. Moreover, during aging, other neuropsychological abilities are known to decline, such as attention, working memory, and episodic memory [2].

Some faculties related to crystalized intelligence might increase over time, such as general knowledge and wisdom [2]. And this amount of additional information, when integrated to crystalized intelligence, can become an advantage. On the other hand, the attentional and working memory decline, related to fluid intelligence, makes it more challenging to solve problems and articulate ideas.

Image studies have shown atrophy in white matter and gray matter, synaptic degeneration, blood flow reduction, and neurochemical alterations [3].

IntechOpen

Those changes are more prominent at the prefrontal cortex; however, older adults that maintain their performance on pair with young adults tend to increase activation in order to keep performance, and this increased activation creates more hemispheric asymmetry in elderly than in youth. Consequently, Cabeza et al. [3] proposed a model called hemispheric asymmetry reduction in older adults (HAROLD), in which an older adult tends to compensate the neuropsychological decline with higher activation at the frontal cortex.

Cognitive training with the intent of increasing abilities and enriching neural networks has been a tendency since the 1960s, when the first behavior protocols sought to train memory using strategies of "chunking" (grouping information bits to be stored as single concepts) and using metacognitive strategies for dealing with complex information. Those strategies to enhance memory capacity were based in conscious and external mechanisms [4].

In the late 1980s, Baltes et al. [1] have demonstrated that older adults may benefit from cognitive training by creating reserve and increasing their performance in cognitive tasks. Afterward, many studies and protocols have been developed to provide cognitive training for the aging population. Some of them are related to strategy making, where the individual has to identify a difficulty level and naturally self-adjust. Reasoning, problem-solving, and goal management also have been used to enhance cognition. Multimodal approaches have also been tried, in which an unrelated task is trained in order to provide skill transfer (e.g., video games or cardiovascular exercise). Lastly, there is the process training, which includes a set of cognitive tasks to be trained heavily and specifically [5].

Recent technological developments have supported new forms of training, nowadays using tools such as computer games to enhance cognitive capacity [6]. Therefore, cognitive training has increasingly become a potential tool to aid healthy individuals with cognitive aging and patients with cognitive decline.

Training working memory—a component of the executive function—is one of the tendencies to enhance cognition and enrich neural networks [7], especially to form cognitive and neuronal reserve in aging people. Most of working memory training is based on computer game protocols, such as Cogmed [4], that might transfer the skill learned to other tasks [5, 8, 9].

Therefore, generally, executive function is trained by two interventional models: behavioral and neuroscientific. The behavioral model focuses on one's acquired ability and trains executive function using computational tasks, with diverse protocols; the neuroscientific model by neuromodulation uses neurofeedback training or neuronal direct stimulation—direct current or magnetic current [10].

Transcranial direct current stimulation (TDCS) is a form of noninvasive neuromodulation based on a small current applied by two electrodes positioned in the scalp in order to create neuronal membrane excitability and enhance neuronal firing. Transcranial magnetic stimulation (TMS) is also noninvasive neuromodulation but instead based on a magnetic field applied to the scalp focused at target areas to create a neuronal action potential to induce firing. Both models provide neuroplasticity at the area applied and, consequently, benefit cognition [10].

2. Working memory model

Working memory is a neuropsychological function that allow us to deal with daily information, such as keeping in mind a telephone number while dialing, organizing the mental operations to accomplish a task in hands, or listening and remembering a sequence of facts in a story in order to understand it.

Working memory can be described as a multimodal system, and Baddeley [11] defines it as a system of temporary storage under attentional control, encompassing our ability for complex thought and comprising diverse neuropsychological constructs. The abilities which working memory allows, although natural to most humans, require a complex cognitive model and several brain areas.

For about 50 years, working memory has been studied to define its main properties. The model adopted in this chapter is based on a construct of Baddeley and Hitch [12], in which working memory orchestrates information received through four components, one attentional and three mnemonic (**Figure 1**).

According to the Baddeley and Hitch model [12], the first component of the working memory is the central executive: an attentional control system that is connected to other three storage systems—the phonological loop, visuospatial sketchpad, and the episodic buffer. The episodic buffer component was included posteriorly [13] and all the components work interconnectedly. Further, each system is limited in capacity [14].

Briefly stating, the phonological loop is able to temporarily keep linguistic expression (e.g., verbal and emotional) and acoustic information, and the visuospatial sketchpad works similarly to the phonological loop, but only for visual and spatial information. Then, the episodic buffer acts as a mechanism that connects perceptual information from the two subsystems to long-term memory, integrating information into a limited number of episodes [11, 15]. Besides that, the phonological loop and the visuospatial sketchpad are considered two slave subsystems of the central executive, a system that accesses long-term memory information by attentional control [14, 15].

The central executive is responsible to keep information in mind while completing a task. Its proposed mechanism is based in frontal lobe patient studies that provided evidence from the connection between the supervisory attentional system (SAS), developed by Norman and Shallice [11], and the central executive [16]. Therefore, according to Baddeley [11], there are four candidates to compound the executive processes: the ability to focus attention, divide attention, change attention, and secure the connection between working memory and long-term memory.

The episodic buffer, completing this model of working memory, is responsible for temporary storage of perceptual information from both the phonological loop and visuospatial sketchpad, combining the information to form long-term memory

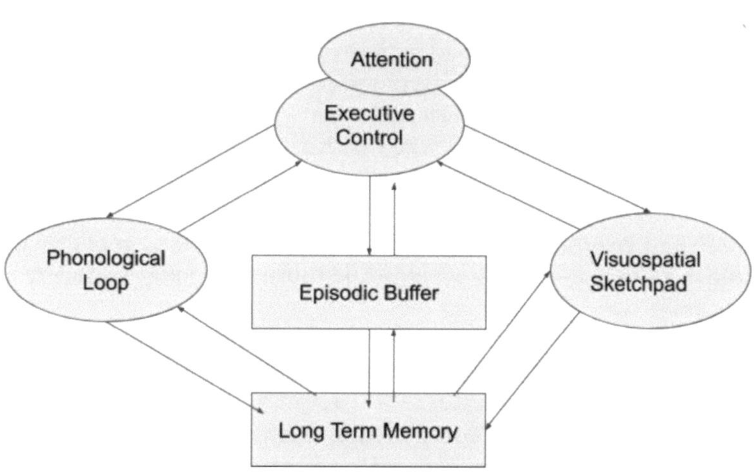

Figure 1.
Working memory model developed by Baddeley and Hitch [12].

content [13]. In conclusion, the function of working memory is to manipulate the information for a limited period of time, and it may increase or decrease in its capacity according to demand and practice [17].

3. Executive function

The executive function consists of multiple top-down neuropsychological functions that enable us to deal with problem-solving in a non-automatic way. It may involve activities demanding attention, such as when writing and remembering a map on way to school [18], as well as activities demanding planning, controlling, and monitoring [19], such as keeping a diet prescription, physical training, or working long hours. All these abilities, also natural to most humans, again require a complex cognitive model that involves inhibition (including self-control), working memory, and flexibility.

Therefore, executive function has three neuropsychological functions associated with it. Firstly, there is inhibitory control, which is the ability to control internal and external stimulus that interfere with thought process while executing an activity that demands attention, filtering out the concurrent stimulus. Inhibition gives rise to what is commonly called self-control, an ability to prevent habits and instinctive behavior to dominate over careful planning [20]. Secondly, there is mental flexibility, which is the capability to alter between stimuli and adjust during the execution of a task in order to complete it [21]. Thirdly, there is a working memory, which has been described in the previous topic.

4. Neurofeedback

Neurofeedback (NF) is a neuromodulation by operant conditioning of brain activity, where physiological signal is acquired by electroencephalogram (EEG), functional magnetic resonance (fMRI), or functional near-infrared spectroscopy (fNIRS), and a computational interface provides a feedback (visual or/and sound) to self-regulation [22].

The neurofeedback works dynamically in the cortex. For instance, when electrical activity is used as parameter, subjects can enhance a brain wave frequency in a region while reducing another brainwave frequency in another region. The Lacroix [23] cognitive model provides a broader view of NF training, as he proposes that a change in a subject's perception of his physiological self-regulation provides a cognitive integration from the conditioned behavior. Consequently, neurofeedback involves a cognitive component associated with a conditioned behavior.

Additionally, the neuronal mechanisms of neurofeedback training are based in the neuromodulation model: the feedback provides a persistent functional brain reorganization and generates neuroplasticity, as pointed out by cortical changes after training in evidence-based studies, while those changes are ruled by a Hebbian learning process [22].

Electroencephalogram is the most common tool for neurofeedback, in which physiological information is collected and fed back to the same individual to induce self-regulation. EEG captures electrocortical activity and decomposes it into brainwaves. Generally it has four components: electrodes, an amplifier, a converter, and software. The electrodes often collect the electrocortical activity from layers III and V at pyramidal cells that occur close to the scalp.

The brain activity is characterized by the postsynaptic potential difference of billions of neurons and captures data closest to the scalp [24]. The potential difference forms a bidimensional (amplitude and frequency) topographic representation of the cortical activity that will be mathematically calculated by the Fourier transformation. Therefore, the Fourier transform makes a decomposition of sinusoidal signals from the cortical depolarization, forming the following frequency band waves: delta, 1–4 Hz; theta, 4–8 Hz; alpha, 8–13 Hz; beta, 13–30 Hz; and gamma, 30–60 Hz.

When applying EEG to neurofeedback, the electrodes are placed according to the international system 10–20, where 10–20 means 10 or 20% distance between electrodes. The placement areas are classified by the distance measured from the middle point between nasion and inion at sagittal direction and right and left temporomandibular disc measurement at coronal direction, placing the vertex at location Cz. From the vertex, a measurement of 10% for the total sagittal and total coronal mark and 20% for the subsequent regions is placed, or in other words, if the distance between nasion and inion is 32 cm, then the vertex is 16 cm, and 10% of each sagittal mark is 3.2 cm. The classification follows the cortical regions F (frontal), C (central), P (parietal), and O (occipital), odds to left hemisphere and evens to right hemisphere [25].

The voltage received by cortical electrodes is very low, around a thousand times lower than cardiac electrical impulse and hundred times lower than muscular activity. Despite capturing a low amplitude, there are further challenges in capturing brain wave signals: electrical information from brain waves must be excluded from many layers of interference, such as the skin, scalp, pia mater, and fluid, beyond external noises and electrical current from electrical apparatus. Therefore, an amplifier and filter must be used to improve the signal [26]. The filters act by reducing noise, leaving mostly the biopotential desired to be converted; the amplifier amplifies the signal to a range of 100–100,000 times the information from electrodes [25]. The converter then changes the analogical signal from the amplifier to digital form. In this process, the analogical signal is decoded as repeated samples over fixed intervals, forming a sampling rate and transforms the signal into a digital information, where the converted resolution has lower amplitude [26]. Lastly, the software presents the digital signal to the experimenter that will be now able to analyze it.

There is a general association between frequency band and cortical activity: higher cortical activity provides higher frequency band waves and is usually involved in higher brain activity. Symmetrically, lower cortical frequency bands are generally associated with lower brain activity. Hence, delta brain waves are associated with sleep, theta and alpha band waves are associated with working memory, attention and creativity, beta and gamma band waves are associated with intense thoughts and stimulus integration [27]. Those associations are based in several evidence-based studies, including the creation of EEG by Berger [28] that firstly divided brain activity into two brain wave frequencies, alpha and beta, and favored the understanding of mental states and electrophysiology, promoting the development of the neurofeedback technique.

Another form to capture brain signal and provide neurofeedback is from functional magnetic resonance image (fMRI) that will offer data of cortical activity from hemodynamic signals—blood-oxygen-level-dependent (BOLD)—in which the magnetic resonance captures changes in blood flow during brain activity. In other words, when there is a neuronal activation, creating a metabolic demand, oxygen venous blood increases to regulate the de-oxygenated arterial blood. This increase of oxy-deoxyhemoglobin also increases the resonance signal around the activated nervous tissue, forming the image. This technique has high spatial resolution but low time resolution, as to capture an image it is necessary to wait for a metabolic process, which may take minutes. Therefore, the protocols used in fMRI neurofeedback must contemplate this temporal delay [29].

The neurofeedback by fMRI is called real-time functional magnetic resonance image (rt-fMRI) and has the advantage of providing training in deeper and specific regions of the brain. Further, although it is a new technique, its results have been significant [30].

Functional near-infrared spectroscopy is similar to magnetic resonance, since the brain activity captured is from BOLD signals. Therefore, the hemodynamic changes are registered by an infrared proximal light spectrum. However, this spectrum only captures activity from layers closer to the scalp [31]. The neurofeedback training by fNIRS is as recent as the rt-fMRI, but it has the advantage of being more accessible, as it involves simpler equipment and less medical environment [32].

5. The EEG neurofeedback

5.1 A brief history of neurofeedback

The first studies that evaluated the association between operant conditioning and cortical changes were conducted by Sterman et al. [32], where he incidentally observed that cats trained to increase their activation in 12–15 Hz at Rolandic cortex were resistant to a convulsion-inducing chemical—hydrazine. Afterward, he conducted this experiment in humans to check if the neurofeedback would be able to inhibit not controlled seizures. This frequency band (12–15 Hz) observed centrally, at the sensorimotor region, became known as the sensorimotor rhythm (SMR).

Another study also related to cortical operant conditioning by neurofeedback is a study conducted by Hardt and Kamiya [33]. The study observed that meditators have higher alpha wave patterns associated with a calm and tranquil state of mind. The study found that increasing alpha wave patterns could successfully reduce symptoms of anxiety.

Afterward, Lubar and Lubar [34] tested the effects of increasing SMR in children with attention deficit hyperactivity disorder with comorbid hyperkinesia and demonstrated that neurofeedback can reduce motor movements and increase attention.

From the mentioned studies, diverse protocols have been developed and applied in order to diminish symptoms of psychiatric disorders, improve cognitive performance, and manage stress. Therefore, neurofeedback has been used since its creation in the 1960s to improve conditions such as convulsion, ADHD, anxiety, depression, and addiction [35–38]. These protocols which have been extensively studied mainly train the central regions of the cortex to change SMR (12–15 Hz) [37].

The SMR occurs precisely over the primary motor cortex. This was observed when cats were operantly conditioned by having the animal press a bar as it waits for a reward. By measuring cortical activity, they found that, when cats increased awareness and reduced movement, this was associated with the activation of 12–15 Hz over primary motor cortex [31].

In humans, the SMR follows the same pattern [39], that is, when there is increased activity (12–15 Hz) over the sensorimotor cortex, there is a suppression of movement and an increased attention.

The mechanism of SMR neurofeedback is through the inhibition of thalamic-cortical circuits, which reduces interference of somatosensorial information [40]. Inhibition caused by the increase of SMR rhythm provides a higher integration of information processing over the cortex, by reducing interference of motor activity on cognitive performance [41].

5.2 Neurofeedback training in the cognitive aging

Cognitive training by neurofeedback has been applied over the last 15 years in healthy subjects. Successful protocols have been established with young populations [42–45]. However, there are fewer studies conducted with elderly populations [7, 46–50].

Angelakis et al. [46] conducted a study with 30 sessions in 6 health elderly subjects in order to test alpha neurofeedback at occipital region measuring their cognitive ability before and after the training. As a result, despite the fact that the training was conducted at the occipital region, changes in alpha production were observed frontally. Moreover, the alpha pick experimental group had an increase at processing speed and executive function, while the increased alpha amplitude is correlated with increase at verbal, visual, and working memory but decreased processing speed and executive function.

Becerra et al. [47] conducted a study for theta suppression at the cortical region that presented a higher-level amplitude at baseline quantitative EEG with 56 health elderly subjects which were evaluated cognitively before and after training. The results have shown that theta suppression promoted changes at absolute power of alpha and, in cognitive terms, there was a significant change at verbal comprehension, verbal IQ at WAIS-III [51], and working memory at Neuropsi [52].

LeComte and Juhel [48] trained four sessions to increase theta centrally (C3-C4) in order to improve memory in healthy elderly. The training happened with 30 subjects evaluated before and after training using the Signoret memory battery [53]. The results have not indicated any memory changes between tested groups. However, it highlighted how important might be the number of neurofeedback sessions to provide cortical changes. Gruzelier [45] has demonstrated it is necessary to have at least 10 sessions to produce an effective training.

Wang and Hsieh [49] conducted a study comparing how neurofeedback might improve attention and working memory in healthy elderly and young subjects. It had 32 subjects randomically assigned to increase theta activity at frontal vertex (Fz) since studies have shown that that working memory tasks require theta activity in this area [54, 55]. Elderly and young subjects showed improvement in attention and working memory even at rest. This study highlighted the question of whether cognitive enhancement performance protocols developed to young people might be applied to elderly as well, although the cortical differences with aging.

A study conducted by Belham et al. [56] suggested that a higher activation in theta centrally in adults and elderly is related to attentional processes as well as cortical integration during mnemonic processes. They also suggested that the mechanism behind brain wave intensity differences observed in elderly in comparison to young people is related to the Compensation-Related Utilization of Neural Circuits Hypothesis (CRUNCH). According to CRUNCH, the elderly brain will recruit higher cognitive resources according to task demand and will have a higher intensity neuronal activity at the beginning and middle of the task, as a way to compensate for the decrease in processing speed and for atrophy. Consequently, elderly will reach the performance ceiling faster, while a young will increase brain activity throughout the task [57].

Another study, conducted by Reis et al. [50], tested the neurofeedback using a short but intensive protocol to increase alpha and theta at several regions (Fp1, Fp2, Fz, and Pz) comparing subjects while they trained their cognitive abilities in working memory tasks. All elderly subjects were tested and retested in order to check for improvement. The results demonstrated that the neurofeedback group increased their working memory significantly, while the group of cognitive training plus neurofeedback had only shown a tendency to improve.

The neurofeedback group was also able to increase theta and alpha frontally (Fz), while neurofeedback with cognitive training presented only a tendency to increase alpha and theta frontally. An interesting result about neurofeedback observed by Reis et al. [50] was that the placebo group was also able to increase their alpha rhythm, as alpha is predominantly involved at attentional tasks, and when a simulation of neurofeedback was presented, the cortical activity was recruited even in a placebo situation. Therefore, the study has demonstrated that neurofeedback was able to change alpha and theta rhythm, consequently improving the performance in working memory task.

6. Neurofeedback training to improve working memory

We conducted a study with 17 healthy elderly subjects in order to increase SMR activity centrally (Cz) in 10 sessions to improve working memory performance, based on the assumption that attentional control is required at the central executive to keep the information continuously accessible [58]. The study conducted was an experimental-placebo randomized study. Quantitative EEG was collected during a working memory task called delayed matching-to-sample (DMTS) task before and after training to check for the cortical changes observed [7].

The DMTS task is a type of match-to-sample task, a pictorial working memory task which subjects are presented with a visual stimulus they are required to remember. It consists of two phases: the first phase presents the subject with an image for 500 ms, and then the image disappears for an interval of 15,000 ms. Then, in the second phase, two images are presented for 2000 ms, one being the same image as in the first phase and another being randomly chosen from a database. The objective is to click using a computer mouse on the picture that was initially presented at the first phase. An auditory feedback is provided (pinched sound to correct answers and bass sound to incorrect or not answered).

The neurofeedback protocol was developed by the authors, where the subjects sit comfortably in front of a computer screen and three cortical electrodes were installed, one at Cz and two other at ears lobes, one for reference and another for grounding. Two other electrophysiological electrodes were installed, one for heart rate frequency and another for breath frequency, both being only for measurement and not analyzed or used as feedback. The objective of the training was to increase SMR in 10% higher of each baseline measurement. The training took 3 min and was divided in three intervals, whereas in every interval it was collected a baseline frequency for 1 min. In other words, the training protocol consisted of 1-min baseline and 3 min of neurofeedback distributed in three blocks.

The equipment used for the neurofeedback training was ProComp Infiniti from Thought Technology, Canada. The amplifier pattern of the ProComp sampled the raw EEG at 256 Hz and converted A/D for live feedback. The software applied an infinite impulse response (IIR) filter to the recorded signal to extract frequency domain information. Spectral amplitude estimates were calculated for the active site (Cz) on raw 1-s EEG segments. A band-pass filter was used to extract the reward EEG frequency band for SMR (12–15 Hz) for feedback.

The EEG equipment used to measure brain wave activity while subject were performing DMTS task was Neuron-spectrum from NeuroSoft, Russia, with a 19 channels WaveGuard Connect cap, ANT Neuro, Deutschland, in a monopolar montage, decoded by Neuron-Spectrum software, NeuroSoft, that capture cortical activity of regions according to the 10/20 system. It was applied a rejection rate of 120 dB established by the program, sample rate of 2000 Hz, higher band filter pass of 0.5 Hz, lower band filter pass of 35 Hz and notch of 60 Hz.

The experimental group did ten sessions of SMR neurofeedback twice a week for 5 weeks. The placebo group did one session and then replayed their first session for the other nine sessions, twice a week for 5 weeks. The control group did the DMTS task firstly, waited 5 weeks, and did another DMTS task, without any contact to neurofeedback.

The results have demonstrated an improvement in working memory performance at the neurofeedback group comparing to placebo group and control. That is, subjects from the experimental group presented a higher number of correct response in the DMTS after neurofeedback training, demonstrating that neurofeedback facilitates attentional process that is critical for a good performance in working memory tasks.

Besides that, a comparison between groups at the pre-training phase has demonstrated that they were not different in performance as a sample ($p > 0.05$ ANOVA). Therefore, there was no performance difference between group compositions that could justify the observed changes. Consequently, the neurofeedback training might be responsible for the change in the performance.

Moreover, the ANOVA between groups after training have demonstrated no difference between experimental group and placebo, although there are differences between experimental and control groups ($p < 0.05$) as well as placebo and control groups ($p < 0.05$) (**Figure 2**). However, the placebo group presented some improvement at their performance on DMTS after training, suggesting that the training procedure, even when without contingency, is capable of facilitating effects over attentional processes that reflect on working memory performance [50].

Therefore, merely being at the office, having the electrodes put on and playing a neurofeedback session that does not give real feedback can exert and facilitate cognitive processes. And although the placebo group also did demonstrate an improvement in performance, it was not statistically significant as in the neurofeedback group.

Thereby, it can be stated that from the principles of operant conditioning, the reward must be contingent to achieve conditioning; however the incontigency of reward can also influence in the results [59], since somehow there is a feedback acting over the subject action. Moreover, it can be observed that none of the participants noticed the placebo condition. That is, even though the training was a repetition of their first session and there is no real feedback, the contingencial expectation over the results interferes in the self-regulation of those subjects [60].

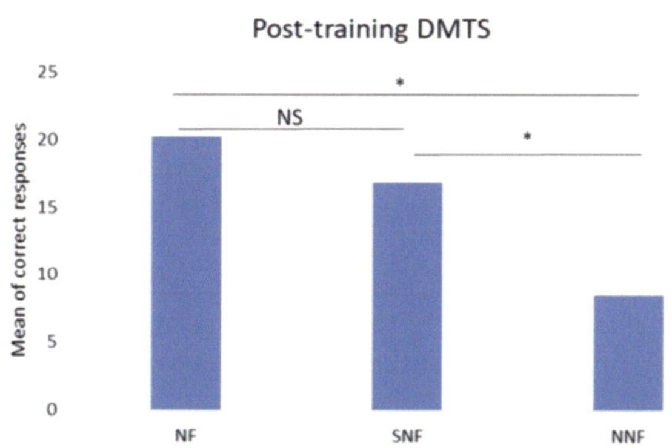

Figure 2.
ANOVA delayed matching-to-sample mean of correct response between groups after neurofeedback training in all groups: NF, experimental group; SNF, placebo group; and NNF, control group. $^*p < 0.05$.

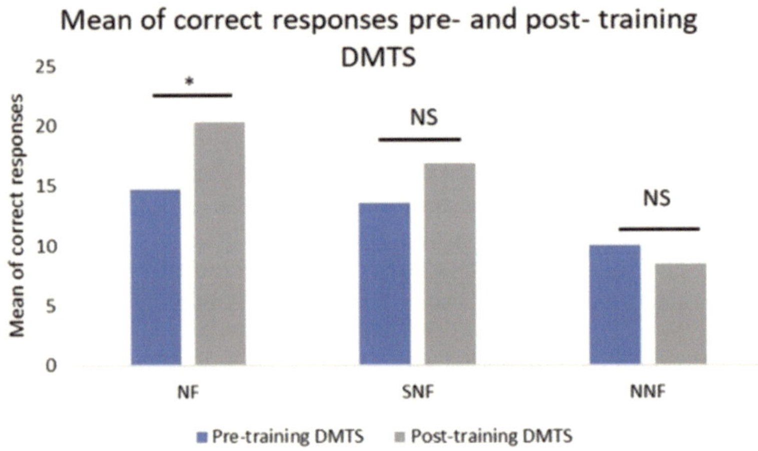

Figure 3.
Mean of the correct responses pre- and post-training at delayed matching-to-sample between condition and groups. NF, experimental group; SNF, placebo group; and NNF, control group. $p < 0.05$.

Hence, if the participant believed the training to be true and received the impression of feedback, even not-contingency over their action, it might be able to modify its self-regulation and consequently obtain an improvement of performance.

Thus, the improvement of working memory does not occur only by the effective training but also by placebo, demonstrating that the exposition to the technique is sufficient to induce a positive changes in cognitive abilities, while the lack of stimulation demonstrate to be deleterious to the participant, as the control group does not present any changes between the conditions (**Figure 3**).

As stated before, the working memory model is multicomponent and involves more than one cortical area: mainly regions of medial temporal lobe and dorsolateral prefrontal cortex. The activation of EEG is superficial, unable to capture neural activity from deeper areas such as hippocampus and inferior parietal cortex. However, in the study, it was possible to observe a higher activation at the pre-training DMTS task from recruited areas associate to working memory task, frontal and central, mainly in alpha and theta frequency band.

It can be also highlighted that at the pre-training condition, all frequency bands had an increased intensity in almost every region measured and, on the other hand, at the post-training there were changes at position with less intensity of some frequency bands. In theta, all cortexes were activated during a DMTS task, but at the post-training, less regions were activated during a DMTS task, with significant difference at the frontal, temporal, central, and occipital areas (**Figure 4**).

For beta band, at the pre-training and post-training, all regions measured presented significant differences, predominantly at the right hemisphere.

It was also possible to observe statistically significant differences at the interaction between the placebo and control groups in gamma activation, at pre- and post-training condition. The activations in both conditions and for all subjects reinforce the role of gamma activity to provide integration at connectivity during working memory tasks [61].

In relation to activation between pre- and post-training, the results of the study have indicated that participants of experimental groups have less activation in all frequency bands at the post-training DMTS task than the placebo group. However, the performance at task increased. Therefore, it can be inferred that the

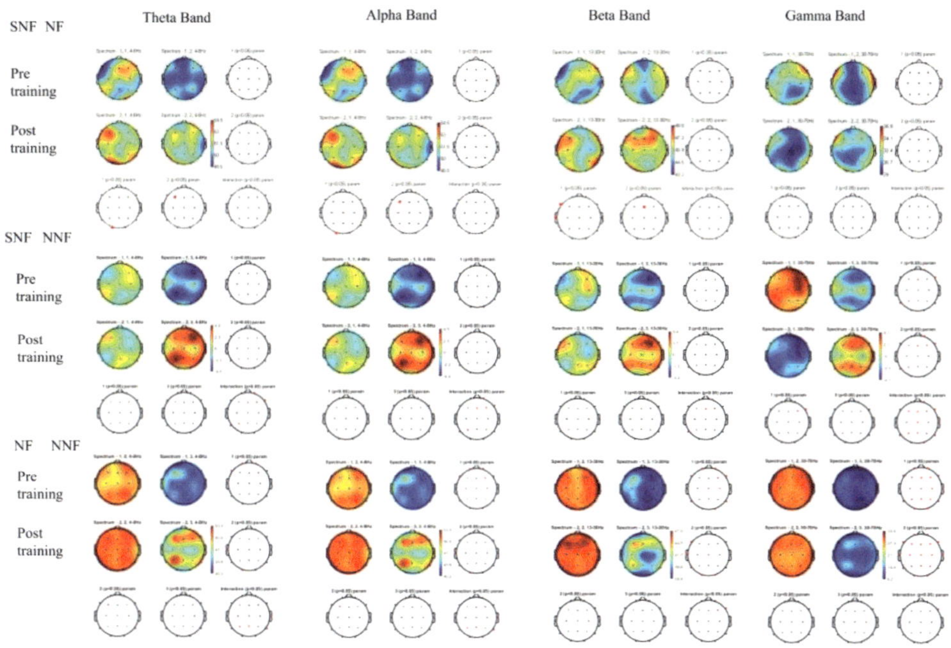

Figure 4.
ANOVA between condition (pre- and post-training) and interaction of theta (4–8 Hz), alpha (8–13 Hz), beta (13–30 Hz), and gamma (30–60 Hz) frequency band (columns). The first role is placebo (SNF) to left and experimental (NF) to right, at pre-training and post-training; second role is placebo (SNF) to left and control (NNF) to right, at pre-training and post-training; and third role is experimental (NF) to left and control (NNF) to right, at pre-training and post-training. The red dots are $p < 0.05$.

neurofeedback training resulted in a less-generalized cortical activation, which is related to a better performance at the working memory task.

In aging populations, cognitive and behavioral changes are evident by neurobiological changes that occur due to volumetric changes in brain structure, and lower efficiency is observed at information processing, including a diminish in speed, working memory, inhibition, and long-term memory [62]. And in compensation for their inefficiency, the elderly increase the intensity of activation during complex task performance, as observed at the placebo group.

Therefore, brain wave changes observed at placebo group as higher activation during DMTS task before and post-training neurofeedback might have occurred to keep performance, which is in line with the CRUNCH hypothesis, previously stated, in which elderly will overcome their difficulty with an increment of brain activity [57]. On the other hand, in the neurofeedback group, the activation was less statistically different from pre- to post-training at DMTS task, but their working memory performance increased. Therefore, the neuromodulation of neurofeedback relies on persistent human functional reorganization and neuroplasticity that is observed in pre- and post-test EEG comparison [63–65]. These changes are based on the combination of Hebbian and homeostatic plasticity [22].

Hence, the neuroplasticity observed at the neurofeedback group is in accordance to the interactive model [66] that is based in two principles:

- First, when a task involves a learning characteristic based on repetition, it is associated with less activation and more specificity of the area.

- On the other hand, if the learning process of a training is based on metacognitive strategies, there is a higher activation of several cortical areas.

Consequently, as the neurofeedback was related to the increase of SMR repeatedly, it was a repeated training, and a reduction of activation was observed and an increase of efficiency.

Afterward, the neurofeedback training even at placebo condition was able to change cortical activity. However, the changes on the experimental group were more precise and specific.

7. Conclusion

The studies mentioned above have demonstrated that the training protocols with elderly involve diverse proposals and sometimes may have inconsistent results. However, despite the diversity of protocols, the studies have demonstrated positive neurophysiological and cognitive effects related to working memory and attention. Therefore, these results suggest that neurofeedback might be an important tool to increase cognitive reserve at aging.

To conclude, since

1. Neurofeedback is an accessible technique for neuromodulation by EEG that provides operant conditioning and cognitive self-perception.

2. Aging individuals experience decline in their neuropsychological abilities.

Techniques and tools that favor the formation of cognitive reserve have become of fundamental importance to society, once the increase in life expectancy leads to a longer period in this later stage of life.

Acknowledgements

We thank Dr. Ana Garcia for assistance in analysis of the data and Psy. Aloysio Campos da Paz Neto for the protocol design and the Laboratory of Neuroscience and Behavior at the University of Brasília, Brazil.

Conflicts of interest

The authors declare no conflict of interest.

Author details

Valeska Kouzak Campos da Paz[1]* and Carlos Tomaz[2]

1 UnB, Brasília, Brazil

2 UniCeuma, São Luís, Brazil

*Address all correspondence to: valeskakcp@gmail.com

References

[1] Baltes PB, Sowarka D, Kliegl R. Cognitive training research on fluid intelligence in old age: What can older adults achieve by themselves? Psychology and Aging. 1989;**4**(2):217-221. DOI: 10.1037/0882-7974.4.2.217

[2] Dumas JA. What is normal cognitive aging? Evidence from task-based functional neuroimaging. Current Behavioral Neuroscience Reports. 2015, 2015;**2**(4):256-261. DOI: 10.1007/s40473-015-0058-x

[3] Cabeza R, Anderson ND, Locantre JK, McIntosh AR. Aging gracefully: Compensatory brain activity in high-performing older adults. NeuroImage. 2002;**17**:1394-1402. DOI: 10.1006/nimg.2002.1280

[4] Klingberg T. Training and plasticity of working memory. Trends in Cognitive Sciences. 2010;**14**(7):317-324. DOI: 10.1016/j.tics.2010.05.002

[5] Lustig C, Shah P, Seidler R, Reuter-Lorenz P. Aging training and the brain: A review and future directions. Neuropsychology Review. 2009;**19**(4):504-522. DOI: 10.1007/s11065-009-9119-9

[6] Green CS, Bavalier D. Exercising your brain: A review of human brain plasticity and training-induced learning. Psychology and Aging. 2008;**23**:692-701

[7] Campos da Paz VK, Garcia A, Campos da Paz Neto A, Tomaz C. SMR neurofeedback facilitates working memory performance in healthy older adults: A behavior and eeg study. Frontiers in Behavioral Neuroscience. 2018;**12**:1-11. DOI: 10.3389/fnbeh.2018.00321

[8] Valenzuela MJ. Brain reserve and the prevention of dementia. Current Opinion in Psychiatry. 2008;**21**:296-302. DOI: 10.1097/YCO.0b013e3282f97b1f

[9] Hosseini SMH, Pritchard-Bermana M, Sosa N, Ceja A, Keslera BSR.Task-based neurofeedback training: A novel approach toward training executive function. NeuroImage. 2016;**134**:153-159. DOI: 10.1016/j.neuroimage.2016.03.035

[10] Enriquez-Gebbert S, Huster RJ, Herrman CS. Boosting brain function: Improving executive functions with behavioral training. International Journal of Psychophysiology. 2013;**88**:1-16

[11] Baddeley AD. Working Memory, Thought, and Action. United Kingdom: Oxford Press; 2007

[12] Baddeley AD, Hitch GJ. Developments in the concept of working memory. Neuropsychology. 1994;**8**(4):485-493

[13] Baddeley AD. The episodic buffer: A new component of working memory. Trends in Cognitive Sciences. 2000;**4**(11):417-423

[14] D'Esposito M, Postle B. The cognitive neuroscience of working memory. Annual Review of Psychology. 2015;**66**:115-142. DOI: 10.1146/annurev-psych-010814-015031

[15] Baddeley AD. Working memory: Looking back and looking forward. Nature Reviews. 2003;**4**:829-839. DOI: 10.1038/nrn1201

[16] Della Salla S, Logie R, Spinnler H. Is primary memory deficit of Alzheimer patients due to a "central executive" impairment? Journal of Neurolinguistics. 1992;7(4):325-346

[17] Eriksson J, Vogel EK, Lansner A, Bergstrom F, Nyberg L. Neurocognitive architecture of working memory. Neuron. 2015;**88**:33-46

[18] Diamond A. Executive functions. The Annual Review of Psychology. 2013;**64**:135-168. DOI: 10.1146/annurev-psych-113011-143750

[19] Seiferth NY, Thienel R, Kirchner T. Exekutive Funktionen. In: Schneider F, Fink GR, editors. Funktionelle MRT in Psychiatrie und Neurologie. Berlin, Heidelberg: Springer-Verlag; 2007. pp. 265-277

[20] MacPherson S, Phillips LH, Della Salla S. Age, executive functions, and social decision making: A dorsolateral prefrontal cortex theory of cognitive aging. Psychology and Aging. 2002;**17**(4): 598-609

[21] Miyake A, Friedman NP, Emerson MJ, Witzki AH, Howerter AM, Wagner T. The unity and diversity of executive functions and their contributions to complex "frontal lobe" tasks: A latent variable analysis. Cognitive Psychology. 2000;**41**:49-100

[22] Sitaram R, Ros T, Stoeckel L, Haller S, Scharnowski F, Lewis-Peacock J, et al. Closed-loop brain training: The science of neurofeedback. Nature Reviews. Neuroscience. 2017;**18**:86-100. DOI: 10.1038/nrn.2016.164

[23] Lacroix JM. Mechanisms of biofeedback control. In: Davidson RJ, Schwartz GE, Shapiro D, editors. Consciousness and Self-Regulation. Springer. Boston, MA: Plenum; 1986. pp. 137-162. DOI: 10.1007/978-1-4757-0629-1_6

[24] Teplan M. Fundamentals of EEG measurement. Measurement Science Review. 2002;**2**:1-11

[25] Schwartz M, Andrasik F. Biofeedback: A Practitioner's Guide. 3o. Edição ed. Nova Iorque, EUA: Guildford Press; 2003

[26] Kaiser DA. Basic principles of quantitative EEG. Journal of Adult Development. 2005;**12**(2/3):99-104

[27] Demos JN. Getting Started with Neurofeedback. Nova York, NY: W.W. Norton and Company; 2005

[28] Berger H. Uber das elektrenkephalogramm des menschen. Arquives Psychiatric Nervenkr. 1929;**87**:527-570

[29] Soares JM, Magalhães R, Moreira PS, Sousa A, Ganz E, Sampaio A, et al. A hitchhiker's guide to functional magnetic resonance. Frontiers in Neuroscience. 2016;**10**:1-15

[30] Sherwood MS, Kane JH, Weisend MP, Parker JG. Enhanced control of dorsolateral prefrontal cortex neurophysiology with real-time functional magnetic resonance imaging (rt-fMRI) neurofeedback training and working memory practice. NeuroImage. 2016;**124**:214-223

[31] Kober SE, Witte M, Stangl M, Väljamäe A, Neuper C, Wood G. Shutting down sensorimotor interference unblocks the networks for stimulus processing: An SMR neurofeedback training study. Clinical Neurophysiology. 2014;**126**:82-95. DOI: 10.1016/j.clinph.2014.03.031

[32] Sterman MB, Howe RC, MacDonald LR. Facilitation of spindle-burst sleep by conditioning electroencephalographic activity while awake. Science. 1970;**167**:1146-1148

[33] Hardt JV, Kamiya J. Anxiety change through electroencephalolographic alphafeedback seen only in high anxiety subjects. Science. 1978;**201**:79-81

[34] Lubar JF, Lubar JO. Eletroct-roencephaloghrafic biofeedback of SMR and beta for treatment of attention deficit disorders in clinical setting. Biofeedback and Self-Regulation. 1984;**9**:1-23

[35] Sterman MB. Phisiological origins and functional correlates of EEG Rythmic activities: Implications for

self-regulation. Biofeedback and Self-Regulation. 1996;**21**:3-33

[36] Thompson M, Thompson L. Neurofeedback combine with training in metacognitive strategies: Effectiveness in student with ADD. Applied Psychophysiology and Biofeedback. 1998;**23**(4):243-263

[37] Monastra VJ et al. Electroencephalographic biofeedback in the treatment of attention deficit/hyperactivity disorder. Applied Psychophysiology and Biofeedback. 2005;**30**(2):95-114

[38] Hammond D. Neurofeedback training for anxiety and depression. Journal of Adult Development. 2005;**12**:131-137

[39] Sterman MB. Basic concepts and clinical findings in the treatment of seizures disorders with EEG operant conditioning. Clinical Electroencephalography. 2000;**31**:45-55

[40] Kober SE, Witte M, Stangl M, Valjamae A, Neuper C, Wood G. Shutting down sensorimotor interference unblocks the networks for stimuling processing: An SMR neurofeedback training study. Clinical Neurophysiology. 2015;**126**(1):82-95

[41] Egner T, Gruzelier J. EEG biofeedback of low beta band components: Frequency specific effects on variables of attention and event- related brain potentials. Clinical Neurophysiology. 2004;**115**:131-139

[42] Vernon D, Egner T, Cooper N, Compton T, Neilands C, Sheri A, et al. The effects of training distinct neurofeedback protocols aspects of cognitive performance. International Journal of Psychophysiology. 2003;**47**: 77-88

[43] Gruzelier J, Egner T, Vernon D. Validating the Efficacy of Neurofeedback for Optimizing Performance. 2006. Available from: http://research.gold.ac.uk/500/1/PSY_Gruzelier_2006a.pdf

[44] Gruzelier J. A theory of alpha/theta neurofeedback, creative performance enhancement, long distance functional connectivity and psychological integration. Research Report - Cognitive process. 2008;**10**:101-109

[45] Gruzelier J. EEG-neurofeedback for optimising performance. I: A review of cognitive and affective outcome in healthy participants. Neuroscience and Biobehavioral Reviews. 2013;**44**:124-141

[46] Angelakis E, Stathopoulou S, Frymiare JL, Green DL, Lubar J, Kounios J. EEG neurofeedback: A brief overview and an example of peak alpha frequency training for cognitive enhancement in the elderly. The Clinical Neuropsychologist. 2007;**21**:110-129

[47] Becerra J, Fernández T, Roca-Stappung M, Díaz-Comas L, Galán L, Bosch J, et al. Neurofeedback in healthy elderly human subjects with electroencephalographic risk for cognitive disorder. Journal of Alzheimer's Disease. 2012;**28**:357-367. DOI: 10.3233/JAD-2011-111055

[48] Lecomte G, Juhel J. The effects of neurofeedback training on memory performance in elderly subjects. Psychology. 2011;**2**:846-852. DOI: 10.4236/psych.2011.28129

[49] Wang JR, Hsieh S. Neurofeedback training improves working memory and attention performance. Clinical Neurophysiology. 2013;**124**(12):1-15

[50] Reis J, Portugal AM, Fernandes L, Afonso N, Pereira M, Sousa N, et al. An alpha and theta intensive and short neurofeedback protocol for healthy aging working memory training. Frontiers in Aging Neuroscience. 2016;**8**:1-11

[51] Wechsler D. Escala de Inteligência Wechsler para adultos -III. São

Paulo, Brasil: Editora Casa do Psicólogo; 2004

[52] Ostrosky-Solis F, Gómez-Perez ME, Matute E, Rosseli M, Ardila A, Pineda D. NEUROPSI Atención y memoria 6 a 85 anos. Manual, instructivo e pontuaciones totales. Cidade do México, México: American Book Store; 2003

[53] Signoret JL. B.E.C. 96: Evaluation des troubles de mémoire et des dêsordres cognitifs associés. Paris, França; 1996

[54] Klimesch W. Memory processes, brain oscillations and EEG synchronization. International Journal of Psychophysiology. 1996;**24**:61-100

[55] Klimesch W, Doppelmayr M, Russengger H, Pachinger T, Schwaiger J. Induced alpha band power changes in human EEG and attention. Neuroscience Letters. 1998;**244**(2):73-76

[56] Belham FS, Satler C, Garcia A, Tomaz C, Gasbarri A, Rego A, et al. Aged-related differences in cortical activity during visuo-spatial working memory task with facial stimuli. PLoS One. 2013;**8**(9):1-8

[57] Reuter-Lorenz PA, Cappell KA. Neurocognitive aging and the compensation hypothesis. Current Directions in Psychological Science. 2008;**17**(3):177-182

[58] Vogel EK, Woodman GF, Luck SJ. The time course of consolidation in visual working memory. Journal of Experimental Psychology. Human Perception and Performance. 2006;**32**(6):1436-1451

[59] Strehl U. What learning theories can teach us in designing neurofeedback treatments. Frontiers in Human Neuroscience. 2014;**8**(894):1-8

[60] Witte M, Kober SE, Nimaus M, Christa N, Wood G. Control beliefs can predict the ability to up-regulate sensorimotor rhythm in neurofeedback training. Frontiers in Human Neuroscience. 2013;**07**:1-8

[61] Constantinidis C, Klingberg T. The neuroscience of working memory capacity and training. Nature Reviews. 2016;**17**(7):438-449. DOI: 10.1038/nrn.2016.43

[62] Park DC, Reuter-Lorenz P. The adaptive brain: Aging and neurocognitive scaffolding. Annual Review of Psychology. 2009;**60**:173-196

[63] Chein JM, Schneider W. Neuroimaging studies of practice-related change: fMRI and meta-analytic evidence of a domain-general control network for learning. Cognitive Brain Research. 2005;**25**:607-623. DOI: 10.1016/j.cogbrainres.2005.08.013

[64] Ghaziri J, Tucholka A, Larue V, Blanchette-Sylvestre M, Reyburn G, Gilbert G, et al. Neurofeedback training induces changes in white and gray matter. Clinical EEG and Neuroscience. 2013;**44**:265-272. DOI: 10.1177/1550059413476031

[65] Scholz J, Klein MC, Behrens TEJ, Johansen-Berg H. Training induces changes in white matter architecture. Nature Neuroscience. 2012;**12**:1370-1371. DOI: 10.1038/nn.2412

[66] Belleville S, Mellah S, de Boysson C, Demonet JF, Bier B. The pattern and loci of training-induced brain changes in healthy older adults are predicted by the nature of the intervention. PLoS One. 2014;**9**:e102710. DOI: 10.1371/journal.pone.0102710

Chapter 4

Feeding and Eating Disorders

Bianca Suciu and Cătălina-Angela Crișan

Abstract

Eating disorders, which are well known as a substantial mental health problem in society, have been reclassified as feeding and eating disorders in DSM-5 and also in the 11th revision of ICD. The new classification includes binge eating disorder and avoidant-restrictive food intake disorder (ARFID), in addition to anorexia and bulimia nervosa. They are considered serious disorders, with high morbidity and mortality risks, that affect the young community in particular. Current research shows increases in all genders and age groups. Various genetic and biologic factors, an insecure personality type, impulsive traits, dysfunctional emotion regulation, and society's ideal of slimness have been found to play a role in the development of these disorders. A dual approach with focus on the symptom and the underlying problems is needed for all types of eating disorders throughout the psychotherapeutic interventions. Assessing comorbid psychiatric and medical symptoms is extremely important. Further research and new directions of treatment are needed with regard to the expanded classifications.

Keywords: eating disorders, anorexia nervosa, bulimia nervosa, binge eating disorder, treatment

1. Introduction

Eating disorders, which are well known as a substantial mental health problem in society, can come across all ages, but anorexia nervosa and avoidant-restrictive food intake are more common in childhood and adolescents, while bulimia nervosa and binge eating disorder are less prevalent in pediatric patients, but also with significant functional impairment [1].

2. Epidemiology

Recently, a systematic review analyzed the lifetime prevalence of eating disorders and found for anorexia nervosa a prevalence of 1.4% for women and 0.2% for men. Bulimia nervosa had higher prevalence scores 1.9% for women and 0.6% for men. Binge eating disorder had the highest prevalence percentage with 2.8% in women and 1% in men. The prevalence for avoidant-restrictive food intake disorder was investigated and was found to be 0.3% [2, 3]. All these results must be cautiously taken into consideration because the real community incidence of eating and feeding disorders is unknown. Other studies found an increasing number of cases diagnosed with bulimia nervosa or binge eating disorder [4, 5]. In the young women's population, anorexia nervosa seems to be the most predominant form of feeding and eating disorders, while binge eating disorder is more common in men [6]. Overall, studies show a higher prevalence of eating disorders among females and the young population [7].

3. Causes

Genetic predisposition is associated with the diagnosis of anorexia nervosa. Studies demonstrated that it is also a vulnerability inherited for anxiety and obsessiveness, by examining the family members of patients suffering from eating disorders and identifying anxiety disorders, obsessive compulsive disorder and autistic spectrum disorders diagnosed in the family members. The families with eating disorders have higher levels of academic achievement, traits of perfectionism and sensitivity, being above the average [8]. On the other hand, some studies explained the onset of anorexic episodes in the context of nonspecific triggers such as puberty, changes of schools or home, exams, conflicts with friends, family members, being bullied and bereavement. The anorexic behavior becomes a mechanism that manifest's in discomfort situations rather than confronting them [9]. A report showed that bulimia and binge eating disorders are being influenced by environmental factors, but theses play also a part in the onset and evolution of anorexia nervosa. In the same study it was mentioned that 17–18 years old was the peak age onset for bulimia and binge eating disorders [10].

4. Symptoms

Typical symptoms describing patients with anorexia nervosa are an obsessive fear of gaining weight, body dysmorphia, voluntary and deliberate purging and over exercising. Purging is a voluntary action, characterized by putting the fingers down the throat to induce vomiting. Because of this repeated action on the knuckles of the right hand appear calluses, known as Russell sign, caused by the repeated pressure from the teeth during purging. In time purging becomes a reflex and patients can vomit without effort, quickly, within seconds. Due to the gastric acidity after vomiting, teeth may become denuded of enamel and the parotid gland becomes enlarged. As a consequence of many hours of physical exercise joint problems can be precipitated and, on the long term, osteoporosis can develop caused by malnutrition and endocrine abnormalities [11, 12].

Specific behaviors usually used by patients in order to lose more weight are represented by avoidance of calorie intake such as a restrictive diet, consuming vegan food, hiding or disposing the food that is served by offering to pets or friends, chewing gum or smoking just to feel the mouth full with something, trying to mimic the feel of fullness by drinking water or diet drinks, always calculating the amount of calories intake by reading all food labels or avoiding medication that can lead to weight gain. Another way to maintain or reduce weight is to overcome the calorie intake by inducing vomiting, using laxatives in excessive doses, exposing the body to cold just for burning more calories, doing exhausting physical exercises, administering pain killers to release pain in order to be able to over exercise, using and buying substances for losing weight. Also, compulsive behaviors of rechecking ones weight, examining oneself in mirrors for hours, seeking to feel their bones through skin, comparing their body to magazines or online pictures can be present [13].

To define compulsive exercises we must assume any form of physical activity that cannot be stopped or cut down even in the presence of detrimental effects on health status [14, 15]. For persons who associate excessive physical exercises, this behavior usually started for healthy issues, prior to the presence of eating symptoms, and patients describe themselves as having greater levels of physical activity than their friends during childhood, or even being athletes during that period [16, 17]. For normal subjects, usually these activities come unplanned and are done in a spontaneous manner, with joy in participating, but for patients with eating disorders activities become carefully planned and self-conscious. A possible explanation of this behavior comes from ancient times, as an evolutionary adaptation; despite weight loss individuals are able to search food in wider areas [18]. Also, a strong emotional involvement is attached to physical activities [19, 20], and it is considered to be the last symptom that resolves [21]. Examples of such exercises are: swimming, running, cycling, all of this done in privet and solitude; go up and down the stairs more than it is required for a task, getting of public transport for walking long distances, standing on feet for longer than it is required or pacing all the time. Studies connect the over activity that is still present after discharge with a more chronic evolution, earlier relapse rates and longer periods of time spent in hospital admissions [22, 23].

Gastrointestinal functional symptoms can also associate in the course evolution of an eating disorder. Patients with anorexia nervosa reported postprandial fullness, abdominal distension and unspecific abdominal pain. On the other hand, for bulimia nervosa more frequent were reported bloating, flatulence and constipation as gastrointestinal functional symptoms [24]. If these symptoms are severe enough and require more investigations, for patients that are malnourished, invasive investigations of the gut such as colonoscopy or upper gastrointestinal endoscopy, could lead to important risks. Patients diagnosed with anorexia nervosa have the gut much thinner than well-nourished patients, and so the risk of tear or perforation is much higher, therefore, less invasive investigation are considered to be safer, such as CT scanning or barium passage [25].

Osteopenia represents a consequence of bone loss after a long period of low weight and sex steroid suppression. This effect may become irreversible in patients with severe anorexia nervosa, and implies a high risk for bone fracture even in young old patients [26].

5. Examination

One of the most important phases in physical examination consists in determining the body mass index, which expresses weight in kilograms reported to height in squared meters (height is greater early in the morning). It is a simple formula to measure the nutritional risk but always needs to be interpreted in the clinical context. Sometimes based on this measurement, the case management plan can be influenced in determining which patient needs the most to be admitted and which can be treated in the community [27]. A so-called normal BMI is considered between the interval of 20–25 kg/m^2, but if this parameter keeps falling as a consequence of inappropriate restriction of food intake, this has to be taken into consideration. Measuring the physical resilience of the patient with a simple screening test can be done by telling the patient to sit up, squat and stand, or by using handgrip for measuring strength [28]. Another important step is measuring pulse, blood pressure, and ECG for investigating the risk of prolonged QTc interval (over 450 ms) that can indicate electrolyte disturbances (hypokalemia, hypomagnesaemia, and hypocalcemia), heart disease (myocardial ischemia and cardiomyopathies), and improper use of drugs such as antipsychotics, antidepressants, antihistamines, antibiotics, and antiarrhythmics. Commonly anorexic patients present cardiovascular instability as bradycardia, showing a pulse under 50 bpm, or resting tachycardia with a pulse over 100 bpm suggesting infection or dehydration [29]. Also, basic screening is necessary. A full blood cell count has to be done, biochemical assays such as transaminase to evaluate liver function, creatinine and urea for determining renal function. Electrolytes abnormalities are common and need to be measured to exclude hyponatremia after an excessive water intake, hypokalemia in the context of excessive purging, or hypocalcaemia, hypomagnesaemia that can indicate the improper use of laxatives. Thyroid function should be checked together with plasma ferritin, folate, and B12 vitamin [30].

Body temperature frequently drops under 36°C in anorexic patients, who voluntary induce hypothermia in order to start shivering, consume energy and lose some more weight. Fever in a patient with low BMI is always significant and can indicate infection, with negative consequences because even minor episodes of sepsis can have a fatal outcome. Other signs present could be pale conjunctives, dry tongue and teguments, muscular weakness, peripheral edema in the context of low-level albumin, hand calluses after self-induced vomiting. It is not uncommon that patients present constipation, as a paradox effect of withdrawing the laxatives that were used for long periods of time in very high doses [31].

6. Making a diagnosis of eating disorder

The ICD-11 restructured the chapter of feeding and eating disorders guided by the principles of more clinical utility and relevance around the world, after 25 years of research and evidence based knowledge. The disorders included in this chapter are not better explained by other health problems, developmentally conditions or cultural context. Moreover, two previous distinct conditions were united in one single block named feeding and eating disorders that combines abnormal eating patterns associated with fear of gaining weight, body image and feeding behaviors that imply limited food intake, eating non-edible substances, or voluntary regurgitation of foods that have been eaten. We could say that this grouping decision enhances the clinical importance of feeding problems during infancy and childhood [32].

The ICD-11 guidelines for Pica have not been changed in a substantial way from the previous version of ICD. Pica is still characterized by a frequent and regular ingestion of non-nutritive substances, like different objects or materials, to a persistent and severe degree that requires special clinical attention, in a subject capable to distinguish between substances that can and cannot be eaten. This type of behavior has severe risks on the health and functioning system of an individual [31, 32].

For the rumination and regurgitation disorder the ICD-11 guidelines are almost the same as in the ICD-10. The main symptoms of the disorder need to be frequent as several times per week and present over a sustained period of at least several weeks. Characteristic symptoms that appear in an individual that reached the age of 2 are represented by regurgitation of food that was previous swallowed or the food that was brought up in the mouth could be re-chewed, re-swallowed or spat out [33].

A new ICD-11 diagnosis is avoidant-restrictive food intake disorder, characterized by a very low and insufficient amount or variety of food in order to supply an adequate level of energy or demands. This course of restriction causes weight loss and nutritional deficiencies but without a preoccupation of body weight and shape [33].

For Anorexia nervosa, the major features of the disorder remained unchanged in the ICD-11, such as a low body weight for an individual's height, age and developmental phase without a better explanation of another condition. The low weight is defined by a body mass index under 18.5 km/m^2 or less than the fifth percentile in children or adolescents, but these should be used as general aspects of reference permitting in some circumstance to diagnose anorexia nervosa at higher levels of weight. A detailed specification was added to anorexia as a severity qualifier indicating that the level of underweight status can influence the prognosis by other health complications determining a high mortality risk or a poorer outcome. This classification consists in significantly low body weight; defined as a BMI between 18.5 and 14.0 kg/m^2 for adult subjects and between the fifth percentile and the 0.3 percentile in children. The next severity step is named as dangerously low body weight and requires a BMI below 14.0 kg/m^2 for adults and for children less than 0.3 percentile. Another important aspect in the ICD-11 is the qualifier anorexia nervosa in recovery with normal body weight, providing a solution for those patients that have regained weight but still need special attention and care. Despite the DSM-5 classifications, ICD-11 emphasizes the behavior patterns (restricting pattern and binge-purge pattern) that are weight related and used by patients in order to lose more weight. In both classification systems, physical symptoms such as amenorrhea, osteopenia are frequent consequences of food restriction, they still occur but they are no longer considered as one of the main criteria for diagnosis. Also, the ICD-11 and DSM-5 do not include as mandatory the presence of a reported fear about gaining weight, considering this symptom as a more culturally based belief. On the other hand, there is a need of modified normal behavior in order to prevent loss weight so that anorexia nervosa diagnosis can be confirmed [32–34].

Bulimia nervosa in the ICD-11 remains characterized by binge eating episodes and compensatory behaviors to prevent weight gain but, different from anorexia nervosa, the patient is not underweight even if they are preoccupied by body shape image. A change in the frequency of the binge eating episodes was made by reducing them to once a week or more over a period of at least 1 month. Also, the time criteria have been shortened admitting the importance of receiving clinical care without any further delay. In parallel, for DSM-5 the time criteria include a period of at least 3 months. A binge eating episode represents a distinct period when an individual has no control over the eating or the amount of food intake. The common type of bulimia is the one without purging but with severe fasting or physical exercises and can be difficult to differentiate from binge eating disorder based solely on the regular compensatory behaviors [35].

A new diagnosis was added to ICD-11, named binge eating disorder, separated by the other eating disorders as a disturbance characterized by recurrent binge eating episodes accompanied by negative emotions and severe distress, without compensatory behaviors to prevent weight gain. This category was previously described in the Appendix of DSM-IV and now forms a new diagnosis in the DSM-5. To assume a correct diagnosis according to DSM-5, 3 out of 5 additional features have to be present, like: eating faster than normal; eating even if the patient does not feel hungry; eating until he feels uncomfortably full; the food intake is done in solitude; and negative emotions such as guilt, disgust or depression can follow the overeating. An important aspect is that ICD-11 guidelines do not require for the binge eating episodes an objective evaluation of the amount of food eaten but suggests the importance of the subjective experience of losing control over eating rather the quantity ingested [36].

While both bulimia nervosa and binge eating disorder associate marked distress in the ICD-11 criteria, the DSM-5 requires marked distress just for binge eating disorder and not in the case of bulimia nervosa. A possible explanation for these differences between the two diagnostic categories would be the presence of the weight-compensatory behaviors that we can assume to reflect severe distress. In ICD-11 disturbances in body shape are required for anorexia and bulimia nervosa;

self-body image concerns can be present in the binge eating disorder or avoidant-restrictive food intake disorder but are not necessary criteria. All in all, the new changes have the purpose to broaden the diagnostic process and facilitate clinical practice with the disadvantage of over diagnosing but also with respect to the course of life evolution [37].

If the criteria of behavior frequency are not fulfilled or other symptoms are considered sub-threshold, those eating disorders are classified in the DSM-5 as unspecified feeding and eating disorders, and in the ICD-11 as poorly specified other feeding and eating disorder [34, 37].

7. Differential diagnosis

Eating disorders must be medically assessed in order to establish if present physical conditions are consequences of the mental illness or different somatic health problems. This strategy allows developing an integrated management plan, because both problems need proper evaluation and treatment and can impact recovery or the quality of life [38].

The most common symptoms in anorexia nervosa are the fear of gaining weight and the excessive preoccupation of being overweight or fat. Despite the fact that they are malnourished, patients try to lose even more weight. In contrast, many gastrointestinal illnesses have as a central symptom the weight loss and in this situation the patient is worried about the loss and tries to regain weight. The main two illnesses with this symptomatology are coeliac disease and inflammatory bowel disease. More family members can be affected by these diseases, but such family predisposition can be present for eating disorders too [39].

On the other hand, functional gastrointestinal disorders cam mimic an eating disorder, but usually they do not associate weight loss and have a long past evolution in the patient's history. Such frequently reported diseases are the irritable bowel syndrome and the non-ulcer dyspepsia, also common in patients with diagnose of eating disorder. Food intolerance and allergies can simultaneously be present in a patient with eating disorders, but in this scenario it is more difficult to precisely discriminate between the two conditions [40]. The loss of appetite is a very common symptom, but nonspecific, in both mental and physical disorders. It can associate with weight lost and needs more investigating. In eating disorders, patients do not lose their appetite, the restriction from food intake has a voluntary component, that is not present in organic disorders, were the loss of appetite is without effort and involuntary. On the other hand, compulsive eating with an increased level of appetite can be present in Prader-Willi syndrome, craniopharyngioma, tumors of the hypothalamus or recovery from acute illnesses. This symptom is characteristic in bulimia nervosa or the binge purge subtype of anorexia [41]. Dysphagia is considered an alarming symptom in old age patients, and needs endoscopy or barium passage, malignancy strictures or achalasia are usually suspected. Other gastrointestinal symptoms that are commonly present include odynophagia, nausea, vomiting, hematemesis or melena, abdominal pain, constipation, diarrhea. Odynophagia described as pain when swallowing can be present in a reflux esophagitis or esophageal candida. Vomiting is a very unspecific symptom usually associated with nausea that can have different causes such as inflammatory bowel disease, side effects of different drugs, a high intracranial pressure, pyloric stenosis, gastro-paresis, but in these circumstances a voluntary control is not present as in eating disorders and it is not hidden [42]. Hematemesis or melena can represent a medical emergency, but frequently represent a consequence of purging and vomiting, with the development of Mallory Weiss tears. For the abdominal pain the doctor should establish the level of intensity, quality and localization of the pain in order to differentiate a peptic ulcer, gallstones, pancreatitis or appendicitis. Constipation, diarrhea, and rectal bleeding are symptoms that need to be integrated with other factors and the most important aspect is the change in bowel habit that can imply Crohn's disease or ulcerative colitis [43].

The age of onset can be a very important clue. Usually, organic conditions, in special malignant illnesses that can manifest with weight loss, become more frequent with old age. If symptoms appear over 50 years, appropriate investigations are required. Moreover, the onset of eating disorders is identified in the teenage years or early adulthood [43].

In order to establish a diagnosis of an eating disorder the patient should be physically examined, the mental state evaluation should be done, all of these supported by a detailed medical history, family history and social context. All symptoms must be placed in a chronological order.

8. Management of eating disorders

International guidelines recommend psycho-behavior therapy for all eating disorders, which can be applied in a form of outpatient care, when the treatment is accepted and the patient accepts to cooperate, with major beneficial effects, being more cost-effective, reducing hospitalizations, making patients feel more secure in their own environment, maintaining social contact with friends and family members, being able to perform other pleasant activities and making the rehabilitation phase much easier. Patients with a BMI over 16 kg/m^2, with bulimia nervosa or binge purge syndrome are usually treated in outpatient or day care units because the risks are less serious on physical harm and this form of outpatient context has been proved to be highly effective [44]. On the other hand, for more severe forms, when patients' symptoms are not improving with home treatment or the patients' physical status is unstable (weight is rapidly diminishing, the BMI is under 14 kg/m^2, low pulse, blood pressure, body temperature decreasing or fever being present, difficulty in performing the basic test of physical strength) more restrictive measures must be taken in a partial or day admission, or even a compulsory treatment would be necessary in order for the patient to improve physical and mentally but also, to limit potential harm behavior [45]. Anorexic patients in general do not want to die, but it is needed to understand the psychological drive of an anorexic patient who has an extreme fear of gaining weight, who is unable to rationally see that their physical state has become critical, and if the weight will continue to drop the result will lead to death [44].

It is highly recommended for these patients to be treated by a multi-disciplinary team with a minimum of a psychological therapist and a family doctor, but in hospital care additional support is required as a registered dietician, specialist physician, psychiatrist, nurses, physiotherapist, occupational therapist and social worker [46]. Nurses and other medical staff represent a key element in the management treatment approach by limiting mobility, imposing bed rest, monitoring fluid balance and physical symptoms (pulse, blood pressure, temperature), supervising mealtimes (observation for at least 1 h after eating), showers, toilets (patients being alone can consider a perfect opportunity to engage in behaviors such as purging, excessive physical exercises or water loading for a false weight gain). Even with the risk of some saying these rules are unethical; protocols like this can avoid numerous unwanted behaviors done by patients in the purpose of resisting the weight gain and destroying the process of recovery. In the context of bed resting for an easier and closer observation it is important to start prophylaxis for deep vein thrombosis with low molecular weight heparin [47]. Also, clothes need to be checked because they can represent means for falsifying weight or transport regurgitated food. Dieticians are also important for the safe management of patients with eating disorders. They need to be consulted for the risk of re-feeding syndrome, must establish a meal plan for proper nutritional requirements, to include all nutrients, carbohydrates, proteins, fats, vitamins and all kinds of minerals, to use supplements if the case imposes, and monitor weight gaining in a correct pace, and also, on the long term, to provide proper education for a balanced nutrition plan and teach patients how to prepare their meals and eat adequately in social situations [46].

The management of over activity can be treated firstly by providing psychoeducation about the advantages and disadvantages of this behavior and to discourage exercise. Also, relaxation and distractions techniques can be helpful, the use of wheelchairs to reduce the level of energy spent, administer Olanzapine with a good effect on the compulsive behavior, providing a calm and warm environment, with a permanent supervision from medical staff [48].

Treatment goals address numerous aspects such as nutritional, physical, social and mental health comorbidities. Some studies were made on healthy subjects, who voluntarily agreed to be starved, and the effect of this demonstrated that even in normal subjects thought processes were slowed, executive functions were impaired, with decision making disturbances, and personality traits accentuated in a manner that persons were more paranoid, depressed or became psychotic. The majority of these symptoms were reversed by re-feeding treatment in normal individuals and similarities were observed for anorexic patients, who had an improvement in thinking, mood stability and improved the engagement level for psychotherapy [49].

For malnourished patients re-feeding may represent the only solution for surviving. It has to be initiated promptly with benefits on the physical strength, cerebral function. It restores the reduced size of internal organs, heart, gut and their functions, offers a better functioning of the immune system, patients being less susceptible for infections. All of these outcomes appear after a slow process, because the body needs to readapt to the increased availability of calories and nutrients [50]. If the patients have a very low BMI, under 16 kg/m^2, or had a rapid loss weight within the last 3–6 months of over 15% of the body weight, had little nutritional intake for more than 10 days or have low levels of potassium, phosphate, magnesium prior to the re-feeding, they are at risk of developing a re-feeding syndrome, according to the NICE guidelines [51]. The re-feeding syndrome can be defined as a consequence of trying to re-establish the normal weight of a very malnourished patient. During this phase, the maximal risk is within 72 h and implies potentially fatal shifts in fluids and electrolytes. The characteristic biochemical abnormality is the hypophosphatemia, but hypokalemia and hypomagnesaemia can also occur. NICE recommends starting re-feeding process at 5 kcal/kg/24 h for those with severe anorexia nervosa, through a nasogastric re-feeding tube and progressively increasing the rate of re-feeding to the target calorie intake over the next 4–7 days. Other studies showed that higher initial re-feeding rates can be applied such as 15 or 20 kcal/kg/24 h, with or without the association of re-feeding syndrome [52].

In order to avoid this kind of situations the patient has to be admitted in special medical units with experience in re-feeding syndrome, to monitor the blood chemistry twice a day, start with caution and increase quickly if the patient tolerates well. A particular aspect is to start giving thiamine before feeding starts, and to continue with it at least 10 days in order to overcome the development of Wernicke's encephalopathy or Korsakoff syndrome. Hypophosphatemia can have fatal effect through numerous clinical features such as cardiac failure, arrhythmias, seizures, tremor, rhabdomyolysis, and respiratory failure. Hypomagnesaemia can also occur and complicate the feeding treatment by cardiac arrhythmia, hypertension crises, tremor, tetany, confusion, seizures and abdominal pain. Hypokalemia can appear as a consequence of staring to feed the anorexic patient, but more common it is present in patients with binge-purge subtype because of vomiting or induced laxative diarrhea. All of these electrolyte deficiencies must be treated properly to offer a safe outcome. Other complications that can occur during re-feeding are elevated transaminase levels with liver failure, coagulation problems, acute tubular renal necrosis, tubular renal nephritis, cardiac Torsade du Pointes, arrhythmias, prolonged QTc, cardiomyopathy [53, 54].

If the patients is in a severe state for the re-feeding process doctors have to decide if an enteral tube feeding is required. For this intervention training and experience is need, because the gut wall in malnourished patients is extremely thin and there is the risk of rupture, a lethal complication. Also after passing the tube, the safety position must be checked before it is used. In order to confirm the placement of the tube, gastric fluid can be aspirated, and the level of acidity can be determined, or an X-ray might be required. Gastrostomy tubes are not advisable to use, they need an endoscopic or radiologic approach, with the risk of peritonitis or other infections. Feeding through a tube is just a temporary solution, as part of an integrated plan, and patients need to be responsible and slowly introduce a full oral intake [55].

For osteopenia the recommended treatment is weight restoration and a normalization of the endocrine hormones. Also hormones substitution with transdermal estrogen, analogue of parathyroid hormone, bisphosphonates, raloxifene and denosumab drugs can be prescribed in this case [56].

Psychotherapy should be the treatment of choice for all eating disorders. The number of sessions required is different in each eating disorder type. In the case of anorexia nervosa no specific psychotherapy has shown clear superiority, but the number of sessions required is the highest, with an average of 40. Adolescents with anorexia nervosa have better outcomes after family therapy. For bulimia nervosa and binge eating disorder psychotherapy should be offered as a first line treatment, especially cognitive behavior therapy, or as an alternative interpersonal psychotherapy, psychodynamic, or family-based therapy in children and adolescent with bulimia nervosa. Usually the number of sessions required is less for bulimia and binge eating disorder, with a medium of 20 weeks [57, 58].

Pharmacological therapies with positive results in controlled trials in eating disorders are second generation of antipsychotics and antidepressants. For anorexia nervosa olanzapine had the most beneficial effects, in the case of bulimia nervosa and binge eating disorder Fluoxetine showed a good outcome, with a small effect from Lisdexamfetamine for binge eating disorder and Mirtazapine for avoidant restrictive eating disorder [59, 60].

9. Evolution and prognosis

Eating disorders characterized by low weight associate high morbidity and mortality rates. A follow-up study which monitored hospitalized patients with anorexia nervosa reported an average life expectancy of 39 years. Studies showed that 1/3 of patients suffering from anorexia nervosa tend to have a full recovery, in same percentage patients have just a partial recovery, and approximately 1/3 will have a chronic evolution or die. On a more optimistic point of view, a full recovery has been shown to be possible but with early intervention plan and sustained treatment over a medium of almost 7 to 9 years [61].

In general the prognosis for bulimia nervosa is good with treatment and assistance, but if the patient associate low self-esteem or different forms of personality disorders these aspects can affect the outcome. Little is known about the prognosis in binge eating disorders or other eating and feeding disorders [62].

For all eating disorders, poor prognostic factors can be considered as: late onset, anxiety in the presence of others when eating, severe weight loss, association of other chronic disorders, difficulties in childhood for social adjustment, being a male, having conflicts with parents or friends, being present binge and purge behaviors, low motivational for change, shame or not having enough money for engaging in psychotherapies sessions, association of concomitant depressed mood and obsessive body imagine preoccupation. Better evolutions have been identified in adolescents than adults, but only in association with family psychotherapy making the majority of these patients partially recovered, with less episodes of relapse. Also, in the young group distribution an onset in adolescents have a much better prognosis than one in early childhood [62].

10. Insight in eating disorders

There is now a general agreement that insight is not an all-or-none phenomenon, but rather a complex, multidimensional concept in psychiatric disorders. It includes different components, like the ability of a patient to recognize the presence of a mental illness, the capacity to accept that some symptoms are pathological and are determined by a mental disorder, the awareness of illness's consequences and compliance with treatment [63].

Lack of insight has been largely demonstrated in schizophrenia, other psychoses and bipolar disorder [64–67]. DSM-5 included an "insight" specifier in OCD, body dysmorphic and hoarding disorder. Also, different levels of lack of insight, from good to absent, have been found in other psychiatric disorders, like depressive and anxiety disorders, specific and social phobias, Alzheimer disease and other neurocognitive disorders, eating disorders [68–71].

Patients with anorexia nervosa (AN) commonly lack insight, at least in the early stages of illness. This element will determine important difficulties in assessment, lack of compliance or avoidance of treatment, frequent relapses and also may limit the identification of eating disorders. These patients have distorted cognitions about body weight and shape and also, they are ambivalent regarding motivation to recover [72]. On the other hand, patients with bulimia nervosa (BN) have typically a bigger level of motivation to recover.

Until now there is not a disorder-specific scale for the assessment of insight in patients with eating disorders. Many researchers use SAI-ED (the Schedule for the Assessment of Insight for EDs), a short self-report questionnaire, which has only seven items. Even if the SAI-ED has not been fully validated, has a significant level of internal consistency [72].

10.1 Factors associated with insight

In their study evaluating the clinical insight in 193 patients with anorexia nervosa, Gorwood et al. observed that 88% of patients (171) had a high level of insight (SAI-ED total score > 4) and 12% of patients (22) had a poor insight (SAI-ED < 4).

The authors drew three important conclusions:

1. Insight was not improved in a vast majority of patients, even if they followed 4 months of specialized care and all clinical and cognitive markers improved.

2. In this study, the only factor that has been demonstrated improving insight was minimum BMI.

3. Premorbid IQ was highly associated with the level of baseline insight.

Other studies revealed other factors correlated with insight (cognitive functions - memory and executive functions), psychiatric and addictive comorbidities, associated personality disorders prescribed psychotropic drugs, social cognitions, use of psychotherapy [72–76].

11. Psychiatric comorbidities in eating disorders

Beside comorbid somatic conditions of eating disorders (anemia, arteriosclerosis, hypertension, high cholesterol, high triglycerides, myocardial infarction, lung problems, stomach ulcer, Bowel problems, liver diseases, fibromyalgia, stroke, epilepsy or seizures, cancer, arthritis, osteoporosis, sleep problems), all three EDs (eating disorders) are associated with other psychiatric conditions, especially mood disorders, anxiety disorders, posttraumatic stress disorder, substance use disorder and personality or conduct disorder [77].

Regarding mood disorders, most common associated with EDs are major depressive disorder, persistent depression, bipolar I [78]. Affective disorders, substance use disorders and anxiety disorders represent the most common predictive factors for suicide. Researchers have reported also that eating disorders are associated with suicide. The meta-analysis of Smith et al. [78], which included 2611 longitudinal studies, concluded that ED diagnosis is significantly associated with an increased risk for suicide attempt (SA) although the rate of SA varied considerably across studies [78]. In the group of patients with anorexia nervosa (AN), the rate of SA was between 3 and 20% [79]; in bulimia nervosa patients (BN), the rate ranged between 25 and 35% [79]; and in BED patients, the rate was 12.5% [78] and 20.8% when combining all EDs [80]. In the study of Udo et al., which included 36,171 respondents in the Third National Epidemiological Survey on Alcohol and Related Conditions (NESARC-III), the prevalence of suicide attempts was 24.8% for AN, 15.5% for anorexia nervosa-restricted type (AN-R), 44.1% for anorexia nervosa binge/purge type (AN-BP), 31.4% for bulimia nervosa, and 22.9% for binge-eating disorder (BID) [77].

Regarding anxiety disorders, most common associated with eating disorders are panic disorder, social anxiety disorder, specific phobias and general anxiety disorder [78]. The association between social anxiety and EDs could be a part of a wider socio-emotional phenotype which it is considered to contribute to the development and maintenance of EDs. SA may be a risk factor for ED, or SA may be secondary to the ED, as a consequence of ED psychopathology or malnutrition [81].

Abuse of substances is common in EDs, the lifetime prevalence being estimated between 23 and 37% [82]. Tobacco, caffeine and alcohol were the most prevalent SUD in the study of Bahji et al., being followed by cannabis and cocaine [83, 84].

Between axis II DSM diagnoses, most common comorbidities in ED are antisocial, borderline and schizotypal personality disorders and conduct disorders [78].

Conflict of interest

The authors declare that they have no conflict of interest.

Author details

Bianca Suciu* and Cătălina-Angela Crișan
Department of Neuroscience, Discipline of Psychiatry and Pediatric Psychiatry, Iuliu Hațieganu University of Medicine and Pharmacy Cluj-Napoca, Romania

*Address all correspondence to: biancabobocel@yahoo.com

References

[1] Hay P. Current approach to eating disorders: A clinical update. Internal Medicine Journal. 2020;**50**(1):24-29

[2] Galmiche M, Déchelotte P, Lambert G, Tavolacci MP. Prevalence of eating disorders over the 2000-2018 period: A systematic literature review. The American Journal of Clinical Nutrition. 2019;**109**:1402-1413

[3] Hudson J, Hiripi E, Pope H, Kessler R. The prevalence and correlates of eating disorders in the National Comorbidity Survey Replication. Biological Psychiatry. 2007;**61**(3):348-358

[4] Hay P, Mitchison D, Lopez Collado AE, González-Chica DA, Stocks N, Touyz S. Burden and health-related quality of life of eating disorders, including avoidant/restrictive food intake disorder (ARFID), in the Australian population. Journal of Eating Disorders. 2017;**5**:21

[5] Udo T, Grilo CM. Prevalence and correlates of DSM-5–defined eating disorders in a nationally representative sample of US adults. Biological Psychiatry. 2018;**84**:345-354

[6] Smink FR, Van Hoeken D, Hoek HW. Epidemiology of eating disorders: Incidence, prevalence and mortality rates. Current Psychiatry Reports. 2012;**14**:406-414

[7] Mulders-Jones B, Mitchison D, Girosi F, Hay P. Socioeconomic correlates of eating disorder symptoms in an Australian population-based sample. PLoS One. 2017;**12**:e0170603

[8] Collier D, Treasure J. The aetiology of eating disorders. The British Journal of Psychiatry. 2004;**185**(5):363-365

[9] Whitney J, Murray J, Gavan K, Todd G, Whitaker W, Treasure J. Experience of caring for someone with anorexia nervosa: Qualitative study. The British Journal of Psychiatry. 2005;**187**(5):444-449

[10] Stice E, Marti C, Durant S. Risk factors for onset of eating disorders: Evidence of multiple risk pathways from an 8-year prospective study. Behaviour Research and Therapy. 2011;**49**(10):622-627

[11] Arcelus J, Witcomb G, Mitchell A. Prevalence of eating disorders amongst dancers: A systemic review and meta-analysis. European Eating Disorders Review. 2013;**22**(2):92-101

[12] Arcelus J. Mortality rates in patients with anorexia nervosa and other eating disorders. Archives of General Psychiatry. 2011;**68**(7):724

[13] Smith J. The Parent' s Guide to Eating Disorders. Oxford: Lion Hutton; 2011

[14] Davis C, Katzman D, Kaptein S, Kirsh C, Brewer H, Kalmbach K, et al. The prevalence of high-level exercise in the eating disorders: Etiological implications. Comprehensive Psychiatry. 1997;**38**(6):321-326

[15] Beumont P, Arthur B, Russell J, Touyz S. Excessive physical activity in dieting disorder patients: Proposals for a supervised exercise program. The International Journal of Eating Disorders. 1994;**15**(1):21-36

[16] Davis C, Kennedy S, Ravelski E, Dionne M. The role of physical activity in the development and maintenance of eating disorders. Psychological Medicine. 1994;**24**(4):957-967

[17] Touyz SW, Beumont PJV, Hook S. Exercise anorexia: A new dimension in anorexia nervosa. In: Handbook of

Eating Disorders: Part 1. Amsterdam: Elsevier; 1987. pp. 143-157

[18] Epling WF, Pierce WD. Activity Anorexia: Theory, Research and Treatment. Lawarence Erlbaum Associates: Mahwan NJ; 1996

[19] Ackard D, Brehm B, Steffen J. Exercise and eating disorders in college-aged women: Profiling excessive exercisers. Eating Disorders. 2002;**10**(1):31-47

[20] Steffen J, Brehm B. The dimensions of obligatory exercise. Eating Disorders. 1999;7(3):219-226

[21] Kron L, Katz J, Gorzynski G, Weiner H. Hyperactivity in anorexia nervosa: A fundamental clinical feature. Comprehensive Psychiatry. 1978;**19**(5):433-440

[22] Solenberger S. Exercise and eating disorders. Eating Behaviors. 2001;**2**(2):151-168

[23] Strober M, Freeman R, Morrell W. The long-term course of severe anorexia nervosa in adolescents: Survival analysis of recovery, relapse, and outcome predictors over 10-15 years in a prospective study. The International Journal of Eating Disorders. 1997;**22**(4):339-360

[24] Norris M, Harrison M, Isserlin L, Robinson A, Feder S, Sampson M. Gastrointestinal complications associated with anorexia nervosa: A systematic review. The International Journal of Eating Disorders. 2015;**49**(3):216-237

[25] Chami T, Nikoomanesh P, Katz P. An unusual presentation of pill-induced esophagitis. Gastrointestinal Endoscopy. 1995;**42**(3):263-265

[26] Miller K. Medical findings in outpatients with anorexia nervosa. Archives of Internal Medicine. 2005;**165**(5):561

[27] Douglas G, Nicol F, Robertson C. Macleod's Clinical Examination. 13th ed. Edinburgh: Churchill Livingstone Elsevier; 2013

[28] Stratton R, Dixon R, Longmore D, Stroud M, Elia M. Effect of recalled weight and height on malnutrition risk. Clinical Nutrition. 2003;**22**:S9-S10

[29] Sachs K, Harnke B, Mehler P, Krantz M. Cardiovascular complications of anorexia nervosa: A systematic review. The International Journal of Eating Disorders. 2015;**49**(3):238-248

[30] Weed LL. Medical Records that Guide and Teach. The New England Journal of Medicine. 1968;278(11):593-600. American Psychiatric Association. Diagnostic and Statistical Manual of Mental Disorders (5th ed.) (DSM-5). Washington DC: American Psychiatric Association; 2013

[31] World Health Organization. International Statistical Classification of Diseases and Related Health Problems, 11th Revision ICD-11. Geneva: World Health Organization; 2019

[32] International Advisory Group for the Revision of ICD-10 Mental Behavioural Disorders. A conceptual framework for the revision of the ICD-10 classification of mental and behavioural disorders. World Psychiatry. 2011;**10**(2):86-92. DOI: 10.1002/j.2051-5545.2011.tb00022.x

[33] Keeley JW, Reed GM, Roberts MC, Evans SC, Medina-Mora ME, Robles R. Developing a science of clinical utility in diagnostic classification systems: Field study strategies for ICD-11 mental and behavioral disorders. American Psychologist Journal. 2016;**71**(1):3. DOI: 10.1037/a0039972

[34] First MB, Reed GM, Hyman SE, Saxena S. The development of the ICD-11 clinical descriptions and diagnostic guidelines for mental and behavioural disorders. World Psychiatry. 2015;**14**(1):82-90. DOI: 10.1002/wps.20189

[35] Uher R, Rutter M. Classification of feeding and eating disorders: Review of evidence and proposals for ICD-11. World Psychiatry. 2012;**11**(2):80-92. DOI: 10.1016/j.wpsyc.2012.05.005

[36] Attia E, Becker AE, Bryant-Waugh R, Hoek HW, Kreipe RE, Marcus MD. Feeding and eating disorders in DSM-5. The American Journal of Psychiatry. 2013;**170**(11):1237-1239. DOI: 10.1176/appi.ajp.2013.13030326

[37] Al-Adawi S, Bax B, Bryant-Waugh R, Claudino AM, Hay P, Monteleone P. Revision of ICD status update on feeding and eating disorders. Advances in Eating Disorders. 2013;**1**(1):10-20. DOI: 10.1080/21662630.2013.742971

[38] Field AE, Sonneville KR, Micali N, Crosby RD, Swanson SA, Laird NM, et al. Prospective association of common eating disorders and adverse outcomes. Pediatrics. 2012;**130**(2):e289-e295. DOI: 10.1542/peds.2011-3663

[39] Fitzsimmons-Craft EE, Ciao AC, Accurso EC, Pisetsky EM, Peterson CB, Byrne CE. Subjective and objective binge eating in relation to eating disorder symptomatology, depressive symptoms, and self-esteem among treatment-seeking adolescents with bulimia nervosa. European Eating Disorders Review. 2014;**22**(4):230-236. DOI: 10.1002/erv.2297

[40] Watson HJ, Fursland A, Bulik CM, Nathan P. Subjective binge eating with compensatory behaviors: A variant presentation of bulimia nervosa. The International Journal of Eating Disorders. 2013;**46**(2):119-126. DOI: 10.1002/eat.22052

[41] Salvioli B, Pellicciari A, Iero L, Di Pietro E, Moscano F, Gualandi S, et al. Audit of digestive complaints and psychopathological traits in patients with eating disorders: A prospective study. Digestive and Liver Disease. 2013;**45**(8):639-644

[42] Aziz Q, Fass R, Gyawali C, Miwa H, Pandolfino J, Zerbib F. Esophageal disorders. Gastroenterology. 2016;**150**(6):1368-1379

[43] Lacy B, Mearin F, Chang L, Chey W, Lembo A, Simren M, et al. Bowel disorders. Gastroenterology. 2016;**150**(6):1393.e5-1407.e5

[44] Hay P, Chinn D, Forbes D, Madden S, Newton R, Sugenor L. Royal Australian and New Zealand College of Psychiatrists clinical practice guidelines for the treatment of eating disorders. The Australian and New Zealand Journal of Psychiatry. 2014;**48**:977-1008

[45] National Institute for Health and Care Excellence (NICE). Eating disorders: Recognition and Treatment Full Guideline. 2017. Available from: https://www.nice.org.uk/guidance/ng69/evidence/full-guideline-pdf-161214767896

[46] Hilbert A, Hoek HW, Schmidt R. Evidence-based clinical guidelines foreating disorders: International comparison. Current Opinion in Psychiatry. 2017;**30**:423-437

[47] Hay PJ, Touyz S, Claudino AM, Lujic S, Smith CA, Madden S. Inpatient versusoutpatient care, partial hospitalization and waiting list for people with eating disorders. Cochrane Database of Systematic Reviews. 2019:CD010827. DOI: 10.1002/14651858.CD010827.pub2

[48] Long C. Assessment and management of eating disordered patients who over-exercise: A four-year follow-up of six single case studies. Journal of Mental Health. 1995;**4**(3):309-316

[49] Thien V, Thomas A, Markin D, Birmingham C. Pilot study of a graded exercise program for the treatment of anorexia nervosa. The International Journal of Eating Disorders. 2000;**28**(1):101-106

[50] Saudek C, Felig P. The metabolic events of starvation. The American Journal of Medicine. 1976;**60**(1):117-126

[51] Boateng A, Sriram K, Meguid M, Crook M. Refeeding syndrome: Treatment considerations based on collective analysis of literature case reports. Nutrition. 2010;**26**(2):156-167

[52] Keys A. The biology of human starvation. The American Journal of Clinical Nutrition. 1978;**31**(2):197-197

[53] Madden S, Miskovic-Wheatley J, Clarke S, Touyz S, Hay P, Kohn MR. Outcomes of a rapid refeeding protocol in adolescent anorexia nervosa. Journal of Eating Disorders. 2015;**3**:8

[54] Schorr M, Klibanski A. Anorexia nervosa and bone. Current Opinion Endocrine and Metabolic Research. 2018;**3**:74-82

[55] Treasure J, Cardi V, Leppanen J, Turton R. New treatment approaches for severe and enduring eating disorders. Physiology & Behavior. 2015;**152**:456-465

[56] Zipfel S, Giel K, Bulik C, Hay P, Schmidt U. Anorexia nervosa: Aetiology, assessment, and treatment. The Lancet Psychiatry. 2015;**2**(12):1099-1111

[57] Dalle Grave R, Calugi S, Sartirana M, Fairburn CG. Transdiagnostic cognitive behaviour therapy for adolescents with an eating disorder who are not underweight. Behaviour Ressearch and Therapy. 2015;**73**:79-82

[58] Schmidt U, Startup H, Treasure J. A Cognitive-Interpersonal Therapy Workbook for Treating Anorexia Nervosa: The Maudsley Model. Abingdon, UK: Routledge; 2018

[59] Attia E, Steinglass JE, Walsh BT, Wang Y, Wu P, Schreyer C. Olanzapine versus placebo in adult outpatients with anorexia nervosa: A randomized clinical trial. The American Journal of Psychiatry. 2019;**176**:449-456

[60] Hilbert A, Petroff D, Herpertz S, Pietrowsky R, Tuschen-Caffier B, Vocks S. Meta-analysis of the efficacy of psychological and medical treatments for binge-eating disorder. Journal of Consulting and Clinical Psychology. 2019;**87**:91-105

[61] Eddy KT, Tabri N, Thomas JJ, Murray HB, Keshaviah A, Hastings E. Recovery from anorexia nervosa and bulimia nervosa at 22-year followup. The Journal of Clinical Psychiatry. 2017;**78**:184-189

[62] Vall E, Wade TD. Predictors of treatment outcome in individuals with eating disorders: A systematic review and meta-analysis. The International Journal of Eating Disorders. 2015;**48**:946-971

[63] Marková IS. Insight in Psychiatry. Cambridge University Press; 2005

[64] David AS. Insight and psychosis. The British Journal of Psychiatry. 1990;**156**:798-808

[65] Amador XF, Strauss DH, Yale SA, Gorman JM. Awareness of illness in schizophrenia. Schizophrenia Bulletin. 1991;**17**:113-132

[66] Amador XF, Strauss DH. Poor insight in schizophrenia. Psychiatric Quarterly. 1993;**64**:305-318

[67] de Assis da Silva R, Mograbi DC, Camelo EVM, Bifano J, Wainstok M, Silveira LAS, et al. Insight in bipolar disorder: A comparison between mania, depression and euthymia using the insight scale for affective disorders. Trends in Psychiatry and Psychotherapy. 2015;**37**(3):152-156

[68] Lee MS, Lee HY, Kang SG, Yang J, Ahn H, Rhee M. Variables influencing antidepressant medication adherence for treating outpatients with depressive disorders. Journal of Affective Disorders. 2010;**123**:216-221

[69] Menzies RG, Harris LM, Jones MK. Evidence from three fearful samples for poor insight type specific phobia. Depression and Anxiety. 1998;**8**:29-32

[70] Vigne P, de Menezes GB, Harrison BJ, Fontenelle LF. A study of poor insight in social anxiety disorders. Psychiatry Reaserch. 2014;**219**:556-561

[71] Konstantakopoulos G, Tchanturia K, Surguladze SA, David AS. Insight in eating disoders: Clinical and cognitive correlates. Psychological Medicine. 2011;**41**:1951-1961

[72] Gorwood P, Duriez P, Lengvenyte A, Guillaume S. Criquillion, on behalf of the FFAB network. Clinical insight in anorexia nervosa: Associated and predictive factors. Psychiatry Research. 2019;**281**:112561

[73] Catapano F, Perris F, Fabrazzo M, Cioffi V, Giacco D, De Santis V, et al. Obssessive-compulsive disorder with poor-insight: a three-year prospective study. Progress in Neuropsychopharmacology and Biological Psychiatry. 2010;**34**(2):323-330

[74] Nair A, Palmer EC, Aleman A, David AS. Relationship between cognition, clinical and cognitive insight in psychotic disorders: A review and meta-analysis. Schizophrenia Research. 2014;**152**(1):191-200

[75] Steinglass JE, Eisen JL, Attia E, Mayer L, Walsh BT. Is anorexia nervosa a delusional disorder? An assessment of eating beliefs in anorexia nervosa. Journal of Psychiatric Practice. 2007;**13**(2):65-71

[76] Yen CF, Hsiao RC, Chen CC, Lin HC, Yen CN, Ko CH, et al. The role of insight to alcohol use disorders in insight to schizophrenia. Comprehensive Psychiatry. 2009;**50**(1):58-62

[77] Udo T, Grilo CM. Psychiatric and medical correlates of DSM-5 eating disorders in a nationally representative sample of adults in the United States. The International Journal of Eating Disorders. 2019;**52**:42-50

[78] Smith AR, Velkoff EA, Ribeiro JD, Franklin J. Are eating disorders and related symptoms risk factors for suicidal thoughts and behaviors? A meta-analysis. Suicide & Life-Threatening Behavior. 2018;**49**(1):221-239

[79] Franko DL, Keel PK. Suicidality in eating disorders: Occurrence, correlates, and clinical implications. Clinical Psychology Review. 2006;**26**(6):769-782

[80] Carano A, De Berardis D, Campanella D, Serroni N, Ferri F, Di Lorio G, et al. Alexithymia and suicide ideation in a sample of patients with binge eating disorder. Journal of Psychiatric Practice. 2012;**18**(1):5-11

[81] Ahn J, Lee J, Jung Y. Predictors of suicide attempts in individuals with eating disorders. Suicide and Life-Threatening Behavior. 2018;**49**(3):789-797

[82] Treasure J, Schmidt U. The cognitive-interpersonal maintenance model of anorexia nervosa revisited: A summary of the evidence for cognitive, socio-emotional and interpersonal predisposing and perpetuating factors. Journal of Eating Disorders. 2013;**1**:13

[83] Hudson JI, Hiripi E, Pope HG, Kessler RC. The prevalence and correlates of eating disorders in the national comorbidity survey replication. Biological Psychiatry. 2007;**61**(3):348-358

[84] Bahji A, Mazhar MN, Hudson CC, Nadkarni P, MacNeil BA, Hawken E. Prevalence of substance use disorder comorbidity among individuals with eating disorders: A systematic review and meta-analysis. Psychiatry Reaserch. 2019;**273**:58-66

Section 2

Medical Aspects

Chapter 5

Neuroprotective Effects of Curcumin and Vitamin D3 on Scopolamine-Induced Learning-Impaired Rat Model of Alzheimer's Disease

Saima Khan and Kaneez Fatima Shad

Abstract

The purpose of this study was to find out the beneficial effects of curcumin and vitamin D3 in rats treated with scopolamine as to generate animal model of tauopathies, i.e., neurodegenerative disorders, including Alzheimer's disease (AD). Abnormal phosphorylation of tau results in the transformation of normal adult tau into paired-helical-filament (PHF) tau and neurofibrillary tangles (NFTs). Our results indicated that scopolamine-treated rats exhibit increased levels of hyperphosphorylated tau protein along with PHF, and curcumin and vitamin D3 lowered the levels of PHF better than donepezil. The effect of abnormal hyperphosphorylation of tau was also detected in the hematoxylin and eosin staining of brain tissues as well as in the western blot analyses in our experimental rat models of AD. This abnormal level of hyperphosphorylated tau probably causes cognitive and memory deficit as observed in different behavioral tests on exploratory groups. Hyperphosphorylated tau may have disrupted the microtubule network in experimental rats. Signs of temporal region dementia noted during behavioral studies may be linked to the neurodegeneration and abnormal hyperphosphorylation of tau observed in our experimental animal model of AD. The curcumin and vitamin D3-treated group presented lower levels of hyperphosphorylated tau and a better behavioral response. Thus, inhibition of abnormal hyperphosphorylation of tau offers a promising therapeutic target for AD and related tauopathies.

Keywords: Alzheimer's disease, memory impairment, inflammation, scopolamine, curcumin, vitamin D3, donepezil

1. Introduction

Alzheimer's disease (AD) is a neurodegenerative disorder, which present mainly in the elderly patients. It is characterized by progressive loss of cognitive functions, amyloid β (Aβ) deposition, and formation of paired-helical-filament (PHF) tau and neurofibrillary tangles (NFTs) in the brain cells. NFTs are formed inside the cell bodies of the neurons. These NFTs cause shrinkage of neurons and resultant loss of cognition and learning [1, 2].

Tau protein is a highly soluble microtubule-associated protein found abundantly in the neuronal cells of the central nervous system (CNS). Tau proteins are the product of alternative splicing from a single gene, designated for microtubule-associated protein tau (MAPT) in humans, located on chromosome 17. There are six isoforms of tau found in the human brain. They can be distinguished by their binding domains. Tau has 79 potential phosphorylation sites on the longest isoform [3]. Tau is the major microtubule-associated protein of a mature neuron. The other two neuronal MAPs are MAP1 and MAP2, which are involved in tubulin interaction and promotion of its assembly into microtubules and stabilization of the microtubule network [4].

Normal adult human brain contains 2–3 moles of phosphorylated tau protein. Hyperphosphorylation of tau decreases its normal function. In Alzheimer's disease, brain tau is approximately three- to fourfold more hyperphosphorylated than the normal adult brain. This hyperphosphorylated state polymerized into paired-helical-filament tau and when mixed with straight filaments (SF) formed neurofibrillary tangles (NFT). The hyperphosphorylated tau in AD brain has the ability to sequester normal tau, MAP1, and MAP2, to disrupt microtubules, and to self-assemble into PHF/SF. Abnormal hyperphosphorylated tau, in the cytosol, does not polymerized into PHF [5]. The cytosolic hyperphosphorylated tau is involved in tubulin assembly but inhibiting its normal assembly and disrupting microtubule [6]. In addition, with hyperphosphorylation of tau, conformational changes and abnormal cleavage of tau may contribute to the pathogenesis of AD [7, 8]. Tau hyperphosphorylation has been reported in AD and other tauopathies; thus, the inhibition of abnormal hyperphosphorylation of tau offers a promising therapeutic target for AD and related tauopathies [9].

Similarly, oxidative stress is also strongly linked to neuronal dysfunction and neuronal cell death [10]. It is suggested that oxidative stress plays a significant role in the pathological conditions of AD by enhancing Aβ deposition, tau phosphorylation, and loss of synapses and neurons [11].

Reactive oxygen species (ROS) are by-products of biochemical and physiological processes in the body and can cause oxidative damage to macromolecules in an uncontrolled manner that may lead to many chronic diseases. Thus, overproduction of ROS is a hallmark of neurodegenerative disorders and other diseases [12, 13].

Neuroinflammation also causes neurodegeneration in the vulnerable regions of the brain such as the hippocampus. Microglia and astrocytes play important roles in neuroinflammation and contribute to neurological disorders [14, 15].

Previous studies showed that curcumin acts as an antioxidant by activating macrophages to remove ROS-like, superoxide anions, H_2O_2, and nitrite radicals. Its anti-inflammatory properties were tested in vivo and in vitro on animals in acute and chronic inflammatory conditions [16]. Moreover, vitamin D also reported to play a part in the cerebral processes of detoxification by interacting with reactive oxygen and nitrogen species in the rat brain and by regulating the activity of glutamyl transpeptidase [17, 18], which is a key enzyme in the metabolism of glutathione. Vitamin D3 is the active form of vitamin D. This study investigated the effects of curcumin and vitamin D3 on memory and learning, by assessing the behavioral responses of scopolamine-induced learning-impaired rats through assays involving the locomotive and maze activities and histological and protein analysis in the rat brain tissues. The findings of this study show that inducing learning impairment in rats by using scopolamine followed by treatment with curcumin and vitamin D3 results in neuroprotection and attenuation of cognitive deficits as shown by reduced brain tissue damage in histoanalysis, decreased accumulation of abnormal proteins with immunoblot analysis and increased in the numbers of correct responses to behavioral stimuli during locomotive and maze tests.

2. Literature review

Aging is the primary risk factor for AD development. Aged population is prone to oxidative stress that results in the degeneration of their brains [19, 20]. Diets containing saturated fat and less intake of vitamin E and C are linked with the risk of AD [20]. AD patients suffer from memory impairment along with other cognitive deficits such as language, visuospatial skills, insight, and apraxia. Most patients may suffer from other symptoms such as depression, hallucination, apathy, and delusions at later stages of AD [21]. Numerous studies have indicated that accumulation of amyloid beta proteins (Aβ) and phosphorylated tau (p-tau) are the key pathological hallmarks of AD [22]. Similarly, oxidative stress changes ionic homeostasis and other biochemical parameters, which ultimately causes neuronal dysfunction and cell death leading to progressive dementia associated with extensive Aβ and tau pathology [23]. Tau is a neuronal microtubule-associated protein that is responsible for maintaining the microtubule dynamics and its function of transportation by axons and neurite outgrowth [24]. Animal models have demonstrated that loss of synaptic plasticity is one of the key components in the neurodegenerative process of AD, and tau is one of the contributing factors for neurodegeneration [25]. Literature indicated that the oxidative stress plays a significant role in the pathology of AD by enhancing Aβ deposition, tau phosphorylation, and loss of synapses and neurons [26].

Vitamin D is a group of fat-soluble secosteroids that helps to absorb calcium, magnesium, phosphate, iron, and zinc. Vitamin D protects the brain from the degenerative processes of AD by binding itself with vitamin D receptors [27]. Vitamin D deficiency has been associated with neurological and psychiatric disorders. Previous studies revealed that it controls Ca^{2+} homeostasis in the hippocampus by regulating intracellular Ca^{2+}. It also controls neurotrophic agents and protects the brain from Aβ-42 accumulation by stimulating phagocytosis. It also protects acetylcholine deficiency by increasing the activity of choline acetyltransferase in the brain. Due to its multiple biological targets, vitamin D can be used as an aide with the standard anti-dementia treatment. Among vitamin Ds, the most important compound is vitamin D3, also known as cholecalciferol. Increasing evidence highlights the impact of vitamin D deficiency as an important factor in various central or peripheral neurological diseases, especially multiple sclerosis and other neurodegenerative diseases, such as amyotrophic lateral sclerosis, Parkinson's disease, and Alzheimer's disease [28].

Curcumin (*Curcuma longa* (Haldi)) was used as a treatment in the animal models of AD. It was observed that curcumin reduced the formation of NFTs, Aβ deposition, and Aβ oligomerization. Curcumin can cross the blood–brain barrier because of its lipophilic nature. It can also inhibit acetylcholinesterase (AChE) activities [29] and can bind with the plaques leading to the alleviation of behavioral impairment [30–31]. Curcumin also acts as an antioxidant by activating macrophages to remove ROS-like radicals, superoxide anions, H_2O_2, and nitrite radicals [32–35].

Donepezil is available with the trade name "Aricept" developed by Eisai Inc. in 1983. It is a reversible AChE inhibitor, used for the treatment of mild to moderate dementia in AD patients. It has a long plasma half-life of 70 h. It is a noncompetitive reversible inhibitor of AChE that improves the function of cholinergic transmission. It increases the concentration of acetylcholine by preventing its hydrolysis. Animal studies have shown its selectivity for brain tissues and inhibition of AChE activities in smooth, striated, cardiac muscles. It can also inhibit AChE in red blood cells similar to its effect at synapses in CNS. AChE inhibition in red blood cells has been used as an indicator of the clinical effectiveness of donepezil in Alzheimer's disease patients [36].

Scopolamine is a tropane alkaloid that acts as a muscarinic receptor antagonist. Scopolamine is used to study memory and cognition in animal model of AD. Studies have shown that scopolamine provides a suitable pharmacological model of memory defect. Scopolamine administration characterizes cognitive deficits resulting in the impairment of verbal learning, spatial learning, and reaction time [37]. Scopolamine can also have an influence on other neurotransmitter systems due to the functional interaction of cholinergic neurons with other neurotransmitter systems [38]. Cholinergic transmission is blocked, resulting in cognitive impairment in a rat model of AD [39]. Histological studies of the brain of Alzheimer's patients have revealed the presence of activated microglia and reactive astrocytes around the Aβ plaques. The chronic activation of microglia secretes cytokines and some reactive substances that exacerbate Aβ pathology; thus, neuroglia plays an important part in the pathogenesis of AD [40]. Curcumin has a lipophilic property that is capable of passing through all cell membranes and thus exerts its intracellular effects. Curcumin has antiproliferative actions on microglia. A minimal dose of curcumin affects the neuroglial proliferation and differentiation. The overall effect of curcumin on neuroglial cells involves decreased astrocytes proliferation, improved myelogenesis, and increased activity and differentiation of oligodendrocytes [40].

3. Aims and objectives of this study

This study was conducted with the following objectives:

1. To determine the effects of curcumin, vitamin D3, and donepezil on behavioral responses of scopolamine-induced memory and learning-impaired rats.

2. To examine the structure of brain tissues obtained from scopolamine-treated rats with and without curcumin or vitamin D3 or donepezil.

3. To investigate the concentration of hyperphosphorylated tau protein in scopolamine-treated rat brain tissues with donepezil, curcumin, or vitamin D3.

4. Material and methods

4.1 Animals

Male Sprague Dawley rats of 200 ± 25 g were obtained from the animal house (PAPRSB Institute of Health Sciences Animal Facility, University Brunei Darussalam). Thirty animals were divided into five groups of six animals per group and reared under a standard laboratory condition with free access to food and water. Rats were acclimatized in a laboratory condition for a minimum of 1 week before undergoing behavioral test. The food was restricted under a daily feeding regime to maintain the weight of the rats.

All experiments were performed during daylight for 27 days, and all groups except group I (saline control) received daily scopolamine injection (2.5 mg/kg) to induce excitotoxicity. Curcumin, vitamin D3, and donepezil were administered to rats orally (**Table 1**). All experiments were conducted in accordance with institutional ethics guidelines for animal care and use (**Table 2**).

Group	Treatment
Group 1	Saline control (0.9% saline)
Group 2	Scopolamine (2.5 mg/kg) injection
Group 3	Scopolamine (2.5 mg/kg) injection and curcumin (80 mg/kg) oral
Group 4	Scopolamine (2.5 mg/kg) injection and donepezil (2.5 mg/kg) oral
Group 5	Scopolamine (2.5 mg/kg) injection and vitamin D3 (0.0179 mg/kg) oral

Table 1.
List of treatments received by each of the five groups of rats.

	Control	Scopolamine	Curcumin	Vitamin D3	Donepezil
Mean	17.42607	176.1054	27.29171	33.8713571	34.12914
SEM	1.261983	71.34413	14.49811	11.5630538	12.12356

Table 2.
Data expressed as mean ± standard error of the mean (SEM), expressed as the mean of time taken by different groups to reach the reward chamber each alternate day for 27 days.

4.2 Experimental design

4.2.1 Behavioral tests

4.2.1.1 Rectangular maze

This test was used to investigate learning and memory. The maze consisted of a rectangular box with an entry and a reward chamber with food, which were placed at the opposite ends of the box (**Figure 1**). All groups were given training in rectangular maze 1 week before drug administration. Each animal was placed in the same spot, recording the time taken by the animal to reach the reward chamber (transfer latency). Five readings were taken for each animal, and the average was calculated as their learning score [41–43].

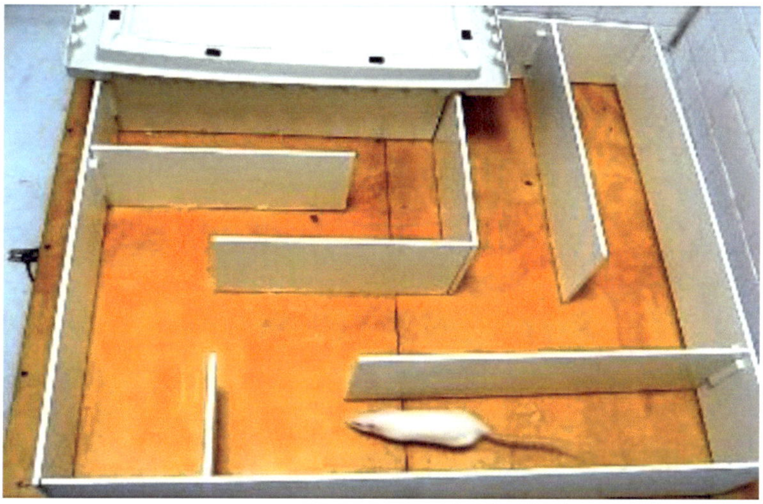

Figure 1.
Rectangular maze test.

4.2.1.2 Locomotor activity

Actophotometer was used to measure the locomotor activity (**Figure 2**). Each animal was treated with their respective compound, was placed in actophotometer, and was given 2 min in activity cage. When the beam of light falling on photocell was cut off due to the movement of the animal, an activity count was recorded. The increase or decrease in locomotor activity was then calculated [42, 43].

4.2.2 Histology

After the behavioral study was conducted, the animals were anesthetized, and their brains were removed and stored in 4% paraformaldehyde (**Figure 3**). The brains were embedded in paraffin and kept in the refrigerator. Paraffin sections (5 μm) were prepared using rotary microtome (**Figure 4**) and stained with hematoxylin and eosin [44]. Photographs were taken for each section.

4.2.3 Estimation of protein concentration

4.2.3.1 Immunoblotting

Curcumin, donepezil, and vitamin D3 reduce tau phosphorylation in the brains of a scopolamine-treated rat model of Alzheimer's disease.

The brain tissues were dissected from the coronal area with clean tools and put on ice as quickly as possible to prevent protein degradation by proteases. The tissues

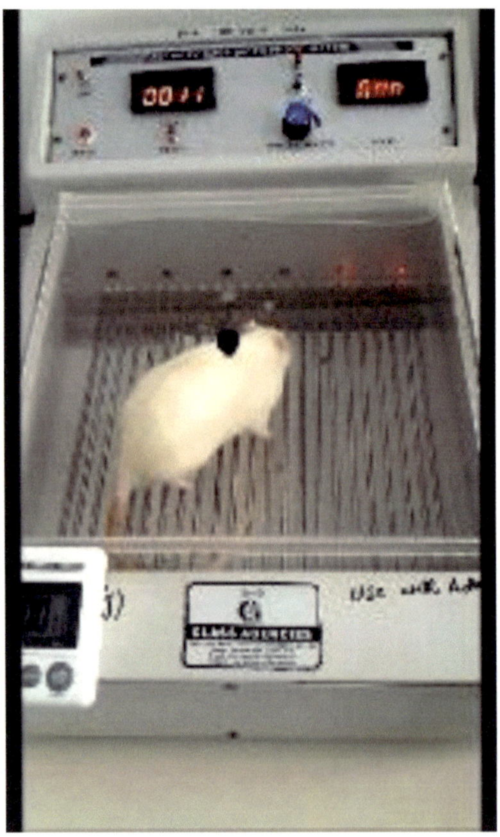

Figure 2.
Actophotometer for locomotor activity.

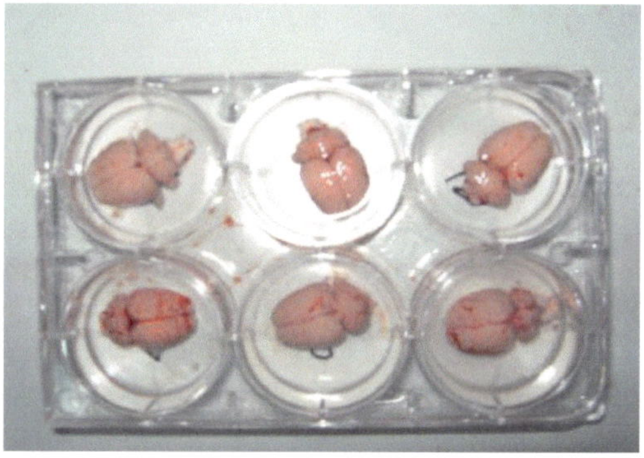

Figure 3.
Freshly dissected rat brains.

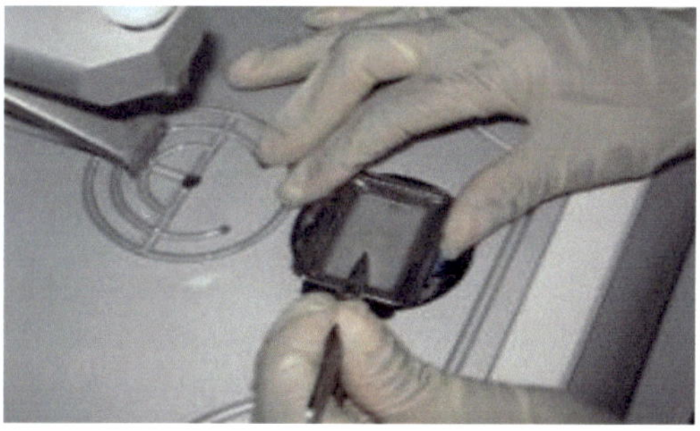

Figure 4.
Paraffin embedding for immunohistochemistry.

were placed in microcentrifuge tubes and immersed in liquid nitrogen to snap-freeze. They were homogenized on ice after adding 1× ice-cold lysis buffer, rinsed twice with the same buffer, and agitated on a shaker for 2 h at 4°C. After centrifugation for 20 min at 12,000 rpm at 4°C, the supernatant was transferred into a fresh tube kept on ice discarding the pellet. A small volume of lysate was sampled to perform a protein quantification assay.

After boiling each cell lysate in Tris-buffered saline, 0.1% Tween 20 (TBST) at 100°C for 5 min, 50 μg of protein was loaded into the wells of the sodium dodecyl sulfate-polyacrylamide gel electrophoresis (SDS-PAGE) gel for immunoblot analysis. After gel running for 1–2 h at 100 V, the proteins were then transferred onto the membrane and blocked for 1 h at room temperature. The membrane was then incubated with 1:1000 dilution of primary antibody in blocking buffer followed by washing three times with TBST for 5 min each wash. The membrane was incubated with the 1:1000 dilution of conjugated secondary antibody in blocking buffer at room temperature for 1 h and washed three times with TBST at 5 min each wash. Excess reagents were removed, and the membrane was covered with transparent plastic wrap. The image was acquired using the darkroom development techniques for chemiluminescence detection.

4.3 Statistical analysis

Data were expressed as mean ± standard error of the mean (SEM). The analysis of variance (ANOVA, single factor) was used to measure transfer latency with statistical significance set at $p < 0.05$.

5. Results

5.1 Rectangular maze test

The effects of curcumin and vitamin D3 on scopolamine-induced rats were investigated using the rectangular maze test comparing the results obtained with that of donepezil, a widely accepted AD standard drug. Rats that were injected with scopolamine showed significantly higher transfer latency, indicating the longer time for rats to reach the food (nearly 200 s). Also, there was no sign of improvement during the successive days (**Figure 5**). Rats treated with curcumin and vitamin D3 displayed significant reduction in transfer latency, which means that treated rats did not take a longer time to reach the food, less than 50 s as shown in **Figure 6**. Furthermore, there was a slight reduction in the latency time from day to day. The effect of these two compounds was also comparable to that of donepezil.

5.2 Locomotor activity

Actophotometer was used to measure locomotor activity by counting total photocell counts per rat for 2 min. Rat injected with scopolamine showed progressive decline in their locomotor activity (**Figure 7**), and average values were shown in **Table 3** and **Figure 8**. Rats treated with curcumin and vitamin D3 showed an initial increase in locomotor activities then slightly declined after 7 days followed by leveling off in the succeeding days. In contrast, rats treated with curcumin and vitamin D3 showed high locomotor activity compared with the non-treated control rats treated with donepezil that exhibited similar response as those treated with curcumin and vitamin D3, suggesting that these two compounds had triggered alertness and excitatory activities in scopolamine-treated rats.

5.3 Histology

Non-treated rats injected with scopolamine revealed prominent degeneration of cells and decrease number of nuclei in their brain tissues as compared to those treated with curcumin and vitamin D3. Moreover, treatment with curcumin, vitamin D3, and donepezil showed similar cell morphology similar to the control group demonstrating brain cells that appeared normal (**Figure 9**).

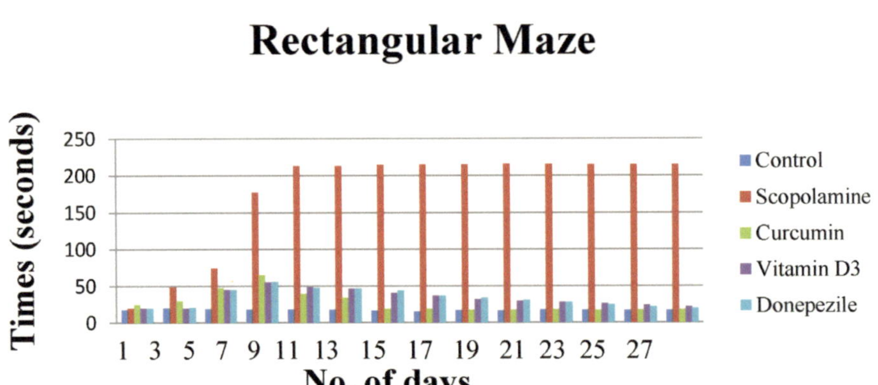

Figure 5.
Effect of curcumin, vitamin D3, and donepezil on latency time compared with the disease control group (mean, n = 6). The histogram shows the mean of latency time in seconds.

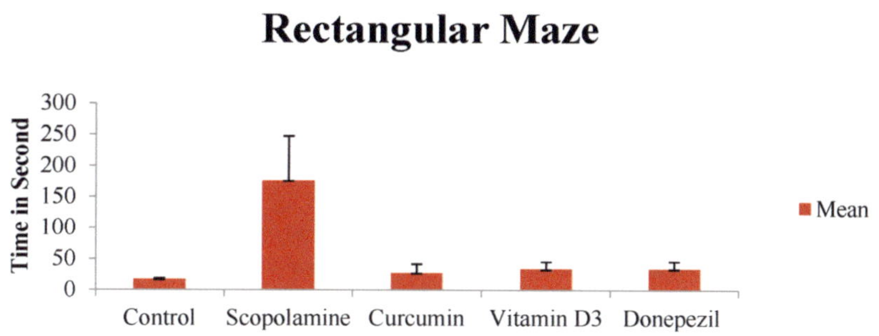

Figure 6.
Time taken to reach the reward chamber in the rectangular maze. Y-axis represents time in second. Data expressed as mean ± SEM.

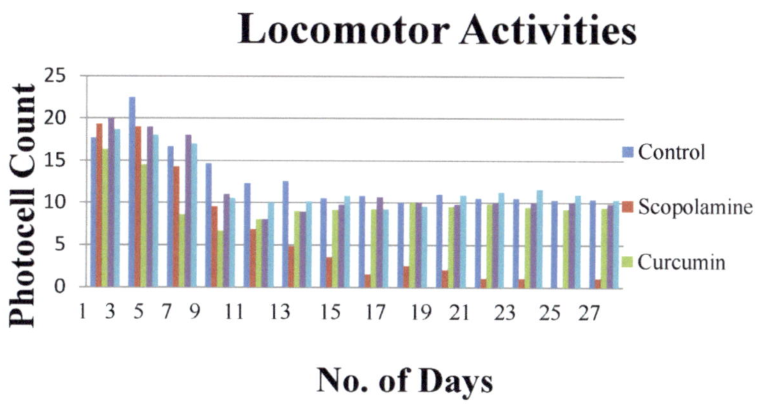

Figure 7.
Effect of curcumin, vitamin D3, and donepezil on latency time compared to scopolamine-treated group (mean, n = 6). Graph shows mean latency time in seconds.

	Control	Scopolamine	Curcumin	Vitamin D3	Donepezil
Mean	12.88686	6.161643	9.911429	11.77929	12.0664286
SEM	3.712271	6.766518	2.502838	3.992999	3.23978538

Table 3.
Data expressed as mean ± SEM for the total number of photocell counts for each group.

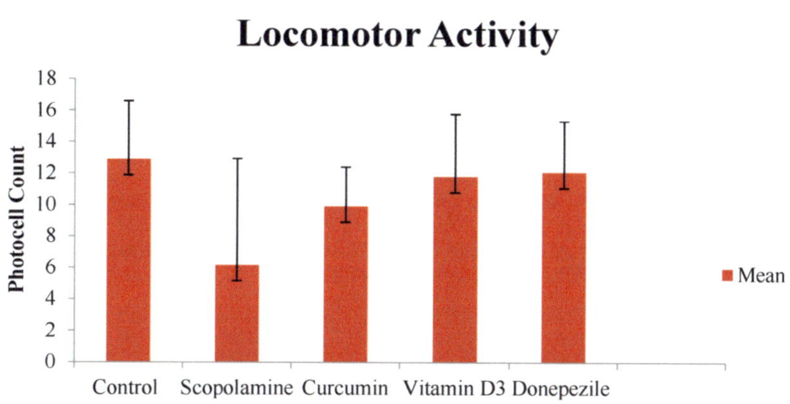

Figure 8.
Locomotor activities of all rats except scopolamine-treated rats in actophotometer showed no significant difference. Data expressed as mean of photocell count (mean ± SEM, n = 6) of animals on each alternate day for 27 days.

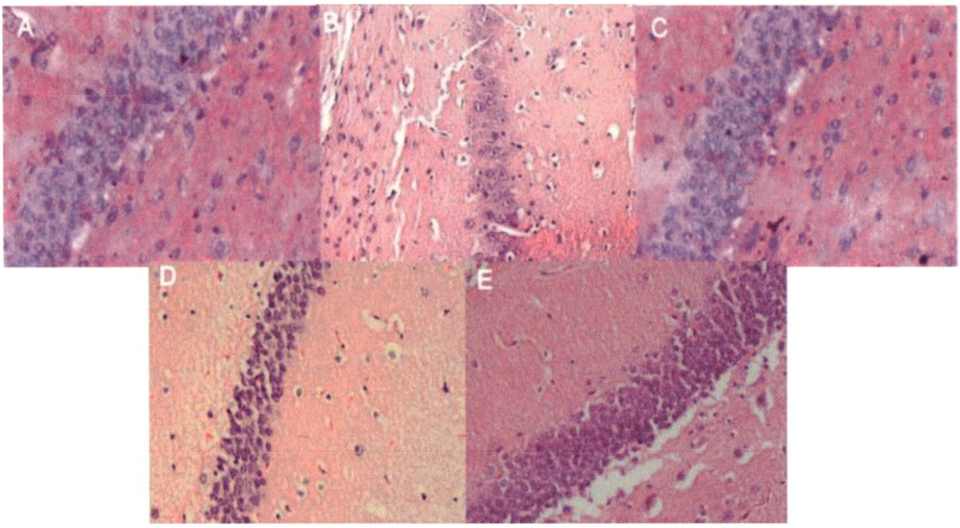

Figure 9.
Hematoxylin and eosin staining of rat brain tissues: A, control; B, scopolamine-induced; C, curcumin-treated; D, vitamin D3-treated; and E, donepezil. The images show no significant difference in the cellular histology of the hippocampal area (cornu ammonis) (CA3) in the experimental groups (curcumin, vitamin D3, and donepezil) as compared with those of scopolamine group, which showed less number of nuclei stained as revealed by H and E staining. Arrows in scopolamine slide B indicated the gaps around the neuronal cells of coronal sections (5 μm) at magnification 40×.

5.3.1 Immunoblotting

See **Figure 10**.

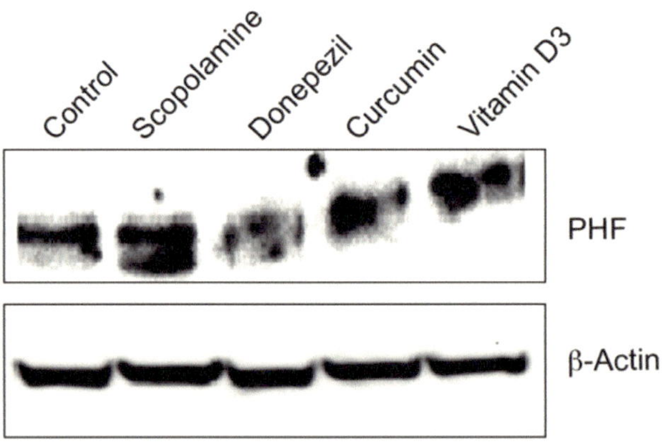

Figure 10.
Western blot analyses of scopolamine-treated and other treatments (curcumin and vitamin D3 and donepezil) groups showing difference in the levels of hyperphosphorylated tau in a rat model of AD. (a) Immunoblot of hippocampus homogenates from treated rats (scopolamine, vehicle, treated with curcumin and vitamin D3) using the PHF monoclonal antibodies and (b) normalized with β actin.

5.3.2 Vitamin D3 + scopolamine

See **Tables 4**, **5** and **Figure 11**.

S/No.	Area	Percent
1	13690.4	17.975
2	22076.4	28.986
3	16481.8	21.641
4	10,292	13.513
5	13,621	17.884

Table 4.
Densitometry data were obtained using image J software, exhibiting relative density of protein from all groups.

S/No.	Area	Percent
1	4240.34	23.631
2	3502.99	19.522
3	1857.51	10.352
4	4913.31	27.381
5	3429.87	19.114

Table 5.
Densitometry data were obtained using image J software. Representing relative density of Tau protein for all groups.

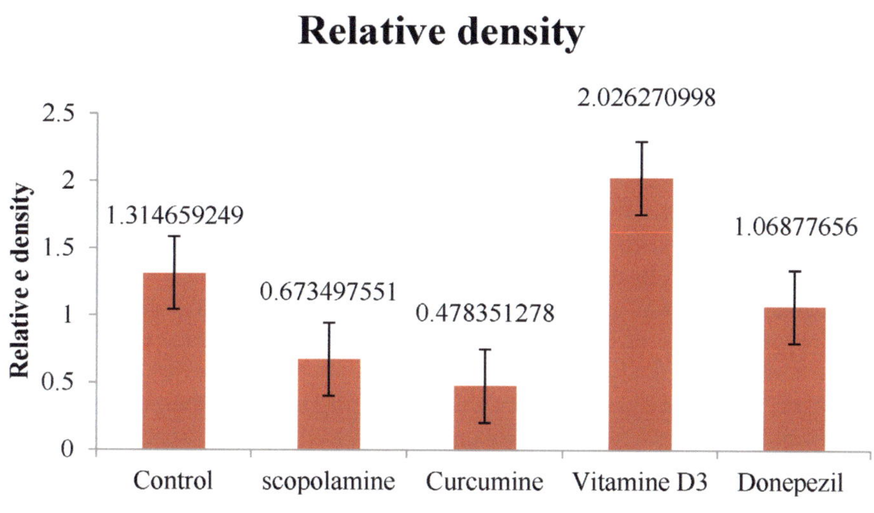

Figure 11.
Densitometry data obtained from image J software, presented as relative density of tau protein present in all groups.

6. Discussion

This study investigated the effects of curcumin and vitamin D3 on learning and memory and locomotion. The first part of the study involved subjecting the rats to several behavioral tests and examining their memory competencies and locomotor responses. Histological studies were also done on rats' brains to observe the changes that have occurred in the brain tissues after various treatments. The results obtained from rats treated with curcumin and vitamin D3 were compared with donepezil-treated rats. Scopolamine (muscarinic cholinergic antagonist) was used to induce memory impairment in rats [45]. Curcumin was selected as the previous research showed that curcumin could be used to recover learning and memory abilities in rats in AD and other inflammatory conditions [46]. Literature also reported that curcumin facilitates learning and memory functions by diminishing or preventing lipid peroxidation in the brains of aged rats [47]. In general, curcumin is a well-known oxygen free radical scavenger [46].

Vitamin D plays an important role in the regulation of numerous neurotransmitters including acetylcholine, dopamine, serotonin, and gamma aminobutyric acid. Several studies have also been reported that vitamin D deficiency is associated with neurological dysfunction and that supplementation of vitamin D may induce a protective effect against neurological disorders [48]. Based on the results of this study, the rats that were injected with scopolamine only revealed a gradual increase in the latency time until day 9, indicating a longer time required for rats to reach the end of the maze where food as a source of attractive stimuli was placed. After the ninth day, the latency time remained high and was three times higher than that of curcumin, vitamin D3, and donepezil. Rats treated with curcumin and vitamin D3 exhibits reduced latency time. A slight increase in time was observed between days 1 and 7 and gradually decreased up to day 27. The daily decrease in the latency time represented the effects of these two compounds on long-term memory. When comparing between curcumin and vitamin D3, rats treated with curcumin had slightly lower latency time than vitamin D3, suggesting that curcumin was comparatively more effective than vitamin D3 and donepezil in improving learning and memory among rats. Rats treated with donepezil initially showed low latency time, but remained constant until the 27 days. The similarity of latency time values obtained among curcumin, vitamin D3, donepezil, and the control suggested that curcumin and vitamin D3 have comparable effects like that of donepezil and may reverse the memory impairment induced by scopolamine.

The locomotor activity of rats was investigated by placing each rat in an actophotometer for 2 min and then assessing their movement as compared with those treated with curcumin and vitamin D3. Furthermore, the results indicated a decline in daily activities suggesting signs of slowing down. Vitamin D3 showed an increase in locomotor activity, which was comparable with those of donepezil and the controls confirming previous studies on the role of vitamin D in motor activities [49].

Curcumin exhibited slightly less action when compared to vitamin D3, donepezil treated, and control rats but was still exhibiting higher movements than scopolamine only. After 9 days, the locomotor activity for each treatment except scopolamine became relatively stable throughout 27 days and did not show any signs of slowing down, indicating that rats treated with vitamin D3 and curcumin exhibited signs of alertness that continued for a longer time.

The effects of each treatment were also histologically examined in rat brains. Sections of the brain tissue from the region of hippocampus were stained to investigate histological appearance before and after the treatment with selected compound. The cells in the brain tissue treated only with scopolamine exhibited less number of nuclei that appeared to be shrunken and smaller than with those of the control group. Treatment with curcumin and vitamin D3 showed no difference as compared with those of the brain tissue treated with donepezil and control group, suggesting that the brain tissues seemed to have recovered after the rats were treated with curcumin and vitamin D3. The difference in the levels of tau protein was also assessed using immunoblotting. In scopolamine-induced group, phosphorylated tau proteins were relatively higher than other groups indicating a state of proliferation in the brain tissues. Previous studies reported that accumulation of phosphorylated tau protein is one of the hallmarks of AD [50].

Western blot images were also assessed visually by making comparisons between bands in different lanes (**Figure 10**). Densitometry data obtained from image J software presented as relative density of tau protein found in all groups (**Tables 4** and **5**). After the rats were treated with curcumin and vitamin D3, the levels of tau proteins were reduced suggesting an attenuation of phosphorylated tau proteins in the rat brains, confirming the earlier studies (**Figures 10** and **11**) [51, 52].

7. Conclusion

We concluded that Alzheimer's disease is a progressive neurodegenerative disorder characterized by gradual memory loss and shrinkage of neuronal cells particularly in the hippocampus and basal forebrain regions. Curcumin and vitamin D3 have biomedical qualities that protect the brain from degeneration associated with AD. In this study, the behavioral tasks involving rectangular maze test and locomotor activity were used to determine if curcumin and vitamin D3 could improve learning and memory among rats subjected to scopolamine-induced impaired cognition. With cognitive impairment, the correct response rate of animals during acquisition and retention period was significantly lower than that of the control group. However, treatment with curcumin and vitamin D3 has increased their correct response rate for both tasks that became equal with those of the control group ($p < 0.05$). Tissue analysis by H and E staining of the rat brain from the scopolamine group showed less number of cells, which was improved upon the treatment with curcumin and vitamin D3, resulting in significantly increase in the number of cells with no gap around them. This was accompanied by reduced level of abnormal tau proteins detected via immunoblot analysis. Together, these findings demonstrate that curcumin and vitamin D3 have the potential to reverse some cognitive deficits, correct memory impairment, and protect the brain from degeneration.

The animal model of AD has shown improvement in learning and memory after exposure to curcumin and vitamin D3 treatment, which slowed down the progress of AD pathologies delaying the onset of AD. With potential as a treatment for AD in future, the active structure and the target of both curcumin and vitamin D3 can be further investigated to elucidate the molecular mechanism by which their beneficial effects can be enhanced for the improvement of AD patients. Vitamin D due to its multiple biological targets can be used as an adjunct to standard anti-dementia treatment in AD. Curcumin has intensively been studied for the improvement of AD symptoms, and existing investigations on inhalable curcumin and ar-turmerone on neural stem cells (NSCs) are currently under clinical trials.

Author details

Saima Khan[1] and Kaneez Fatima Shad[2]*

1 Institute of Health Sciences Universiti Brunei Darussalam, Gadong, BE, Brunei Darussalam

2 University of Technology, Sydney, Australia

*Address all correspondence to: ftmshad@gmail.com

References

[1] Iqbal K, Liu F, Gong C-X, Grundke-Iqbal I. Curr Alzheimer Res. 2010;7(8):656-664

[2] Brady S, Siegel G, Albers RW, Price D. Basic Neurochemistry: Molecular, Cellular and Medical Aspects. Academic Press; 2005

[3] Billingsley ML, Kincaid RL. Regulated phosphorylation and dephosphorylation of tau protein: Effects on microtubule interaction, intracellular trafficking, and neurodegeneration. The Biochemical Journal. 1997;**323**(3):577-591

[4] Kopke E, Tung YC, Shaikh S, Alonso AC, Iqbal K, Grundke-Iqbal I. Microtubule-associated protein tau. Abnormal phosphorylation of a non-paired helical filament pool in Alzheimer disease. Journal of Biological Chemistry. 1993;**268**:24374-24384

[5] Alonso AD, Zaidi T, Grundke-Iqbal I, Iqbal K. Role of abnormally phosphorylated tau in the breakdown of microtubules in Alzheimer disease. Proceedings of the National Academy of Sciences of the United States of America. 1994;**91**:5562-5566

[6] Iqbal K, Grundke-Iqbal I, Zaidi T, Merz PA, Wen GY, Shaikh SS, et al. Defective brain microtubule assembly in Alzheimer's disease. Lancet. 1986;**2**:421-426

[7] Li B, Chohan MO, Grundke-Iqbal I, Iqbal K. Disruption of microtubule network by Alzheimer abnormally hyperphosphorylated tau. Acta Neuropathology (Berl). 2007;**113**: 501-511

[8] Wang JZ, Gong CX, Zaidi T, Grundke-Iqbal I, Iqbal K. Dephosphorylation of Alzheimer paired helical filaments by protein phosphatase-2A and -2B. The Journal of Biological Chemistry. 1995;**270**:4854-4860

[9] Alonso A, Zaidi T, Novak M, Grundke-Iqbal I, Iqbal K. Hyperphosphorylation induces self-assembly of tau into tangles of paired helical filaments/straight filaments. Proceedings of the National Academy of Sciences of the United States of America. 2001;**98**(12):6923-6928

[10] Nunomura A, Castellani RJ, Zhu X, Moreira PI, Perry G, Smith MA. Involvement of oxidative stress in Alzheimer disease. Journal of Neuropathology & Experimental Neurology. 2006;**65**(7):631-641

[11] Chen Z, Zhong C. Oxidative stress in Alzheimer's disease. Neuroscience Bulletin. 2014;**30**(2):271-281

[12] Moreira PI, Smith MA, Zhu X, Nunomura A, Castellani RJ, Perry G. Oxidative stress and neurodegeneration. Annals of the New York Academy of Sciences. 2005;**1043**(1):545-552

[13] Folli F, Corradi D, Fanti P, Davalli A, Paez A, Giaccari A, et al. The role of oxidative stress in the pathogenesis of type 2 diabetes mellitus micro-and macrovascular complications: Avenues for a mechanistic-based therapeutic approach. Current Diabetes Reviews. 2011;**7**(5):313-324

[14] Lee Mosley R, Benner EJ, Kadiu I, Thomas M, Boska MD, Hasan K, et al. Neuroinflammation, oxidative stress, and the pathogenesis of Parkinson's disease. Clinical Neuroscience Research. 2006;**6**(5):261-281

[15] Rohl C, Armbrust E, Herbst E, Jess A, Gulden M, Maser E, et al. Mechanisms involved in the modulation of astroglial resistance to oxidative stress induced by activated microglia: Antioxidative systems, peroxide elimination, radical generation, lipid

peroxidation. Neurotoxicity Research. 2010;**17**(4):317-331

[16] Kumar A, Dora J, Singh A. A review on spice of life *Curcuma longa* (turmeric). International Journal of Applied Biology and Pharmaceutical Technology. 2011;**2**(4):371-379

[17] Garcion E, Sindji L, Nataf S, Brachet P, Darcy F, Montero-Menei CN. Treatment of experimental auto-immune encephalomyelitis in rat by 1,25-dihydroxyvitamin D3 leads to early effects within the central nervous sys- tem. Acta Neuropathologica. 2003;**105**:438-448

[18] Garcion E, Wion-Barbot N, Montero-Menei CN, Berger F, Wion D. New clues about vitamin D functions in the nervous system. Trends in Endocrinology and Metabolism. 2002;**13**:100-105

[19] Coyle JT, Puttfarcken P. Oxidative stress, glutamate, and neurodegenerative disorders. Science. 1993;**262**(5134): 689-695

[20] Barnard ND, Bush AI, Ceccarelli A, Cooper J, de Jager CA, Erickson KI, et al. Dietary and lifestyle guidelines for the prevention of Alzheimer's disease. Neurobiology of Aging. 2014;**35**:S74-S78

[21] Murman DL, Colenda CC. The economic impact of neuropsychiatric symptoms in Alzheimer's disease. PharmacoEconomics. 2005;**23**(3): 227-242

[22] Selkoe DJ. Cell biology of protein misfolding: The examples of Alzheimer's and Parkinson's diseases. Nature Cell Biology. 2004;**6**(11):1054-1061

[23] Haass C, Selkoe DJ. Soluble protein oligomers in neurodegeneration: Lessons from the Alzheimer's amyloid β-peptide. Nature Reviews Molecular Cell Biology. 2007;**8**(2):101-112

[24] Johnson GV, Stoothoff WH. Tau phosphorylation in neuronal cell function and dysfunction. Journal of Cell Science. 2004;**117**(24):5721-5729

[25] Crimins JL, Pooler A, Polydoro M, Luebke JI, Spires-Jones TL. The intersection of amyloid beta and tau in glutamatergic synaptic dysfunction and collapse in Alzheimer's disease. Ageing Research Reviews. 2013;**12**(3):757-763

[26] Chen Z, Zhong C. Oxidative stress in Alzheimer's disease. Neuroscience Bulletin. 2014;**30**(2):271-281

[27] Gezen-Ak D, Atasoy IL, Candas E, Alaylioglu M, Yılmazer S, Dursun E. Vitamin D receptor regulates amyloid beta 1-42 production with protein disulfide isomerase A3. ACS Chemical Neuroscience. 2017;**8**(10):2335-2346

[28] Kalueff AV, Tuohimaa P. Neurosteroid hormone vitamin D and its utility in clinical nutrition. Current Opinion in Clinical Nutrition and Metabolic Care. 2007;**10**:12-19

[29] Ahmed T, Gilani A. Inhibitory effect of curcuminoids on acetylcholinesterase activity and attenuation of scopolamine induced amnesia may explain medicinal use of turmeric in Alzheimer's disease. Pharmacology Biochemistry and Behavior. 2009;**91**(4):554-559

[30] Ono K, Hasegawa K, Naiki H, Yamada M. Curcumin has potent anti-amyloidogenic effects for Alzheimer's β-amyloid fibrils in vitro. Journal of Neuroscience Research. 2004;**75**(6):742-750

[31] Yang F, Lim GP, Begum AN. Curcumin inhibits formation of amyloid β oligomers and fibrils, binds plaques, and reduces amyloid in vivo. Journal of Biological Chemistry. 2005;**280**(7):5892-5901

[32] Akinyemi AJ, Oboh G, Oyeleye SI, Ogunsuyi. Anti-amnestic effect

of curcumin in combination with donepezil, an anticholinesterase drug: Involvement of cholinergic system. Neurotoxicity Research. 2017;**31**(4): 560-569. ISSN: 1476-3524

[33] Ma Q-L, Zuo X, Yang F. Curcumin suppresses soluble tau dimers and corrects molecular chaperone, synaptic, and behavioral deficits in aged human tau transgenic mice. The Journal of Biological Chemistry. 2013;**288**(6):4056-4065

[34] Menon VP, Sudheer AR. Antioxidant and anti-inflammatory properties of curcumin. Advances in Experimental Medicine and Biology. 2007;**595**:105-125. DOI: 10.1007/978-0-387-46401-5_3

[35] Ray B, Lahiri DK. Neuro-inflammation in Alzheimer's disease: Different molecular targets and potential therapeutic agents including curcumin. Current Opinion in Pharmacology. 2009;**9**(4):434-444

[36] Pakaski M, Feher A, Juhasz A, Drotos G, Fazekas OC, Kovacs J, et al. Serum adipokine levels modified by donepezil treatment in Alzheimer's disease. Journal of Alzheimer's Disease. 2014;**38**(2):371-377

[37] Preston GC, Brazell C, Ward C, Broks P, Traub M, Stahl SM. The scopolamine model of dementia: Determination of central cholino-mimetic effects of physostigmine on cognition and biochemical markers in man. Journal of Psychopharmacology. 1988;**2**(2):67-79

[38] Flood JF, Cherkin A. Scopolamine effects on memory retentionin mice: A model of dementia? Behavioral and Neural Biology. 1986;**45**:169-184

[39] Goverdhan P, Sravanthi A, Mamatha T. Neuroprotective effects of meloxicam and selegiline in scopolamine-induced cognitive impairment and oxidative stress. International Journal of Alzheimer's Disease. 2012;**2012**(8). Article ID 974013. DOI: 10.1155/2012/974013

[40] Mishra S, Palanivelu K. The effect of curcumin (turmeric) on Alzheimer's disease: An overview. Annals of Indian Academy of Neurology. 2008;**11**(1):13

[41] Indumathy S, Kavimani S, Raman KV. The role of angiotensin antagonists in memory enhancement. International Journal of Pharma and Bio Sciences. 2010;**1**(3):1-4

[42] Moghaddam AH, Zare M. Neuroprotective effect of hesperetin and nano-hesperetin on recognition memory impairment and the elevated oxygen stress in rat model of Alzheimer's disease. Biomedicine & Pharmacotherapy. 2018;**97**:1096-1101

[43] Shahidi S, Zargooshnia S, Asl SS, Komaki A, Sarihi A. Influence of N-acetyl cysteine on beta-amyloid-induced Alzheimer's disease in a rat model: A behavioral and electrophysiological study. Brain Research Bulletin. 2017;**131**:142-149

[44] Jahanshahi M, Golalipour MJ, Afshar M. The effect of *Urtica dioica* extract on the number of astrocytes in the dentate gyrus of diabetic rats. Folia Morphologica. 2009;**68**(2):93-97

[45] Sunderland T, Tariot PN, Cohen RM, Weingartner H, Mueller EA, Murphy DL. Anticholinergic sensitivity in patients with dementia of the Alzheimer type and age-matched controls: A dose-response study. Archives of General Psychiatry. 1987;**44**(5):418-426

[46] Pan R, Qiu S, Lu DX, Dong J. Curcumin improves learning and memory ability and its neuroprotective mechanism in mice. Chinese Medical Journal. 2008;**121**:832-839

[47] Sun CY, Qi SS, Zhou P, Cui HR, Chen SX, Dai KY. Neurobiological and

pharmacological validity of curcumin in ameliorating memory performance of senescence-accelerated mice. Pharmacology, Biochemistry, and Behavior. 2013;**105**:76-82

[48] Annweiler C, Karras SN, Anagnostis P, Beauchet O. Vitamin D supplements: A novel therapeutic approach for Alzheimer patients. Frontiers in Pharmacology. 2014;**5**:6

[49] Burne TH, Johnston AN, McGrath J, Mack-ay-Sim A. Swimming behavior and post-swimming activity in vitamin D receptor knockout mice. Brain Research Bulletin. 2006;**69**:74-78

[50] Harrison RS, Sharpe PC, Singh Y, Fairlie DP. Amyloid peptides and proteins in review. Reviews of Physiology, Biochemistry and Pharmacology. 2007;**159**:1-77

[51] Huang HC, Tang D, Xu K, Jiang ZF. Curcumin attenuates amyloid-β-induced tau hyperphosphorylation in human neuroblastoma SH-SY5Y cells involving PTEN/Akt/GSK-3β signaling pathway. Journal of Receptors and Signal Transduction. 2014;**34**(1):26-37

[52] Das TK, Jana P, Chakrabarti SK, Hamid A, Mas RW. Curcumin downregulates GSK3 and Cdk5 in scopolamine-induced Alzheimer's disease rats abrogating Aβ 40/42 and tau hyperphosphorylation. Journal of Alzheimer's disease reports. 2019;**3**(1):257-267

Chapter 6

Attention Deficit Hyperactivity Disorder

Sophia Bakhtadze, Tinatin Tkemeladze and Tinatin Kutubidze

Abstract

Attention deficit hyperactivity disorder (ADHD) is a mental disorder of the neurodevelopmental type. The disorder represents one of the common causes of referral for behavioral problems in children to medical and mental health doctors all around the world. The diagnosis can be done by DSM-V criteria. According to DSM-V, there are three main subtypes of ADHD: ADHD-inattentive type, ADHD-hyperactive-impulsive type, and ADHD-combined type. The etiology of ADHD is not definitively known. A genetic imbalance of catecholamine metabolism in the cerebral cortex appears to play a primary role. Various environmental factors may play a secondary role. Cognitive impairments in a variety of domains have been found in ADHD as well as impairment in overall intellectual function. A meta-analysis of children and adolescents with ADHD showed impairments in several aspects of executive functioning. The most important part of any intervention plan for a child with ADHD is the physical, behavioral and neuromotor/neuropsychological examination. Medication should be started with one of the stimulants. Both d-amphetamine and methylphenidate have been shown to be effective for improvement of hyperactivity, concentration problems, learning disorders, and other comorbidities.

Keywords: ADHD, inattention, hyperactivity, impulsivity, behavioral therapy

1. Introduction

Attention deficit hyperactivity disorder (ADHD) is a mental disorder of the neurodevelopmental type. It is characterized by difficulty paying attention, excessive activity and acting without regards to consequences, which are otherwise not appropriate for a person's age. The disorder represents one of the common causes of referral for behavioral problems in children to medical and mental health doctors all around the world. It is one of the most prevalent psychiatric conditions in children affecting 5% of children and adolescents worldwide. Symptoms which are specific for ADHD could decrease with age as almost 65% of children with ADHD have partial resolution of signs but 15% of ADHD children exhibit complete disappearance of clinical picture in adulthood [1].

A meta-analysis of 175 research studies worldwide on ADHD prevalence in children aged 18 and under found an overall pooled estimate of 7.2% [2].

The number of children with ADHD can reach millions. According to data received in 2016 from USA almost 6.1 million of children have ADHD (9.4%). About

388,000 children are 2–5 years of age; 4 million children are 6–11 years; and 3 million children aged 12–17 years. Boys are more likely to be diagnosed with ADHD than girls [3]. The prevalence age for diagnosis is 2–17 years.

Centers for Disease Control and prevention (CDC) uses datasets from parent surveys and healthcare claims to understand diagnosis and treatment patterns for ADHD. Estimates for diagnosis and treatment can vary depending on the source [4]. The methods used for ADHD assessment are also different.

Coexisting disorders are common in children with ADHD. According to a national 2016 parent survey every 6 in 10 children with ADHD could have at least one other mental, emotional or behavioral disorder; almost half of the children with ADHD have coexisting behavioral and conduct disorders. One third of ADHD children could exhibit anxiety disorders as well. Depression, autism spectrum disorder and Tourette syndrome are also common disorders accompanying ADHD [2].

The first information about ADHD appeared in 1865 while German doctor Heinrich Hoffman described hyperactive child ("Fidgety Phil"). The enormous scientific contribution was done by George Still and Alfred Tregold who were the first authors to emphasize those clinical clues which still persist [5]. In 1922, the condition was called as "postencephalic behavior disorder", later in 1947, it was changed with "brain-injured child," then in 1963 it was renamed as "perceptually handicapped child" and ending with "minimal brain dysfunction" in 1966 [6]. Two years after in 1968 Diagnostic and Statistical Manual (DSM) recognized it as a syndrome under the term "hyperkinetic reaction of childhood or adolescence." In late 80s DSM-III recognized two subtypes of attention deficit disorder *(ADD) with hyperactivity and ADD without hyperactivity.* DSM-III revised the term ADD and changed it with "attention-deficit hyperactivity disorder (ADHD)." Finally DSM-IV identified three subtypes of the syndrome: ADHD-inattentive type, ADHD-hyperactive-impulsive type, and ADHD-combined type [7]. The DSM-V shared the same clinical forms of ADHD and identified strict diagnostic criteria for each [8].

2. DSM-5 diagnostic criteria

A. A persistent pattern of inattention and/or hyperactivity-impulsivity that interferes with functioning or development as characterized by (1) and/or (2):

1. **Inattention:** Six (or more) of the following symptoms have persisted for at least 6 months to a degree that is inconsistent with developmental level and that negatively impact directly on social and academic/occupational activities.

Note: The symptoms are not solely a manifestation of oppositional behavior, defiance, hostility or failure to understand tasks or instructions. For older adolescents and adults (age 17 and older) at least five symptoms are required.

a. Often fails to give close attention to details or make careless mistakes in schoolwork, at work or during other activities (e.g., overlooks or misses details, work is inaccurate).

b. Often has difficulty sustaining attention in tasks or play activities (e.g., has difficulty remaining focused during lectures, conversations or lengthy reading).

c. Often does not seem to listen when spoken to directly (e.g., mind seems elsewhere, even in the absence of any obvious distraction).

d. Often does not follow through on instructions and fails to finish schoolwork, chores, or duties in the workplace (e.g., starts tasks but quickly loses focus and is easily sidetracked).

e. Often has difficulty organizing tasks and activities (e.g., difficulty managing sequential tasks; difficulty keeping materials and belongings in order, messy, disorganized work; has poor time management; fails to meet deadlines).

f. Often avoids, dislikes or is reluctant to engage in tasks that require sustained mental effort (e.g., schoolwork or homework; for older adolescents and adult, preparing reports, completing forms, reviewing lengthy papers).

g. Often loses things necessary for tasks or activities (e.g., school materials, pencils, books, tools, wallets, keys, paperwork, eyeglasses, mobile telephones).

h. Is often easily distracted by extraneous stimuli (for older adolescents and adults may include unrelated thoughts).

i. Is often forgetful in daily activities (e.g., doing chores, running errands; for older adolescents and adults returning calls, paying bills, keeping appointments).

2. **Hyperactivity and impulsivity:** Six (or more) of the following symptoms have persisted for at least 6 months to a degree that is inconsistent with developmental level and that negatively impacts directly on social and academic/occupational activities:

Note: The symptoms are not solely a manifestation of oppositional behavior, defiance, hostility or a failure to understand tasks or instructions. For older adolescents and adults (age 17 and older) at least five symptoms are required.

a. Often fidgets with or taps hands or feet or squirms in a seat.

b. Often leaves seat in situations when remaining seated is expected (e.g., leaves his or her place in the classroom, in the office or other workplace or in other situations that require remaining in place).

c. Often runs about or climbs in situations where it is inappropriate (Note: In adolescents or adults may be limited to feeling restless).

d. Often unable to play or engage in leisure activities quietly.

e. Is often "on the go" acting as if "driven by a motor" (e.g., is unable to be or uncomfortable being still for extended time as in restaurants, meeting; may be experienced by others as being restless or difficult to keep up with).

f. Often talks excessively

g. Often blurts out an answer before a question has been completed (e.g., complete people's sentences; cannot wait for turn in conversation).

h. Often has difficulty waiting his or her turn (e.g., while waiting in line).

i. Often interrupts or intrudes on others (e.g., butts into conversations, games or activities; may start using other people's things without asking or receiving permission; for adolescents and adults, may intrude into or take over what others are doing).

B. Several inattentive or hyperactive-impulsive symptoms were present prior to age 12 years.

C. Several inattentive or hyperactive-impulsive symptoms are present in two or more setting (e.g., at home, school or work; with friends or relatives; in other activities).

D. There is clear evidence that the symptoms interfere with or reduce the quality of social, academic or occupational functioning.

E. The symptoms do not occur exclusively during the course of schizophrenia or another psychotic disorder and are not better explained by another mental disorder (e.g., mood disorder, anxiety disorder, dissociative disorder, personality disorder, substance intoxication or withdrawal).

Specify whether

314.01 (F90.2) Combined presentation: If both criterion A1 (inattention) and criterion A2 (hyperactivity-impulsivity) are met for the past 6 months.

314.00 (F90.0) Predominantly inattentive presentation: If criterion A1 (inattention) is met but criterion A2 (hyperactivity-impulsivity) is not met for the past 6 months.

314.01 (F90.1) Predominantly hyperactive/impulsive presentation: If criterion A2 (hyperactivity-impulsivity) is met but criterion A1 (inattention) is not mere over the past 6 months.

Specify if:

In partial remission: When full criteria were previously met, fewer than the full criteria have been met for the past 6 months and the symptoms still result in impairment in social, academic or occupational functioning.

Specify current severity:

Mild: Few if any symptoms in excess of those required to make the diagnosis are present and symptoms result it only minor functional impairments.

Moderate: Symptoms or functional impairment between "mild" and "severe" are present and symptoms result in only minor functional impairments.

Severe: Many symptoms in excess of those required to make the diagnosis or several symptoms that are particularly severe, are present or the symptoms result in marked impairment is social or occupational functioning.

2.1 Etiology

The etiology of ADHD is not definitely known. A genetic imbalance of catecholamines in the cerebral cortex appears to play a primary role. A genetic contribution to the pathogenesis of ADHD is supported by the increased risk of ADHD in the first-degree relatives of patients with ADHD and twin studies from different countries that consistently provide heritability estimates of approximately 75% [1].

Various environmental factors may play a secondary role; the significance of environmental factors is controversial. Dietary influences, sleep deficiency, prenatal medications, prematurity, iron deficiency, iodine deficiency and etc.

2.1.1 Dietary influences

The influence of diet on attention, hyperactivity, and behavior is controversial. Some children may demonstrate mild adverse behavioral effects of diets containing food additives, artificial colors, excess sugar, or reduced intake of essential fatty acids and minerals.

2.1.2 Food additives

Food additives were first suggested as potential cause of hyperactive behavior in the 1970. Systematic reviews and the meta-analyses of randomized trials with methodological limitations suggest that some children with ADHD respond favorably to elimination diets [9, 10]. However, this conclusion is not universally accepted, and the issue remains controversial.

2.1.3 Refined sugar

Adverse behavior effects including hyperactivity are commonly attributed to excess sugar intake by parents and teachers. Parent of children with ADHD frequently note a worsening of hyperactivity after consuming high carbohydrate meal. There are proposed mechanisms: sensitivity to refined sugar and functional reactive hypoglycemia (which triggers release of stress hormones such as adrenaline) after ingesting sugar [11].

There is no evidence that sugar effects the behavior and/or cognitive performance [11]. Future studies are necessary to confirm the effect on even a small subset of children.

2.1.4 Food sensitivity

Food allergy is proposed as a possible factor in the cause of ADHD. There are few well-designed trials evaluating the potential association between food sensitivity (allergy or intolerance) and behavior. Demonstration of such association requires removal of the suspect food(s) from child's diet (elimination diet). Followed by challenge with suspected food(s) versus placebo. The role of food sensitivity as a cause of ADHD is difficult to document, cooperation on neurologist, allergist and dietician being essential. The hypoallergic diet deserves further study [4].

2.1.5 Iron deficiency

The role of iron deficiency in the ADHD has not clearly defined. A comparison of clinical characteristics of children with the lowest serum ferritin levels (20ng/ml) and those with highest serum ferritin levels (60ng/ml) show no significant difference in severity or frequency of ADHD and comorbid symptoms [4]. In addition, there appears to be an overlap between restless leg syndrome (which is associated with iron deficiency) and ADHD symptom in children [12].

2.1.6 Zinc deficiency

The role of zinc in ADHD is also controversial. Several studies have been conducted to find out the role of zinc in the etiology of ADHD. Study by Arnold and colleagues [13] did not show that the zinc alone could improve the ADHD symptoms. In another study zinc was a part of the treatment [14]. In conclusion, zinc is tolerated well in children with ADHD. However, further evidences are required to indicate whether zinc is effective for treating children with ADHD. It is recommended to replicate the randomized well-controlled trials [15].

2.1.7 Prenatal exposure to tobacco smoke

Prenatal exposure to tobacco smoke is consistently associated with development of ADHD in case-control and cohort studies [16]. Smoking during pregnancy increased the risk of offspring ADHD. The risk of ADHD was greater for children whose mothers were heavy smokers than for those mothers were light smokers. The authors suppose that there can be relationship between maternal smoking and ADHD in children but could not clarify if other confounding risk factors can affect on this causality. Thus it is necessary to perform more studies in order to detect association between maternal smoking and ADHD in offsprings.

2.1.8 Iodine deficiency and children with ADHD

Correlation of the Iodine deficiency and ADHD in children is of high interest. Thyroid hormones are necessary for the normal metabolic function and the Iodine is important element in the synthesis and regulation of thyroid hormones. It is well known that Iodine deficiency (ID) can lead to mental retardation although preventable and the most critical period for this is fetal development. Maternal thyroid function and Iodine concentration of infant are strongly correlated and the group of disorders due to disturbances in this correlation are called ID disorders. According to Hope Abel and colleagues [17] maternal ID during pregnancy has direct association with severe ADHD symptoms in offsprings at eight years of age. Although it is not recommended maternal iodine intake in order to avoid ADHD risk in child especially as it is known iodine supplementation in the first trimester is associated with an increased health risks

2.1.9 Lead exposure and ADHD

Lead (Pb) has as a neurotoxic effect leading to abnormal behavior in children. There are plenty of studies attempting to detect correlation between exposure to heavy metals and other harmful environmental factors in the pathogenesis of behavioral disorders. In 1991 recommended level of lead in children's blood (BLL) by CDC is set to 10 micrograms of lead per deciliter of blood (μg/dL) and it has not been changed since then. Donzelli et al. [18] performed systematic review of 17 studies assessing the correlation of lead level and ADHD. According to their results there is a direct correlation between low lead level of lead in ADHD children's blood and severity of ADHD symptoms. However, we need more high quality clinical studies to prove this relationship.

Although evidence shows that ADHD is a worth recognizing disorder many environmental risk factors such as exposure to heavy metals, dietary factors, environmental exposure to different substances could intensify or accelerate the progression of this disease. The efforts for early diagnosis of the disease is crucial, and identifying the contributing factors is of prime importance to prevent ADHD.

Although evidence shows that ADHD is a worth recognizing disorder many environmental risk factors such as exposure to heavy metals, dietary factors, environmental exposure to different substances could intensify or accelerate the progression of this disease. The efforts for early diagnosis of the disease is crucial, and identifying the contributing factors is of prime importance to prevent ADHD.

2.2 Genetic factors

It has been implicated that genetic factors play a critical role in the etiology of ADHD as well as its comorbidities. Based on multiple familial, twin, adoption and single epidemiological studies ADHD is considered as one of the psychiatric disorders which shows the strongest genetic basis. Several twin studies have revealed that concordance in monozygotic (MZ) twins is higher than in dizygotic (DZ) twins with heritability estimates of approximately 75–80%. Large numbers of linkage studies, genome wide association studies (GWAS) and meta-analyses have been conducted and numbers of susceptibility variants, genes and chromosomal regions have been reported to be associated with ADHD. Moreover, number of studies also shows that about one third of ADHD's heritability is due to a polygenic component encompassing many common variants, where each variant individually has small effect but their cumulative effect contributes to the development of the condition. Investigation of copy number variants (CNVs) has also shown that rare insertions or deletions contribute to the part of ADHD's heritability. Recent progress in identifying ADHD susceptibility genes underlines new biological pathways that may have implication for prevention and treatment development.

According to the literature the mean heritability across multiple twin studies of ADHD is 74–80% [19, 20] and it is similar in ADHD males and females [21]. According to one study, where 894 probands with ADHD and their 1135 siblings were studied, there was nine-fold increased risk of ADHD in siblings of ADHD probands compared with siblings of controls. Several adoption studies also indicate that ADHD is greater among the biological relatives of non-adopted ADHD children than adoptive relatives of adopted ADHD children and the risk for ADHD in adoptive relatives is similar to the risk in relatives of control children. Additionally, adoption studies suggest that the familial aggregation of ADHD is defined more by genetic factors rather than common environmental factors. Based on the largest longitudinal study to date on familial aggregation of ADHD, the closer was the relatedness of probands and their relatives the higher was the familial aggregation [20]. Consistently, among full siblings, the familial aggregation did not differ significantly by index person's sex. Moreover, it is expected that genetic factors play more important role in explaining familial aggregation than shared environmental factors [22], given that the familial aggregation is remarkably higher in MZ twins than in DZ twins and similar between DZ twins and nontwin full siblings.

Genetic linkage was the first genome-wide method applied to ADHD. This method looks through the genome to find evidence that a segment of DNA is transmitted with a disorder within families. According to the literature there is no clear-cut evidence about which chromosomal regions are linked to ADHD and so far none of the findings met genome-wide significance, suggesting that common DNA variants having a large effect on ADHD may not exist [23].

Genome-wide association studies (GWAS) scan the entire genome to detect common (frequency more than 1%) DNA variants that have very small etiologic effects. The early GWAS of ADHD did not discover any DNA variants that achieved genome-wide significance. However, recent studies have implicated contribution of some genes with relevant biological roles in ADHD. For example *USP6* is involved in regulation of dopamine levels in the synapses and regulates neurotransmitter homeostasis. Certain variants in *LINC00461* are associated with educational attainment and *ST3GAL3* and *MEF2C* are associated with ID and psychiatric disorders [24]. The GWAS analyses also showed that polygenic effects may also contribute to ADHD's heritability, where multiple common risk variants each with very small effects contribute to the development of the disease as a cumulative effect. The polygenic nature of ADHD was confirmed by evaluating polygenic risk scores and revealing that it predicted ADHD, in a dose-dependent manner. The discovery of a polygenic susceptibility to ADHD does not show which DNA variants comprise the susceptibility, however significant findings implicate that genes involved in biological processes such as synaptic plasticity, catecholamine metabolic processes, G-protein signaling pathways, cell adhesion, neuronal morphogenesis and neuron migration were over-represented in ADHD. Moreover, many of these genes show considerable interactions with genes identified as trending towards significance in GWAS [25].

It has been known for a long time that rare DNA variants can lead to ADHD. Because chromosomal deletions and duplications often delete or duplicate a large segment of DNA which may include part of a gene or even several genes, they often have clear implications for gene functioning. Several studies indicate that there is a greater burden of large, rare CNVs among ADHD patients compared with controls [26]. Despite the fact that deletions and duplications are equivalently over-represented in ADHD individuals, statistical significance for ADHD is observed only for duplications, as well as in schizophrenia and ASDs [27] Several well-known syndromes and chromosomal abnormalities may be associated with multiple medical and psychiatric problems along with ADHD. Among these are Klinefelter syndrome, Turner syndrome, 22q11 deletion syndrome, fragile-X syndrome, tuberous sclerosis, neurofibromatosis, Williams syndrome, as well as translocations involving *SLC9A9*, duplication of 7p15.2-15.3 and deletion of 15q13. It is noteworthy to mention that such larger chromosomal rearrangements show increased incidence of ADHD along with global developmental delay (GDD), intellectual disability (ID) and ASD [28]. Beside chromosomal abnormalities there is increasing evidence of single-gene contribution to ADHD, including inactivating mutation in *TPH2*, duplication of *CHRNA7* and pathogenic changes in *PARK2*, *FBXO33* and *RNF122* [29]. New technologies like next generation sequencing (NGS) and whole exome sequencing (WES) revealed several novel rare variants in candidate genes, among them *TBC1D9*, *DAGLA*, *QARS*, *CSMD2*, *TRPM2*, and *WDR83*, *NT5DC1*, *SEC23IP*, *PSD*, *ZCCHC4*, and *BDNF* [30].

It is clear that certain DNA variants increase the risk for ADHD. It is not common that only a single genetic alteration may cause ADHD in the absence of other DNA variants. At the same time it is clear that there are no common DNA variants that are necessary and sufficient causes of ADHD. GWAS show that a genetic susceptibility to ADHD encompasses of many common DNA variants, but yet we do not know exactly which variants or how many of them contribute to the polygenic nature. The heritability that cannot be explained by main effects of rare or common variants is likely due to gene-gene and gene-environment interactions.

The accumulating evidence for ADHD risk factors genes does not exclude the environmental etiological factors which likely work through epigenetic mechanisms, but these yet have barely been studied in ADHD. In the coming years, we can expect breakthroughs in the genetics of ADHD. Unraveling the genetics of ADHD will not be easy, but with rapid development of technologies and with wider application and better interpretation of whole exome and whole genome sequencing (WGS) data the knowledge and significance of various rare and common variants will increase dramatically. Such advances will enable us to understand the etiology of ADHD and set forth opportunities to diagnose and treat the disorder.

2.3 Biological basis

Attention problems manifested in ADHD are due to dysfunction of ventral catecholaminergic pathways projecting to prefrontal and frontal cortex. More than thirty structural and functional neuroimaging studies in ADHD brain have been reported. The main area in the brain implicating in ADHD is prefrontal cortex and its innervations of subcotrical regions such as caudate-putamen, nucleus accumbens, and amygdala. Reduced size of corpus callosum has been detected in some children with ADHD and typically larger corpus callosum in the human female brain may be protective against ADHD. Cerebellum has been implicated in cognition and emotion besides the well-known role in coordination and maintaining body posture, suggesting a possible role contributing to ADHD that is consistent with reports of disorders of fine motor movements in ADHD children. Hippocampus as an important site for memory is also can be considered as possible participant in pathogenesis of ADHD. Structural brain imaging could not confirm the structural abnormalities of hippocampus but functional imaging found reduced cerebral glucose metabolism in hippocampus in adolescents with ADHD [31].

2.4 Neurobiology

The neurotransmitter dopamine has been recognized to play a role in attention and cognition especially executive functioning and reward processing [32]. It is a key contributor to behavioral adaptation.

Dopamine transporter is the most important molecule in the regulation of dopamine signaling in most areas of the brain-is the main target of stimulants like Methylphenidate and also dexamphetamine-drugs for ADHD treatment. These drugs block the dopamine transporter and lead to an increase in dopamine concentration particularly in the parts of the basal ganglia that are highest in the expression of the transporter, the striatum [33]. Positron emission tomography (PET) shows that people with ADHD have more dopamine transporter activity compared with healthy controls [34]. Besides genetic studies reveal that disorders in dopamine signaling could occur due to alteration in dopamine receptors which also has to be seen by PET. Meta analyses have shown significant involvement of dopamine transporter protein (DAT) and its gene- *DAT1* gene 3'-regulatory region in a larger group of patients with ADHD suggested association of this set of genes with severity of symptoms in children with this disorder [35].

Norepinephrine signaling is related with dopamine system as norepinephrine is a downstream product of metabolism of dopamine. Innervation of the prefrontal cortex by norepinephrine pathways is very important to understand ADHD. Norepinephrine and dopamine signaling are linked in prefrontal cortex thus influencing each other in organizing prefrontal cortex performance in cognitive tasks [36]. The role of norepinephrine can be explained by the fact that

Methylphenidate and dexamphetamine inhibit the norepinephrine transporter together with DAT [36]. It is proved that altering norepinephrine signaling can improve ADHD symptoms but there is lack of evidence to link it with ADHD neurobiology [37].

Serotonin has been studied closely in animal models of ADHD. It was found that serotonin-potentiating agents can inhibit effects on motor hyperactivity [38]. Serotonin neurotransmission may modulate the severity of ADHD symptoms rather than being related to ADHD onset [39]. Other position means that it may be the comorbidity especially with conduct disorder, obsessive compulsive disorder and aggression and mood disorders rather than the core symptoms of ADHD which is influenced by serotonin [40]. Although serotonin receptor gene HTR1B and gene encoding the serotonin transporter (SLC6A4, 5-HTT, SERT) have been implicated in ADHD the effect of environment on ADHD symptoms may explain some of the observed inconsistency across studies especially the effect of stress on ADHD seems to be influences by genetic variation in the serotonin transporter gene [37]. In experimental models serotonin may be critically involved in mediating the behavior inhibiting effects of stimulants [41]. All these suggest that serotonin may play a role in pathogenesis in some circumstances but do not establish serotonin-enhancing drugs as useful treatment.

2.5 Main cognitive finding associated with ADHD

Cognitive impairments in a variety of domains have been found in ADHD as well as impairment in overall intellectual function. Deficit in executive function are common in children with ADHD. Executive functioning are the group of cognitive processes which are responsible for purposeful, goal-directed and problem solving behavior. A meta-analysis of children and adolescents with ADHD showed impairments in several aspects of executive functioning.

2.5.1 Intellectual function

Visuospatial abilities (block-design subtest) and general knowledge (vocabulary subtest) on the Wechsler Intelligence Scale for Children-III (WISC-III) have to be changed in children with ADHD compared with healthy controls. Children with predominantly inattention without hyperactivity have disorders of visuospatial abilities. In contrast, the ADHD group predominantly with hyperactivity have the same evidence in visuospatial abilities or vocabulary as their healthy teens [1].

2.5.2 Language

Language can be impaired in ADHD children. A meta-analysis of children with ADHD found impairments in verbal fluency especially in phenomic fluency compared with semantic fluency [42]. Sometimes in adolescents with ADHD the disorders with object naming also can be revealed [43].

2.5.3 Learning and memory

Working memory is considered to be the most central executive function. Working memory disorders are quite variable in ADHD children. Mainly working memory is impaired and becomes the core feature of ADHD with the strongest impairments reported for the spatial domain of working memory as opposed to the verbal or phonological domain [44]. Visuospatial working memory is provided predominantly by inferior and superior parietal areas together with dorsolateral prefrontal regions [45–48, 49], Cerebellum also can be activated during visuospatial working memory tasks [50, 51]. Learning disorders also can be seen in ADHD children. Children with learning disorders and ADHD have more severe learning problems than children who have only ADHD. Learning disorder and attention problems are on continuum, are interrelated and usually coexist [52]. Comorbidity with learning disorders is a modifying factor in the health related quality of life of children with ADHD [4]. It was found that 5% of children have ADHD without learning disorder, 5% have learning disorder without ADHD and 4% have both conditions. Boys are more likely those girls to have each diagnosis. In 2006 approximately 4.5 million school aged children have ever been diagnosed with ADHD and 4.6 million children with learning disorders [53, 54]. Thus ADHD associated learning and language disabilities are important comorbidities. Neurological assessment is recommended in children with learning disorder who fail to make academic progress despite appropriate educational intervention. The adolescents with ADHD experienced written expression impairment (17.2–22.4%) at a similar rate to reading impairment (17.0–24.3%) and at a slightly lower rate than mathematics impairment (24.7–36.3%) [4]. Dyslexia occurs in 5–10% of school children; it overlaps with ADHD and shows similar genetic characteristics but different brain localizations [4].

Another part of executive disorder is **impairment of response inhibition.** Response inhibition specifically is the ability to control oneself by suppressing or altering intended actions that are no longer required or appropriate. Thus normal response inhibition enables people to adapt properly to changes in the environment. Impaired response inhibition is central to theoretical models of ADHD [55]. According to Barkley [56] response inhibition is a central deficit of ADHD affecting top-down multiple executive functions including working memory, self-regulation, internalization of speech and reconstitution. A large community study showed that ADHD symptoms in children and adolescents are associated with worse response inhibition and slower response latency [57]. Response inhibition deficit in ADHD is proved by magnetic resonance imaging (MRI). Healthy children activate core network of brain regions involved in response inhibition including a frontal-striatal and frontal-parietal network. Children and adolescents with ADHD show decreased activation in frontal, medial and parietal regions during inhibition compared with healthy teens [58].

Willcut et al [59] found impairments in other domains of executive functioning like planning and vigilance in addition to response inhibition and working memory. They noted that while impairment in executive functioning are closely associated with ADHD such deficits do not explain all of the cognitive impairments observed in ADHD suggesting that executive dysfunction is only one part of the cognitive impairments associated with ADHD [1].

Another frequently described comorbidity is disorder of **cognitive flexibility**. It is clear that ADHD children are more likely to respond with overlearned and automatic responses when faced with problem-solving situations or context that demand the thoughtful formation of strategies and the flexible shifting of thought [60]. Barkley et al [60] suggested that **behavioral or verbal creativity** can be impaired in children with ADHD as a consequence of their poor verbal inhibition.

Decision making can be considered as important part of executive functioning. ADHD children and adolescents have specific decision making deficits. ADHD people have no impaired learning rate per se as it was suggested before [61]. ADHD individuals exhibit less comprehensive decision process and more frequent exploration activity compared with controls. This feature could occur due to impaired reward prediction processing in the medial prefrontal cortex which is considered as an integrative hub in the brain responsible for decision making and learning. The deficit in decision making in adolescents and adults was similar in severity to the deficits in attention in individuals with ADHD [62].

Reward sensitivity is an evolutionary important part of executive functioning. Rewards are accompanied by positive feeling and they reinforce reward linked behavior [37]. This process of reinforcing behavior forms the basic principle of learning [63]. Individuals with highly sensitive to rewards shows maladaptive behavior like risky behavior and addictions [37]. Theoretical model of ADHD consider altered reward sensitivity as a main cognitive mechanism [64], Children and adolescents with ADHD are performing risky and suboptimal decisions. ADHD population with impaired reward processing and impulsivity show increased activations in the anterior cingulated and anterior frontal cortex as well as in orbitofrontal cortex and nucleus accumbens [65]. Other studies in ADHD adolescents have reported less triatal activation during reward compared with healthy teens [66].

Specific motor deficits may be found in children with ADHD but like other measures of neuropsychological functioning, such difficulties are not specific predictors of the presence of ADHD [67]. Commonly difficulties can be seen in coordination. When both attention and coordination deficits co occur in conjunction with perceptual problems the term "deficit in attention, motor control and perception (DAMP)" can be applied [68]. The concept of DAMP is fairly controversial and the label is more widely used in Scandinavian countries than in UK or USA.

2.5.4 Treatment

The most important part of any intervention plan for a child with ADHD is the physical, behavioral and neuromotor/neuropsychological examination followed by oral and written information of parents, child, teacher about the type of problems the child exhibits and their possible etiology.

Special education- many children with ADHD need special educational measures. In order to acquire some academic skill some children will need individualized education lasting for several hours every day [69].

The two most commonly used behavioral interventions are:

1. Creating and maintaining a well structured environment to compensate for poor stimulus control

2. Parent training

It is very important to organize the school environment with minimal distractions and with seating that is somewhat isolated and close to the front of the classroom in front of the teacher. Common triggers that can easily distract child are instructional demand, withholding of a desired object or activity and withdrawal of parental attention.

Behavior therapy can be considered as the best method for treatment of ADHD children and youths regarding the improvement of behavior, self-control and self-esteem. It is recommended for parents of children younger than 12 years of age to start training in behavior therapy. For children less than 6 years of age it is better to start behavior therapy before prescribing ADHD medicine. Behavior therapy helps parents to learn skills and strategies to improve their children academic achievement at school, behavior at home and improve their social interaction. Although studying and practicing of behavioral therapy needs time and effort from parents the sequence benefit for the child and family could last for a long period of time.

Parent training in behavior management is also known as parent behavior therapy, behavioral parent training or just parent training. If possible, families should look for a therapist who focuses on training parents. Some therapists will have training or certification in a parent training program that has been proven to work in young children with ADHD.

The following are the main goals for therapist while working with parents:

- Parents need to know how to make positive reinforcement, how to construct and control child's behavior. Thus they need to acquire these skills and strategies.
- Parents need to be aware how to interact and communicate with their ADHD children
- Therapists needs to teach parents practical skill how to work with their child
- Therapist needs to meet with family members to observe the progress in their activity and to provide support
- Therapist needs to re-evaluate treatment strategy and method and in case if it is needed to change strategy plans.

3. What can parents expect?

It is recommended for parents to attend eight or more session with a therapist who can work with groups of parents or only with one family. It is necessary to work on a regular basis in order to monitor progress of parents and to change the working strategy in case if it needed. Parents' role in treatment planning and implementing is extremely crucial as they can have greatest influence on their child's behavior. There are many treatment options for therapist for working with ADHD children. Play therapy and talk therapy could be considered as one of the best treatment option. Talk therapy uses verbal communication between ADHD child and therapist in order to improve child's emotional state. Although behavioral therapy needs time and effort its effect could last for long period of time [70].

Successful treatment for ADHD means both behavior therapy and medication. For children 6 years of age and older, the American Academy of Pediatrics (AAP) recommends both behavior therapy and medication. For children under 6 years of age behavior therapy is recommended as the first line of treatment [71].

Medication should be start with one of the stimulants. Both d-amphetamine (10–40 mg/day given in 2–5 dosed with 3-hour intervals in order to last through the school day) and methylphenidate (20–80 mg/day given in the same fashion) have been shown to be effective for improvement of hyperactivity, concentration problems, learning disorders and other comorbidities. Both drugs have minimal side effects. "Long-acting," "slow-release" preparations of methylphenidate have also been shown to have good effects and they can sometimes be dosed (18–54 mg/day or 10–60 mg/day depending on preparation) only once daily. Relatively common side effects are loss of appetite, a tendency to increase the likelihood of tics and stereotypies, reduced mimicry and hallucinations. They can easily stop with drug discontinuation. There are some evidence that long-term methylphenidate treatment should be as effective as the combination of methylphenidate and behavioral therapy and considerably more effective than behavioral therapy alone [72]. Combination of methylphenidate and behavioral therapy is the best choice for improving both ADHD and ADHD plus depression and anxiety. Doctor should be careful for monitoring the child's height, drug dependency while treating the child with stimulants for long term period although they appear rare compared with tricyclic antidepressants.

The noradrenergic reuptake inhibitor atomoxetine has also been shown to have beneficial effects on ADHD as a second line treatment in children with ADHD. Although clinical effects appear to be less effective than with methylphenidate but the advantage if this medication is that it can be used only once daily and it is not stimulant [69].

Author details

Sophia Bakhtadze[1*], Tinatin Tkemeladze[2] and Tinatin Kutubidze[3]

1 Department of Paediatric Neurology, Tbilisi State Medical University, Tbilisi, Georgia

2 Department of Molecular and Medical Genetics, Tbilisi State Medical University, Tbilisi, Georgia

3 Department of Child and Adolescent Medicine, Tbilisi State Medical University, Tbilisi, Georgia

*Address all correspondence to: sophiabakhtadze@yahoo.com

References

[1] Hedges D et al. The Brain at Risk. Springer Nature Switzerland AG: Springer International Publisher; 2019

[2] Danielson ML, Bitsko RH, Ghandour RM, et al. Prevalence of parent-reported ADHD diagnosis and associated treatment among US children and adolescents, 2016. Journal of Clinical Child and Adolescent Psychology. 2018;**47**(2):199-212

[3] Thomas R et al. Prevalence of attention-deficit/hyperactivity disorder: A systematic review and meta-analysis. Pediatrics. 2015;**135**(4):e994-e1001

[4] Millichap G. Attention Deficit Hyperactivity Disorder Handbook: A Physician's Guide to ADHD. 2nd ed. New York: Springer-Verlag; 2010

[5] Still G. Some abnormal psychical conditions in children. Lancet. 1902;**1**: 1008-1012

[6] Stewart M. Hyperactive children. Scientific American. 1970;**222**:94-98

[7] Psychiatric Association (APA). Diagnostic American and Statistical Manual of Mental Disorders. 4th ed. Washington, DC: APA; 1994

[8] Psychiatric Association (APA). Diagnostic American and Statistical Manual of Mental Disorders. 5th ed. Washington, DC: APA; 2013

[9] Schab D, Trinh NH. Do artificial food colors promote hyperactivity in children with hyperactive syndromes? A meta-analysis of double-blind placebo-controlled trials. Journal of Developmental and Behavioral Pediatrics. 2004;**25**(6):423

[10] Krummel DA, Seligson FH, Guthrie HA. Hyperactivity: is candy causal? Critical Revue of Food Science and Nutrition. 1996;**36**(1-2):31

[11] Wolraich M, Wilson D, White J. The effect of sugar on behavior or cognition in children. A meta-analysis. JAMA. 1995;**274**(20):1617-1621

[12] Cortese S, Konofal E, Lecendreux M, Arnulf I, Mouren MC, Darra F, et al. Restless legs syndrome and attention-deficit/hyperactivity disorder: A review of the literature. Sleep. 2005;**28**(8):1007

[13] Arnold LE, Disilvestro RA, Bozzolo D, Bozzolo H, Crowl L, Fernandez S, et al. Zinc for attention-deficit/hyperactivity disorder: Placebo-controlled double-blind pilot trial alone and combined with amphetamine. Journal of Child and Adolescent Psychopharmacology. 2011;**21**:1-19

[14] Akhondzadeh S, Mohammadi MR, Khademi M. Zinc sulfate as an adjunct to methylphenidate for the treatment of attention deficit hyperactivity disorder in children: A double blind and randomized trial. BMC Psychiatry. 2004;**4**:9

[15] Ghanizadeh A, Berk M. Zinc for treating children and adolescents with attention-deficit hyperactivity disorder: A systematic review of randomized controlled clinical trials. European Journal of Clinical Nutrition. 2013;**67**:122-124

[16] Huang L, Wang Y, Zhang L, et al. Maternal smoking and attention-deficit/hyperactivity disorder in offspring: A meta-analysis. Pediatrician. 2018;**141**(1):piie20172465

[17] Hope Abel M, Ystrom E, et al. Maternal Iodine intake and offspring attention-deficit/hyperactivity disorder: Results for a large prospective cohort study. Nutrients. 2017;**9**(11):1239

[18] Gonzelli G, Carducci A, Llopis-Gonzalez A, Verani M,

Llopis-Morales A, Cioni L, et al. The association between lead and attention-deficit/hyperactivity disorder: A systematic review. Journal of Environmental Research and Public Health. 2019;**16**(3):piiE382

[19] Faraone S, Larsson H. Genetics of attention deficit hyperactivity disorder. Molecular Psychiatry. 2019;**24**(4): 562-575

[20] Chen Q, Brikell I, Lichtenstein P, Serlachius E, Kuja-Halkola R, Sandin S, et al. Familial aggregation of attention-deficit/hyperactivity disorder. Journal of Child Psychology and Psychiatry. 2017;**58**:231-239

[21] Larsson H, Lichtenstein P, Larsson JO.Genetic contributions to the development of ADHD subtypes from childhood to adolescence. Journal of the American Academy of Child and Adolescent Psychiatry. 2006;**45**:973-981

[22] Lee SH, Ripke S, Neale BM, Faraone SV, Purcell SM, Perlis RH, et al. Genetic relationship between five psychiatric disorders estimated from genome-wide SNPs. Nature Genetics. 2013;**45**:984-994

[23] Faraone SV, Mick E. Molecular genetics of attention deficit hyperactivity disorder. Psychiatry Clinics of North America. 2010;**33**:159-180

[24] Demontis D, Walters RK, Martin J, Mattheisen M, Als TD, Agerbo E, et al. Discovery of the first genome-wide significant risk loci for ADHD. Submitted for publication, bioRxiv. 2017;**14558**:1-43

[25] Groen-Blokhuis MM, Middeldorp CM, Kan KJ, Abdellaoui A, van Beijsterveldt CE, Ehli EA, et al. Attention-deficit/hyperactivity disorder polygenic risk scores predict attention problems in a population-based sample of children. Journal of the American Academy of Child and Adolescent Psychiatry. 2014;**53**:1123-1129 e6

[26] Yang L, Neale BM, Liu L, Lee SH, Wray NR, Ji N, et al. Psychiatric GWAS Consortium: ADHD Subgroup. Polygenic transmission and complex neuro developmental network for attention deficit hyperactivity disorder: genome-wide association study of both common and rare variants. American Journal of Medical Genetics and Biological Neuropsychiatric Genetics. 2013;**162B**(5):419-430

[27] Thapar A, Martin J, Mick E, Arias Vasquez A, Langley K, Scherer SW, et al. Psychiatric gene discoveries shape evidence on ADHD's biology. Molecular Psychiatry. 2015;**21**:1202-1207

[28] Lo-Castro A, D'Agati E, Curatolo P. ADHD and genetic syndromes. Brain & Development. 2011;**33**(6):456-461

[29] Jarick I, Volckmar AL, Putter C, Pechlivanis S, Nguyen TT, Dauvermann MR, et al. Genome-wide analysis of rare copy number variations reveals PARK2 as a candidate gene for attention-deficit/hyperactivity disorder. Molecular Psychiatry. 2012;**19**:115-121

[30] Faraone SV, Larsson H. Genetics of attention deficit hyperactivity disorder. Molecular Psychiatry. 2019;**24**:562-575

[31] Taylor E. People with Hyperactivity: Understanding and Managing Their Problems. London: Mac Keith Press; 2007

[32] Nieoullon A. Dopamine and the regulation of cognition and attention. Progress in Neurobiology. 2002;**67**(1):53-83

[33] Kuczenski R, Segal DS. Stimulant actions in rodents: Implications for attention-deficit/hyperactivity disorder treatment and potential substance abuse. Biological Psychiatry. 2005;**57**(11):1391-1396

[34] Fusar-Poli P, Rubia K, Rossi G, Sartori G, et al. Striatal dopamine transporter alterations in ADHD: pathophysiology or adaptation to psychostimulants? a meta-analysis. The American Journal of Psychiatry. 2012;**169**(3):264-272

[35] Bralten J, Franke B, Waldman I, et al. Candidate genetic pathways for attention-deficiti/hyperactivity disorder (ADHD) show association to hyperactive/impulsive symptoms in children with ADHD. Journal of American Academy of Child and Adolescent Psychiatry. 2013;**52**(11):1204-1212.e.l

[36] Arnsten AF, Pliszka SR. Catecholamine influences on prefrontal cortical function: relevance to treatment of attention deficit/hyperactivity disorder and related disorders. Pharmacology, Biochemistry, and Behavior. 2011;**99**(2):211-216

[37] Rohde LJ, Gerlach M, Buitelaar J. The World Federation of ADHD Guide. Santana, Sao Paulo: Artmed Editora LTDA; 2019

[38] Bishop C, Kamdar DP, Walker PD. Intrastiatal serotonin 5-HT2 receptors mediating dopamine D1-induced hyperlocomotion in 6-hydroxydopamine-lesioned rats. Synapse. 2003;**50**:164-170

[39] Bralten J, Franke B, Waldman I, Rommelse N, Hartman C, Asherson P, et al. Candidate genetic pathways for attention-deficit/hyperactivity disorder (ADHD) show association to hyperactive/impulsive symptoms in children with ADHD. Journal of American Academy of Child and Adolescent Psychiatry. 2013;**52**(11):1204-1212.e1

[40] Banerjee E, Nandagopal K. Does serotonin deficit mediate susceptibility to ADHD? Neurochemsitry International. 2015;**82**:52-68

[41] Gainetdinov RR, Wetsel WC, Jones SR, et al. Role of serotonin in the paradoxical calming effect of psychostimulants on hyperactivity. Science. 1999;**283**:397-401

[42] Walshaw P, Alloy L, Sabb F. Executive function in pediatric bipolar disorder and attention-deficit hyperactivity disorder: In search of distinct phenotypic profiles. Neuropsychological Reviews. 2010;**20**:103-120

[43] Rucklidge J, Tannock R. Neuro-psychological profiles of adolescents with ADHD: Effect of reading difficulties and gender. Journal of Child Psychology and Psychiatry. 2002;**43**:988-1003

[44] Martinussen R, Hayden J, Hogg-Johnson S, Tannock R. A meta-anaylsis of working memory impairements in children with attention-deficit/hyperactivity disorder. Journal of American Child and Adolescent Psychiatry. 2005;**44**(4):377-384

[45] Awh E, Jonides J. Overlapping mechanisms of attention and spatial working memory. Trend in Cognitive Sceince. 2001;**5**(3):119-126

[46] Smith E, Jonides J, Koeppe R. Dissociating verbal and spatial working memory using PET. Cerebral Cortex. 1996;**6**(1):11-20

[47] Thomas K, King S, Franzen P, Welsh T, Berkowitz A, Noll D, et al. A Developmental functional MRI study of spatial working memory. NeuroImage. 1999;**10**(3 Pt):327-338

[48] Zurowski B, Gostomzyk J, Gron G, Weller R, Schirrmeister H, Neumeier B, et al. Dissociating a common working memory network from different neural substrates of phonological and spatial stimulus processing. NeuroImage. 2002;**15**(1):45-57

[49] Booth J, Burman D, Meyer J, Lei Z, Trommer B, Davenport N, et al. Larger deficits in brain networks for response inhibition than for visual selective attention in attention-deficit hyperactivity disorder (ADHD). Journal of Child Psychology and Psychiatry. 2005;**46**(1):94-111

[50] Leung H, Oh H, Ferri J, Yi Y. Load response functions in the human spatial working memory circuit during location memory updating. NeuroImage. 2007;**35**(1):368-377

[51] Middleton F, Strick P. Basal ganglia and cerebellar loops: motor and cognitive circuits. Brain Research Reviews. 2000;**31**(2-3):236-250

[52] Kasper L, Alderson R, Hudec K. Moderators of working memory deficits in children with attention-deficit/hyperactivity disorder (ADHD): A meta-analytic review. Clinical Psychology Review. 2012;**32**:605-617

[53] Mayes S, Calhoun S, Crowel E. Learning disabilities and ADHD: overlapping spectrum disorders. Journal of Learning Disabilities. 2000;**33**: 417-424

[54] Bloom B, Cohen R. Summary health statistics for US children: National health Interview Survey. National Center for Health Statistics. Vital and Health Statistics. 2007;**10**(234)

[55] Molitor S, Joshua M, et al. The written expression abilities of adolescents with Attention-Deficit/Hyperactivity Disorder. Research in Developmental Disabilities. 2016;**51-52**:49-59

[56] Oosterlaan J, Logan G, Sergeant J. Response inhibition in AD/HD, CD, comorbid AD/HD+CD, anxious, and control children: A meta-analysis of studies with stop task. Journal of Child Psychology and Psychiatry. 1998;**39**(3):411-425

[57] Barkley R. Behavioral inhibition, sustained attention, and executive functions: constructing a unifying theory of ADHD. Psychological Bulletin. 1997;**121**(1):7-12

[58] Crosbie J, Arnold P, Paterson A, Swanson J, Dupuis A, Li X, et al. Response inhibition and ADHD traits: correlates and heritability in a community sample. Journal of Abnormal Child Psychology. 2013;**41**(3):497-507

[59] Hart H, Radua J, Nakao T, Mataix-Cols D, Rubia K. Meta anaylisis of functional magnetic resonance imaging studies of inhibition and attention in attention-deficit/hyperactivity disorder: exploring task-specific, stimulant medication and age effect. JAMA Psychiatry. 2013;**70**(2):185-198

[60] Willcut E, Doyle A, Nigg J, Faraone S, Pennington B. Validity of the executive function theory of attention – deficit/hyperactivity disorder: A meta-analytic review. Biological Psychiatry. 2005;**57**:1336-1346

[61] Barkley R. Attention -Deficit Hyperactivity Disorder. A handbook for diagnosis and treatment. 3rd ed. New York, London: The Guilford press; 2006

[62] Tobias U, Hauser P, Iannaccone M, et al. Role of the medial prefrontal cortex in impaired decision making in juvenile attention-deficit/hyperactivity disorder. JAMA Psychiatry. 2014;**71**(10):1165-1173. DOI: 10.1001/jamapsychiatry.2014;1093

[63] Blaukopf C, DiGirolamo G. Reward, context and human behavior. The Scientific World Journal. 2007;7:626-640

[64] Luman M, Tripp G, Scheres A. Identifying the neurobiology of altered reinforcement sensitivity in ADHD:

a review and research agenda. Neuroscience and Behavior Review. 2010;**34**(5):744-754

[65] Plichta M, Scheres A. Ventral-striatal responsiveness during reward anticipation in ADHD and its relation to trait impulsivity in the healthy population: A meta-analysis review of the fMRI literature. Neuroscience and Biobehavioral Reviews. 2014;**38**:125-134

[66] Paloyelis Y, Mehta M, Faraone S, Asherson P, Kuntsi J. Striatal sensitivity during reward processing in attention-deficit/hyperactivity disorder. Journal of American Academy of Child and Adolescent Psychiatry. 2012;**51**(7):722-732.e.9

[67] Mowinckel A, Lund Pedersen M, Eilertsen E, Biele G. A meta-analysis of decision making and attention in adults with ADHD. Journal of Attention Disorders. 2015;**19**:355-367

[68] Kadesjo B, Gillberg C. Attention deficits and clumsiness in Swedish 7-year old children. Developmental Medicine and Child Neurology. 1988;**40**: 796-804

[69] Aicardi J. Diseases of the Nervous System in Childhood. 3rd ed. London: Mac Keith Press; 2009

[70] Centers for Disease Control and Prevention. 2019. Available from: https://www.cdc.gov/ncbddd/adhd/behavior-therapy.html

[71] Wolraich M, Hagan J, et al. Clinical practice guideline for the diagnosis, evaluation and treatment of attention-deficit/hyperactivity disorder in children and adolescents. American Academy of Paediatrics. 2019;144(4)e20192528. DOI: 10.1542/peds.2019-2528. Available from: www.aappublications.org/news

[72] Arnold L, Abikoff H, Cantwell D, et al. National Institute of Mental Health Collaborative Multimodal Treatment Study of Children with ADHD (the MTA). Design challenges and choices. Archives of General Psychiatry. 1997;**54**: 865-870

Chapter 7

Suicide Attempts from Height and Injury Patterns: An Analysis of 64 Cases

Stamatios A. Papadakis, Dimitrios Pallis, Spyridon Galanakos, Konstantinos Kateros, Grigorios Leon, George Machairas and George Sapkas

Abstract

Falls from height are a common cause of death and disability. A majority of free falls occur accidentally and only a minority result from suicidal behaviour. Adolescents in many countries show high rates of suicide attempts and their repetition is a common feature. We describe the demographic characteristics of these patients, their psychiatric diagnosis at the time of the attempt and the injury patterns. We present 64 patients who sustained injuries as a result of a fall from height. They were divided into those without mental disorders (n = 32, group I) and those with mental disorders (n = 32, group II). The mean height from which the fall occurred was 5.4 m (range, 3–25 m). The mean injury severity score was 19 (range, 6–58) for all fall victims. Upper extremity fractures were found in 37 patients, while pelvic and lower extremity fractures were found in 198 cases. Spinal fractures were noted in 32 patients. Head injuries were revealed by CT scan in 16 patients. Patients following a suicidal high fall mostly had lower limb fractures, pelvis fractures, spinal fractures and head injuries.

Keywords: attempted suicide, spinal cord injury (SCI), limb and spinal fractures

1. Introduction

Falls from height cause significant death and disability worldwide, due to the severe traumatic load inflicted on their victims [1–4]. According to the WHO, the yearly mortality due to suicide worldwide is approximately 800,000 people. What is more important is the fact that it affects mainly young people, suicide being the primary cause of death in the age group of 25–34 years [5]. The mean incidence of suicides across Europe in 2013 was of 11.7 deaths per 100,000 people. Low rates, under 8 deaths per 100,000 inhabitants were recorded in Italy, Malta, Cyprus and the United Kingdom. The lowest incidence was observed in Greece (4.8 cases per 100,000 people) [6]. There was a lag between the beginning of the economic crisis in Europe, and the manifestation of its effects on the Greek population. These became evident 3 or 4 years later, in the form of a reduction of household income and an increase in the rate of unemployment [7–9].

Causes for this mechanism of injury include both accidental falls and deliberate suicide attempts [10]. The latter constitutes a major social problem, with implications for the entire society, but particularly for the affected family. The psychological profile of people committing suicide is complex and unique for each case [11]. Thus, identifying contributing factors that may lead to suicide and establishing strategies for the safekeeping of mental health in communities are of paramount importance.

The type of injuries incurred after a fall constitute a unique pattern of blunt trauma, with a characteristic distribution of damage (multiple lesions in a variety of body areas) [1, 12, 13]. The most common form of trauma are fractures, followed by other areas, such as the head, the thorax, the abdomen as well as the retroperitoneum, being injured by varied degrees [14]. The quantity and the quality of traumatic load absorbed depend on factors like the height from which the fall occurred, the part of the patient's body that had the first impact, the surface where the impact occurred and the victim's age, taking into account the associated comorbidity, and reduced physiologic reserve that advanced age implies [15–17]. Anticipation and prediction of the exact areas being injured are not possible, because of the multitude of factors involved, and the exact unpredictability of the fall's kinematic [18, 19].

As aforementioned, one can infer that the differential diagnosis of falls from height from other types of blunt trauma (for example, a road-traffic-collision with expulsion of the occupants from the vehicle) is difficult. Thus, a high index of suspicion must be maintained concerning the initial cause in cases of polytrauma in victims with an unknown history [20]. An array of papers have dealt with injury-related deaths in general, while others have differentiated between unintentional and intentional injury-related deaths [21–24]. There are few studies though that have looked into patients with intentional or unintentional injuries, due to a fall from height, at a single centre [13, 25].

As noted by research in the past, self-harm due to a fall is a rare phenomenon, being responsible for 4–7% of deaths from suicide in the developed world [26–29]. On the other hand, studies have shown that psychiatric disorders are a frequent finding in patients suffering trauma [30–32]. Nevertheless, the connection between mental disorders and specific injury patterns has not been adequately described. Furthermore, the elucidation of patterns of injury incurred after accidental falls and after intentional suicide jumps, might be of help to forensic pathologists while investigating the circumstances of a death after a fall from height.

2. Materials and methods

From January 1990 to October 2012, 64 patients (15 males and 49 females) were studied as a result of falls from height. Fall from height $\geq$ 3 m is classified as high energy trauma in accordance to ATLS guidelines [33]. The mean patient age was 34 years (range 16–65 years). These 64 cases comprised our series and, for comparison, were divided into those without mental disorders (n = 32, group I) and those with mental disorders (n = 32, group II). Group II cases were further stratified according to their psychiatric diagnosis.

The principles of Advanced Trauma Life Support were followed in the management of all patients. Basic laboratory screening included haemoglobin level, prothrombin time, type and crossmatch and arterial blood gas analysis. Data collected included age, gender, associated trauma, injury severity score (ISS), Glasgow Coma

Scale (GCS), haemodynamic status (systolic blood pressure less than 90 mm Hg on arrival), length of intensive care unit (ICU) and hospital stay.

Also, the following trauma variables were analysed: specific intracranial injuries (epidural, subdural and subarachnoid haemorrhage and brain contusion), spinal injuries (cervical, thoracic and lumbar spine), thoracic injuries, specific intra-abdominal injuries (liver, spleen, kidney, and hollow viscus) and specific fractures (pelvis, femur and tibia). The diagnosis of mental disorder was ascertained by psychiatric specialists using the criteria of the International Classification of Disease Ninth Version Clinical Modification (ICD-9CM).

3. Results

The mean height of fall was 5.4 m (range, 3–25 m). The patients were separated in two groups: group I, without mental disorders (n = 32), and group II, with mental disorders (n = 32). The demographic data, including age, gender, height of fall, ISS, GCS, initial shock (SBP <90 mm Hg), hospital stay (days), ICU stay (days) and deaths are summarized in **Table 1**. The mean hospital stay was 29 days (range 19–45) and the mean ICU stay was 9 (range, 5–13) (**Table 1**).

Concerning their background psychiatric disorder in group II, the diagnosis was schizophrenia in 32 patients, depression in 12, drugs or alcohol abuse in 3, personality disorder in one, manic depression in one, another psychiatric condition in one and 14 cases without a specific diagnosis (generally marital or work related).

Data	Patients
Age	35 (18–65)
Gender (M:F)	15:49
ISS	20 (12–58)
GCS	9 (6–13)
Haemodynamic status-SBP <90 mmHg	34
Hospital stay (days)	29 (19–45)
ICU stay (days)	9 (5–13)
Deaths	13

Table 1.
Comparisons of demographic data of patients with suicide attempts from height.

4. Socioeconomic factors

Patients due to suicide attempts from height comprised of 15 males and 49 females with a mean of age 35 years (range: 18–65 years). Of those, 16 were single, 14 were married and 2 were divorced. Thirty-three patients were employed, 6 were housewives, 7 were unemployed, 3 were students/pupils and 15 had various occupations. As far as religion was concerned, 48 were Christian Orthodox, one Roman Catholic, one Jewish, one Muslim and 13 of other religions.

Regarding their family status: 20 had children, 6 had only their parents, 3 had only their spouse, 2 had a step family, 2 had parents who were divorced, 6 had parents and/or siblings, one had both parents and children and 24 had no family at all.

5. Mechanism of fall, severity of injuries and associated lesions

The falls had occurred from a roof or balcony in 39 cases, from a window in 12, from a bridge in 7 and inside the house in 6. The mean injury severity score (ISS) was 20 (range 12–58) for all victims of fall. Sixteen patients arrived at the emergency department in shock. The most common body region having sustained severe trauma were the fractured extremities and/or spine, followed by the chest, the head and the abdomen for both groups (**Table 2**).

Head injuries were revealed by CT scan in 16 patients. The mean GCS was 9 (range 6–13) for both groups. The most common intracranial injury was brain contusion and subarachnoid haemorrhage, followed by subdural hematoma and epidural hematoma. The incidence of subarachnoid haemorrhage in the suicide group was significantly higher than in the accidental group.

Associated abdominal injuries were present in 4 patients. The most common injury was liver laceration, followed by kidney and spleen laceration. One died with an operative finding of a large central retroperitoneal haematoma due to a vena cava rupture. In the remaining 3 patients, ultrasonography showed minimal intraperitoneal blood and these patients were not operated on. Thoracic injuries were present in 32 patients. The most common of these were rib fractures—26 cases. Twelve of these patients had a haemopneumothorax and 6 had a sternum fracture. Conservative treatment with assisted ventilation was necessary in these cases (**Table 3**).

Upper extremity fractures were found in 37 patients, while pelvic and lower extremity fractures were found in 198 cases. Spinal fractures were noted in 32 patients. As far as the level of injury was concerned, in 16 cases, it was in the lumbar level, in 9 cases in the cervical, in 5 cases in thoracic and in 2 cases the sacral vertebrae were concerned. Regarding the neurologic deficit, in 23 cases, the injury was incomplete (14 with ASIA C and 9 with ASIA D), and in 9 cases, it was complete (4 with ASIA A and 5 with ASIA B). Further details with our data of 32 patients with spinal cord injury as a result of deliberate self-harm have been published previously [34]. It seems that the neurological complications of spinal injuries were correlated with the increase of the height from which the fall occurred.

Patients with psychiatric disorders were more frequently shocked on arrival at the emergency department than those in the accidental group, the most common reason for death being head injury. Fatalities were more common when patients fell from greater heights (over 4 m), or when their head hit a hard surface, such as concrete.

Fall from	**Patients**
Roof/balcony	39
Window	12
Bridge	7
Inside the house	6
Associated injuries	
Abdominal trauma	4
Thoracic trauma	32
Head injuries	16
Extremity fractures	199
Spinal fractures	32

Table 2.
Location where the fall occurred and associated injuries.

	Patients
Skull, thorax and upper extremities	
Skull	16 (25%)
Shoulder	4 (6.2%)
Scapula	6 (9.3%)
Sternum	6 (9.3%)
Ribs	26 (40.6%)
Humerus	8 (12.5%)
Elbow joint	8 (12.5%)
Distal radius	7 (10.9%)
Hand	4 (6.2%)
Spinal fractures	32 (50%)
Pelvis	27 (42.1%)
Lower extremities	
Acetabulum	9 (14%)
Femoral neck	38 (59.3%)
Femur	18 (28.1%)
Knee joint	17 (26.5%)
Tibia	19 (29.6%)
Ankle joint	36 (56.2%)
Calcaneum	34 (53.1%)

Table 3.
The distribution of fractures in percentage across body region for the two groups of patients.

The final causes of inpatients' death were: head injury in 8 cases, multiple organ failure in 3 cases, pneumonia in one case and cardiac complications in another one. The majority of patients who died of organ failure had sustained significant head injury. In one case, death occurred after a second suicide attempt 2 years later.

6. Medical management—outcome

Each patient underwent a psychiatric evaluation by a consulting psychiatrist as soon as his condition and cooperation permitted. The assessment comprised of an interview. Regarding the type of treatment for the spinal fracture—dislocations, instrumentation devices included titanium rods, transpedicular screws, sacral bars and bone grafting in all patients. No new suicide attempt was recorded during the hospital stay.

All patients were discharged from hospital approximately 6–8 weeks after the operation with a custom-made thermoplastic thoracolumbar or lumbosacral orthosis for another 8 weeks and instructions for physical therapy and rehabilitation programs. The mean follow-up was 6 years (12 months to 10 years range). At follow-up, 27 patients were available for evaluation due to the death of 5 patients, 1–3 years post initial injury, because of suicide in one case (patient 7 of group II) and medical complications in 4 cases [renal failure in 3 cases (patients 8, 14 and 30 in group II) and pneumonia in one (patient 21)]. In the remaining patients, new unsuccessful attempts were recorded in 2 cases (7%) due to psychiatric disorders, 1–3 years after the first attempt (patients 10 and 24). All survivors received psychiatric follow-up. The overall mortality was significantly higher in those patients who fell from more than 10 m.

7. Discussion

Suicides and suicide attempts constitute a major concern for public health services, with implications for both families and society [35]. Trauma incurred due to falls from height poses a great burden on health services due to its severity. This is particularly important if we take into account the fact that this is a largely preventable mechanism of injury. Prior knowledge of the possible traumatic patterns incurred after a fall from height can prove helpful in the initial evaluation of this group of patients. From an epidemiologic point of view, trauma due to falls may occur across all age groups, but it is the two extremes, the very young and elderly, which are particularly susceptible to it [36].

In this study, we have considered two groups of patients. Group I represented patients with no mental disorders and group II with mental disorders. It is quite difficult to identify someone who is prone to committing suicide. In addition, the observed number of suicides and suicide attempts being committed at a younger age (i.e. adolescence) has been a cause of concern worldwide and particularly in Europe [37]. The male-female ratio of suicide attempts varies across age groups. Thus, in the younger age group (15–24 years old), it is 1:1.9; and in the middle age group (45–54 years old) it is 1:1.7. This ratio further decreases for those older than 55 years to 1:1.4 [38]. In this study, the male-female ratio was 1:3. The female sex was associated with an increased likelihood of death due to a higher amount of energy involved in their attempted fall.

According to other studies [39, 40], young males tend to repeat suicide attempts more frequently than females and the methods used by them lead to an increased mortality. A suicide attempt in the past is a red flag for a possible attempt in the future; so, there is a strong correlation between suicide attempts and deaths from suicide both regionally and nationally, and particularly in young males [41]. Also, there is a strong correlation between repeated attempts and completed suicide, especially in the group of males who have used a violent method [42, 43].

The study by Dickson et al. had the aim of establishing a correlation between mortality and various factors, such as the patients' injury severity score (ISS), the height from which the fall took place, the patient's intention and the body regions that were injured. In addition, the height of the fall strongly correlated with the patient's ISS and was an important predictor of mortality [44]. Head and/or chest injuries, if due to a fall from height, were strongly associated with an increased incidence of death. According to the authors, this mechanism of injury should be a triage priority when tasking ambulances. In addition, the best way of treating these injuries is their prevention. No other significant predictors of mortality were found in this study.

In the case series by Kent and Pearce, 282 suicide attempts were studied, 13 of which were completed. Of those, 8 happened at home, all patients were older than 49 years; and in 7 out of 8 deaths, ladders were implicated [45]. The retrospective study by Petratos et al. analysed in detail the musculoskeletal traumatic pattern resulting from falls from height, and focused particularly on the correlation between specific fracture patterns and the height from which the fall happened, as well as on the causation of the fall (suicide attempt vs. accident). According to their findings, with an increase in the height from which the fall occurred, the frequency of limb, thoracic and pelvic fractures also increased. Such a correlation was not evident for head injuries. Nevertheless, the anatomical regions having sustained fractures (including the cranium) varied in accordance with the height of the fall. Thus, we can infer a mechanism of injury that is varying proportionately to the height of the fall. There was no significant difference between the patients who attempted suicide and those who fell by accident as far as the number of fractures incurred or the regions having been injured were concerned. Nevertheless, with regard to our results that have been published previously, patients who attempted suicide had a significantly greater number of bilateral lower limb fractures than their accidental fall counterpart. In addition, logistic regression analysis shows a significant correlation between the cause of the fall and the presence of lower limb fractures. According to the authors, further research is necessary in order to establish a correlation between incurred traumatic pattern, the height of the fall and the patient's intention [46].

Choi et al. in his recent study attempted to differentiate the characteristics of traumatic pattern between intentional and non-intentional falls [47]. In addition, he attempted to determine prognostic factors for suicide attempt-related injury and promote adequate measures for the prevention and management of such injuries. In this study, 8992 patients with an accidental fall (non-intentional group) and 144 patients who committed a suicide attempt (intentional group) were included. Falls from a height greater than 4 metres were more frequently encountered in the intentional group. Death prior to patient's arrival in the accident and emergency department occurred in 54.9% of the cases of suicide attempt. Patients within the intentional group, having sustained increased traumatic load, had fallen from higher, were older and were more likely to be of lower educational level (high-school graduates, instead of college). Due to the fact that injuries sustained after an intentional fall were more likely to have a reserved outcome, the authors highlighted the importance of prevention. Such measures include telephone support and counselling lines, the installation of signs advising against suicide in high risk areas for an intentional fall, such as bridges, along with suggestions for government-coordinated programs aiming for the education of the public and the improvement of social conditions generally and the support of the community and family in particular.

The reasons behind a suicide attempt are multifactorial, hard to quantify and unique in every case. Nevertheless, the study of multiple suicide attempts puts into evidence some risk factors that would lead to such a decision. These are common across all age groups and include: the presence of mental illness, either currently or in the past, a history of alcohol or drug dependence, as well as the presence of depression [10]. Epidemiologically, one out of five persons who have attempted suicide will try once more within a year, and 10% of them will succeed in the end. Drug ingestion is the most common mechanism for a suicide attempt. Violent mechanisms such as hanging, falls from height and use of weapons are not common [48]. The persons who have attempted suicide by falling from height usually become polytrauma patients. The types of injuries incurred are two: deceleration injuries due to inertial phenomena, usually at viscera with vascular pedicles, and direct impact injuries [49].

The severity of fractures incurred will depend on factors like the area over which the impact is applied [50]. The smaller the area of spread of the impact, the greater the local load. Therefore, patients landing on their legs tend to suffer more severe injuries than those who have landed on their flanks, or prone, or supine [51]. Patients due to accidental falls mostly suffered spinal fractures and upper extremities fractures in an attempt to protect themselves. Patients due to suicidal high falls attempts suffered mostly of lower limb fractures, pelvis, spinal fractures and head injuries. Distal radius and hand was the most common affected region in upper extremities in patients with non-intentional falls, in an attempt to protect mainly the head and grab something stable to prevent further fall. In patients with intentional falls, kinetic energy is absorbed mainly by the lower limbs, pelvis, spine and head, leading to characteristic fracture patterns [52]. The most common cause for death is head injury [51, 53, 54] and this is accordance to our results. Turk and Tsokos reviewed 68 medicolegal autopsy cases (22 females, 46 males, age range 13–89 years) of fatal falls from height from 1997 to 2001 [55]. The cause of instant death was head trauma in 24 (35%), internal blood loss in 9 (13%) and polytrauma in 30 (44%) cases. Other causes of death, when the individuals survived the trauma for a longer period, included septic multiple organ dysfunction syndrome and pulmonary embolism. In general, suicides were from greater heights than accidents (mean height 22.7 m for suicides and 10.8 m for accidents, respectively). Strikingly, severe head injuries predominantly occurred in falls from heights below 10 m (84%) and above 25 m (90%). Head trauma was the cause of death in 11 of the 19 cases that were from 9 m or less (58%). Of all cases, 51 (75%) died within a few minutes. A survival time of several hours up to 1 day was observed in 8 cases. Nine patients survived for several days (up to 16 days). Five of them fell from heights below 10 m. Patients with intentional fall from height have a higher early mortality than patients due to accidental fall from height [56].

The easiest way to underline the suspicion that the mode is suicide is if a suicide note is found at the jumping site; this is, however, closer to being the exception than the rule. Analysing the distance of the body from the site of descent may sometimes also help us determine the manner of death. The distance of the body from the site of descent includes the falling height and the horizontal distance. The falling height in suicide was statistically higher than that in accident [57, 58]. For similar heights, Wischhusen et al. have demonstrated that in passive falls, the horizontal distance is usually farther than jumps [59]. From a mechanical point of view, during a fall from height, potential (dynamic) energy is converted into kinetic and this leads to fractures upon impact. Another important factor of the severity of injuries is the height of fall, as the kinetic energy is increasing due to acceleration during the fall and is maximum at the time of impact [60]. In suicide falls, kinetic energy is absorbed mainly by the lower limbs, pelvis and spine, leading to characteristic fracture patterns. In accidental falls, patients most probably extend their arms and flex their hips, which lead to a damping effect that protects the spine [61]. Hence, the most important determinant of survival after a free fall is the position of the body at the time of impact [49]. There were only 3 patients (cases 1, 22 and 31) in group II who have sustained solely upper extremity fractures. The most common body position at the time of impact is with the patient standing and landing with the lower extremities first. This usually leads to calcaneal or pilon fractures, as well as thoracolumbar fractures. If the impact takes place with the patient seated, then higher thoracic or cervical injuries are more likely to happen, which are associated with a higher rate of mortality. Finally, an unpredictable fracture pattern takes place when the victim suffers multiple secondary impacts, in various postures, after bouncing from the primary impact. The amount of injury incurred will depend on the rate of dissipation and absorption of energy, through the patient's body.

According to the paper by Teh et al., there is a difference to the traumatic pattern incurred by jumpers compared to fallers [13]. Namely, the jumpers tend to impact their dominant lower limb first, as well as sustaining right sided thoracic injuries in the process. We did not confirm the above-mentioned findings in our study. The severity of spinal cord injuries was more important in the suicide than the accidental group [52]. This was in accordance with studies performed in the past, which also showed the early neurologic involvement in such cases. As far as prognosis of spinal cord injury is concerned, complete injuries will be unaltered both in level and extent in a year's time. On the other hand, incomplete injuries may show signs of improvement for a period of 2 years after the impact [62]. Our results regarding prognosis for ambulation in ASIA A patients and for functionality in ASIA C patients are in accordance with current knowledge [63].

Anderson et al. performed a retrospective study, regarding the rehabilitation outcome of patients with spinal cord injury, as a result of deliberate self-harm (DSH) [29]. According to them, spinal fractures in the DSH group were mainly the result of falls from height. Underlying causes were revealed, such as psychiatric disorders and substance abuse, necessitating formal psychiatric review. There was no difference in short-term rehabilitation results between the DSH and accidental spinal cord injury group. In addition, DSH seemed to impact the length of stay only in patients with a spinal fracture, but without cord injury.

According to the literature, there are three studies on the subject of acute spinal cord injury following a suicide attempt that stand apart. The first is by Stanford et al. In his paper, 56 cases were followed over a period of 30 years (1970–2000). Fifty five cases were due to a fall from height and one open injury, through the use of a gun. Follow-up of 8 years on average was available for 47 cases (84%). The vertebral levels most frequently injured were C5 and L1. About 23 patients suffered from a complete spinal cord injury and 32 had a severe traumatic load (ISS > 15). The psychiatric background of these patients included personality disorder in 27, schizophrenia in 16, depression in 14 and substance abuse/dependence in 20. Of these patients, 4 were successful in subsequent suicide attempts [28].

The following two studies on this subject are from the UK [26] and Denmark [27]. Both of those are observational and retrospective, with a long follow-up. According to the latter, there is an increasing incidence of suicide attempts and associated spinal cord injury from 1965 to 1987. Approximately one third of the patients who attempted suicide suffered from schizophrenia. According to other papers [64, 65], schizophrenia is strongly correlated with falls from height (from bridges in particular). There were 7 patients in our study who have sustained a fall from a bridge. Damage control surgery principles are followed initially for the treatment of life-threatening injuries and for both limb and spinal trauma [66]. The primary goals of fracture fixation are timely mobilization and safe transfer to psychiatric services. Conservative treatment measures are not usually recommended for this group of patients.

Our findings are in accordance with relevant bibliography [67, 68], regarding the psychiatric background of patients who attempt suicide by falling from height. The spectrum of conditions encountered encompasses bipolar disorder, substance dependence and abuse, personality disorder and schizophrenia.

From an epidemiological point of view, schizophrenia is encountered in 5–10% of cases of suicide attempt. These patients may have well planned their suicide or even suffered from an active self-harm ideation. From the above-mentioned, we gather that management of these patients from a trauma point of view must take into consideration their psychiatric needs. The latter may cause significant disturbance in the delivery of medical care [69]. Most of the patients in this study had a positive response following adequate psychiatric intervention. Hence, we gather that prevention and early identification of persons at risk for a suicide attempt with the use of appropriate screening tools by health care professionals are invaluable.

Education of medical and nursing staff regarding the demands and particularities of care of this population, suffering from both spinal cord injury and psychiatric disorders, cannot be overemphasized. Regular follow-up with multidisciplinary team input and future research are necessary for the provision of high-quality care to this population.

8. Conclusions

According to the literature, it has been difficult to obtain comparable international data on suicide attempts, owing to disparities in definitions, survey designs and study methods, because the combination of free falls and mental disorders produces a unique group of patients. It has been our experience that psychiatric conditions, and especially the suicidal risk, should be evaluated and treated as early as possible during the orthopaedic or surgical hospitalization. Management requires both psychopharmacological therapy and psychotherapy. It has to be directed towards the achievement of symptomatic relief and, if possible, towards the remission of the primary psychiatric disorder.

The management of these patients in the orthopaedic or surgical ward is difficult, because of restlessness, non-cooperation of the patient and the problem of staff inexperienced in handling the psychiatric patient. When prolonged orthopaedic and rehabilitation management are necessary, it is suggested that the patient be transferred to a psychiatric hospital while continuing the necessary orthopaedic treatment. The outcome data provide critical information concerning those individuals who have attempted suicide and suggests future methods for the identification of suicidal factors.

Conflicts of interest

The authors declare that they have no conflicts of interest.

Author details

Stamatios A. Papadakis[1]*, Dimitrios Pallis[1], Spyridon Galanakos[1], Konstantinos Kateros[2], Grigorios Leon[3], George Machairas[1] and George Sapkas[4]

1 Department of Orthopaedics, KAT General Hospital of Attica, Athens, Greece

2 Department of Orthopaedics, "G. Gennimatas" General Hospital, Athens, Greece

3 Private Forensic Pathology Practice, Athens, Greece

4 Department of Orthopaedics, Metropolitan Hospital, Athens, Greece

*Address all correspondence to: snapmd@gmail.com

References

[1] World Health Organization Preventing Suicide: A Global Imperative. Geneva, Switzerland: World Health Organization; 2014

[2] Eurostat. Causes of deaths statistics. Retrieved from: http://ec.europa.eu/eurostat/statisticsexplained/index.php/Causes_of_death_statistics [Last accessed: 27 October 2016]

[3] Kentikelenis A, Karanikolos M, Reeves A, McKee M, Stuckler D. Greece's health crisis: From austerity to denialism. Lancet. 2014;**383**:748-753

[4] Economou M, Madianos M, Peppou LE, Theleritis C, Patelakis A, Stefanis C. Suicidal ideation and reported suicide attempts in Greece during the economic crisis. World Psychiatry. 2013;**12**:53-59

[5] Kontaxakis V, Papaslanis T, Havaki-Kontaxaki B, Tsouvelas G, Giotakos O, Papadimitriou G. Suicide in Greece: 2001-2011. Psychiatriki. 2013;**24**:170-174

[6] Isbister ES, Roberts JA. Autokabalesis: A study of intentional vertical deceleration injuries. Injury. 1992;**23**:119-122

[7] Lewis WS, Lee AB, Grantham SA. "Jumpers syndrome": The trauma of high free fall as seen at Harlem hospital. The Journal of Trauma. 1965;**5**(6):812-818

[8] Mathis RD, Levine SH, Phifer S. An analysis of accidental free falls from a height: The "spring break" syndrome. The Journal of Trauma. 1993;**34**(1):123-126

[9] Steedman DJ. Severity of free-fall injury. Injury. 1989;**20**:259-261

[10] Castle K, Duberstein PR, Meldrum S, Conner KR, Conwell Y. Risk factors for suicide in blacks and whites: An analysis of data from the 1993 National mortality followback survey. The American Journal of Psychiatry. 2004;**161**:452-458

[11] Scalea T, Goldstein A, Phillips T, et al. An analysis of 161 falls from a height: The "jumper syndrome". The Journal of Trauma. 1986;**26**(8):706-712

[12] Velmahos GC, Demetriades D, Theodorou D, Cornwell EE, Belzberg H, Asensio J, et al. Patterns of injury in victims of urban free-falls. World Journal of Surgery. 1997;**21**:816-821

[13] Teh J, Firth M, Sharma A, Reznek R, Chan O. Jumpers and fallers: A comparison of the distribution of skeletal injury. Clinical Radiology. 2003;**58**:482-486

[14] Fang JF, Shih LY, Lin BC, Hsu YP. Pelvic fractures due to falls from a height in people with mental disorders. Injury. 2008;**39**:881-888

[15] Agalar F, Cakmakci M, Sayek I. Factors effecting mortality in urban vertical free falls: Evaluation of 180 cases. International Surgery. 1999;**84**:271-274

[16] Demetriades D, Murray J, Brown C, et al. High-level falls: Type and severity of injuries and survival outcome according to age. The Journal of Trauma. 2005;**58**:342-345

[17] Bertocci GE, Pierce MC, Deemer E, et al. Influence of fall height and impact surface on biomechanics of feet-first free falls in children. Injury. 2004;**35**:417-424

[18] Adamec J, Jelen K, Kubovy P, Lopot F, Schuller E. Forensic biomechanical analysis of falls from height using numerical human body

models. Journal of Forensic Sciences. 2010;**55**(6):1615-1623

[19] Guyomarc'h P, Campagna-Vaillancourt M, Chaltchi A, Sauvageau A. Skull fracture with brain expulsion in a one-level jumping-fall. Journal of Forensic Sciences. 2009;**54**(6):1463-1465

[20] Fracasso T, Schmidt S, Schmeling A. Commentary on: Kremer C, Racette S, Dionne CA, Sauvageau A. Discrimination of falls and blows in blunt head trauma: Systematic study of the hat brim rule in relation to skull fractures. Journal of Forensic Sciences. May 2008;**53**(3): 716-719. Journal of Forensic Sciences. 2011;**56**(6):1662. Author reply 1663

[21] Hong J, Lee WK, Park H. Change in causes of injury-related deaths in South Korea, 1996-2006. Journal of Epidemiology. 2011;**21**:500-506

[22] Im JS, Choi SH, Hong D, Seo HJ, Park S, Hong JP. Proximal risk factors and suicide methods among suicide completers from national suicide mortality data 2004-2006 in Korea. Comprehensive Psychiatry. 2011;**52**:231-237

[23] Lee CA, Choi SC, Jung KY, et al. Characteristics of patients who visit the emergency department with self-inflicted injury. Journal of Korean Medical Science. 2012;**27**:307-312

[24] Rockett IR, Regier MD, Kapusta ND, et al. Leading causes of unintentional and intentional injury mortality: United States, 2000-2009. American Journal of Public Health. 2012;**102**:e84-e92

[25] Richter D, Hahn MP, Ostermann PA, Ekkernkamp A, Muhr G. Vertical deceleration injuries: A comparative study of the injury patterns of 101 patients after accidental and intentional high falls. Injury. 1996;**27**:655-659

[26] Kennedy P, Rogers B, Speer S, Frankel H. Spinal cord injuries and attempted suicide: A retrospective review. Spinal Cord. 1999;**37**(12):847-852

[27] Biering-Sorensen F, Pederson W, Giortz Muller P. Spinal cord injury due to suicide attempts. Paraplegia. 1992;**30**(2):139-144

[28] Stanford RE, Soden R, Bartrop R, Mikk M, Taylor TKF. Spinal cord and related injuries after attempted suicide: Psychiatric diagnosis and long-term follow-up. Spinal Cord. 2007;**45**(6):437-443

[29] Anderson J, Allan DB. Vertebral fracture secondary to suicide attempt: Demographics and patient outcome in a Scottish spinal rehabilitation unit. The Journal of Spinal Cord Medicine. 2011;**34**(4):380-387

[30] Zatzick DF, Kang SM, Kim SY, et al. Patients with recognized psychiatric disorders in trauma surgery: Incidence, inpatient length of stay, and cost. The Journal of Trauma. 2000;**49**:487-495

[31] Demetriades D, Gkiokas G, Velmahos GC, et al. Alcohol and illicit drugs in traumatic deaths: Prevalence and association with type and severity of injuries. Journal of the American College of Surgeons. 2004;**199**:687-692

[32] Schecter WP, Klassen C, O'Connor P, et al. The unmet challenge of the trauma system. Archives of Surgery. 2005;**140**:902-904

[33] The ATLS Subcommittee and the International ATLS Working Group AC of SC on T. Advanced trauma life support (ATLS®): The ninth edition. Journal of Trauma and Acute Care Surgery. 2013;**74**:1363-1366

[34] Papadakis SA, Galanakos S, Apostolaki A, Kateros K, Antoniadou O, et al. Spinal cord injuries following

suicide attempts. Topics in paraplegia. ed. Yannis Dionysiotis, IntechOpen. 2nd July 2014. pp. 53-70. Chapter 3

[35] American Spinal Injury Association. International Standards for Neurological Classification of Spinal Cord Injury, Revised 2002. Chicago: American Spinal Injury Association; 2002

[36] Lambert DA, Sattin RW. Deaths from falls, 1978-1984. MMWR. CDC Surveillance Summaries. 1988;**37**(1):21-26

[37] Hultın A, Jiang G-X, Wasserman D, Hawton K, Hjelmeland H, et al. Repetition of attempted suicide among teenagers in Europe: Frequency, timing and risk factors. European Child & Adolescent Psychiatry. 2001;**10**:161-169

[38] Petronis KR, Samuels JF, Moscicki EK, Anthony JC. An epidemiologic investigation of potential risk factors for suicide attempts. Social Psqchiatry and Psychiatric Epidemiology. 1990;**25**:193-199

[39] Beautrais AL. Serious suicide attempts in young people: A case control study. American Journal of Psychiatry. 1996;**153**:1009-1014

[40] Li G, Ling J, Di Scala C. Characteristics and outcomes of self inflicted paediatric injuries: The role of method of suicide attempt. Injury Prevention. 1997;**3**:115-119

[41] Hawton K, Arensman E, Wasserman D, et al. Relation between attempted suicide and suicide rates among young people in Europe. Journal of Epidemiology and Community Health. 1998;**52**:191-194

[42] Granboulan V, Rabain D, Basquin M. The outcome of adolescent suicide attempts. Acta Psychiatrica Scandinavica. 1995;**91**:265-270

[43] Hawton K, Fagg J, Platt S, Hawkins M. Factors associated with suicide after parasuicide in young people. British Journal of Psychiatry. 1993;**306**:1641-1644

[44] Dickinson A, Roberts M, Kumar A, Weaver A, Lockey DJ. Falls from height: Injury and mortality. Journal of the Royal Army Medical Corps. 2012;**158**(2):123-127

[45] Kent A, Pearce A. Review of morbidity and mortality associated with falls from heights among patients presenting to a major trauma Centre. Emergency Medicine Australasia. 2006;**18**(1):23-30

[46] Petaros A, Slaus M, Coklo M, Sosa I, Cengija M, Bosnar A. Retrospective analysis of free-fall fractures with regard to height and cause of fall. Forensic Science International. 2013;**226**(1-3):290-295

[47] Choi JH, Kim SH, Kim SP, Jung KY, Ryu JY, Choi SC, et al. Characteristics of intentional fall injuries in the ED. The American Journal of Emergency Medicine. 2014;**32**(6):529-534

[48] Crandall M, Luchette F, Esposito TJ, West M, Shapiro M, Bulger E. Attempted suicide and the elderly trauma patient: Risk factors and outcomes. The Journal of Trauma. 2007;**62**(4):1021-1027

[49] Maull KI, Whitley RE, Cardea JA. Vertical deceleration injuries. Surgery, Gynecology & Obstetrics. 1981;**153**(2):233-236

[50] Snyder RG. Human tolerance to extreme impacts in free-fall. Aeroscace Medicine. 1963;**34**:695-709

[51] Layton TR, Villella R, Kelly EG. High free fall with survival. The Journal of Trauma. 1981;**21**(11):983-985

[52] Pallis D, Georgiou DF, Abadiotaki M, Galanakos S, Sapkas G, Macheras G, et al.

Comparison of traumatic pattern between accidental falls from height and suicide attempts. In: Presented orally at 20th Congress Efort. Lisbon; 2019

[53] Turgut K, Sarihan ME, Colak C, Güven T, Gür A, Gürbüz S. Falls from height: A retrospective analysis. World Journal of Emergency Medicine. 2018;**9**(1):46-50

[54] Kohli A, Banerjee KK. Pattern of injuries in fatal falls from buildings. Medicine, Science, and the Law. 2006;**46**(4):335-341

[55] Turk EE, Tsokos M. Pathologic features of fatal falls from height. The American Journal of Forensic Medicine and Pathology. 2004;**25**:194-199

[56] Kiran Kumar KV, Srivastava AK. Pattern of injuries in fall from height. Journal of Indian Academy of Forensic Medicine. 2013;**35**(1):47-50

[57] Goren S, Subasi M, Tyrasci Y, Gurkan F. Fatal falls from heights in and around Diyarbakir, Turkey. Forensic Science International. 2003;**137**:37-40

[58] Mao SW, Liu XJ, Su CP, Zhang M, Mu ZQ, et al. Analysis of 574 cases of high-fall death. Fa Yi Xue Za Zhi. 2009;**25**:276-278

[59] Wischhusen F, Patra S, Braumann M, Turk EE, Puschel K. Analysis of jumping/falling distance from a height. Forensic Science International. 2006;**156**:150-153

[60] Piazzalunga D, Rubertà F, Fugazzola P, Allievi N, Ceresoli M, Magnone S, et al. Suicidal fall from heights trauma: Difficult management and poor results. European Journal of Trauma and Emergency Surgery. 2019

[61] Cifu D, Wehman P, Mckinley W. Determining impairment following spinal cord injury. In: Rondinelli R, Katz R, editors. Disability evaluation. Physical Medicine and Rehabilitation Clinics of North America. 2001;**12**(3):603-612

[62] Kirshblum S, O'Connor K. Levels of spinal cord injury and predictors for neurologic recovery. Physical Medicine and Rehabilitation Clinics of North America. 2000;**11**(1):1-27. Edited by Hammond M. Topics in spinal cord injury medicine

[63] Whiteneck G, Tate D, Charlifue S. Predicting community reintegration after spinal cord injury from demographic and injury characteristics. Archives of Physical Medicine and Rehabilitation. 1999;**80**(11):1485-1491

[64] Abel SM, Ramsey S. Patterns of skeletal trauma in suicidal bridge jumpers: A retrospective study from the southeastern United States. Forensic Science International. 2013;**231**(1-3): 399.e1-399.e5

[65] Cetin G, Günay Y, Fincanci SK, Ozdemir Kolusayin R. Suicides by jumping from Bosphorus bridge in Istanbul. Forensic Science International. 2001;**116**(2-3):157-162

[66] Burri C, Kreuzer U, Limmer J. Principles and practice of fracture treatment in the multiply injured patient. Injury. 1982;**14**(1):44-50

[67] Sims A, O'Brien K. Autokabalesis: An account of mentally ill people who jump from buildings. Medicine, Science, and the Law. 1979 Jul;**19**(3):195-198

[68] Prasad A, Lloyd GG. Attempted suicide by jumping. Acta Psychiatrica Scandinavica. 1983;**68**(5):394-396

[69] Katz K, Gonen N, Goldberg I, Mizrahit J, et al. Injuries in attempted suicide by jumping from a height. Injury. 1988;**19**:371-374

Chapter 8

Advances in Emotion Recognition: Link to Depressive Disorder

Xiaotong Cheng, Xiaoxia Wang, Tante Ouyang and Zhengzhi Feng

Abstract

Emotion recognition enables real-time analysis, tagging, and inference of cognitive affective states from human facial expression, speech and tone, body posture and physiological signal, as well as social text on social network platform. Recognition of emotion pattern based on explicit and implicit features extracted through wearable and other devices could be decoded through computational modeling. Meanwhile, emotion recognition and computation are critical to detection and diagnosis of potential patients of mood disorder. The chapter aims to summarize the main findings in the area of affective recognition and its applications in major depressive disorder (MDD), which have made rapid progress in the last decade.

Keywords: emotion recognition, computational modeling, machine learning, depressive disorder

1. Introduction

Making computers capable of emotional computing was first proposed by Minsky (one of the founders of artificial intelligence) of the MIT. In his book *The Society of Mind* he proposed that "The question is not whether intelligent machines can have any emotions, but whether machines can be intelligent without emotions" [1]. Picard [2] proposed the concept of affective computing (AC) in 1995. Her monograph "Affective Computing" published in 1997 defined affective computing as "calculation related to, derived from or capable of emotions." She divided the research content of affective computing into nine aspects: mechanism of emotion, acquisition of emotion information, recognition of emotion pattern, modeling and understanding of emotion, synthesis and expression of emotion, application of emotion computing, interface of emotion computer, transmission and communication of emotion, and wearable computer. Among these aspects, the practical research of emotion recognition is largely based on theories of mechanism of emotion and acquisition of emotion information.

The mechanism of emotion is based on phenomenal and mechanistic views of emotion. The phenomenal views typical involved two approaches: discrete and dimensional views of emotion. The former proposed that emotion can be labeled as a limited set of basic emotions which could be combined into complex emotions. This method is problematic because the labels for emotions may be too restrictive to reflect complex emotions. Additionally, these labels may be culture dependent which could not reflect common substrates of different affective labels.

The latter proposed that emotions can be distributed in a multidimensional space which continuously evolves. Two common dimensions are valence (pleasantness) and arousal (activation level). The emotion recognition algorithms using emotion representation based on emotional labels are intuitive which are ambiguous for computer processing. Additionally, recognition of emotion pattern involves the classification of emotional data according to a large group of labels. For these reasons, researchers developed a number of dimensional model of emotions, such as Russell's circumplex model, Whissell's evaluation-activation space model, and Plutchik's wheel of emotions [3].

According to the mechanistic views of emotion, emotion pattern recognition not only relies on semantic labels but also physiological signals which originate in the peripheral nervous system (PNS) and central nervous system (CNS) dynamics [3]. (1) *The PNS emotion patterns*. The PNS included the autonomic and the somatic nervous systems (ANS and SNS). According to Schachter and Singer's peripheral theories of emotion (or cognition-arousal theory), people assess their emotional state by physiological arousal. Emotion states are inherent in these physiological dynamics and feasibly recognized by using PNS physiological data, according to the work from the lab led by Picard. Ekman and colleges provided the first evidence of PNS differences (including hand temperature, heart rate, skin conductance, and forearm tension) among four negative emotions [4]. However, their algorithms are based on intentionally expressed emotion and are user dependent, which may restrict generalization to other users [5]. (2) *The CNS emotion patterns*. The large majority of computational models of emotion stem from appraisal theory of emotion, which emphasized the CNS process of emotion. Frijda criticized the arousal theory of emotion and proposed that awareness of autonomic responding is not prerequisite for emotional experience or behavior. The differentiation of the emotions is explained as the result of the sequential appraisal for affective stimulus. Scherer suggests that there may be as many emotions as there are different appraisal outcomes. Thus there exists the minimal set of appraisal criteria necessary to the differentiation of primary emotional states. However, it should be noted that physiological changes is not only determined by appraisal meaning but also by factors outside of the appraisal or emotion realm. Therefore, there is not adequate evidence for consistent and specific PNS response during emotional episodes [6].

Practically, the acquisition of emotional information is required for emotion recognition. Emotional information characteristics included a variety of physiological or behavioral reactions concurrent with emotional state changes, including internal and external emotional features. (1) *Internal emotional information*. It refers to physiological reactions that cannot be detected from the outside of human body, such as the electrical or mechanical/chemical output of human brain activity (EEG), heart muscle activity(ECG, heart rate, pulse), skeletal muscle activity (EMG), breathing activity (respiration), and blood vessel activity (blood pressure, hemangiectasis). (2) *External emotional information*. It refers to the reactions that can be directly observed from the appearance, such as facial expression, speech, and posture. The extraction of common features for highly individualized emotion information constitutes the fundamental basis of emotion recognition. A great amount of features could be extracted from internal and external emotional signals, by calculating their mean, standard deviation, transformation, wave band power and peak detection, and others.

2. Methods for emotion recognition

The main methods for emotion recognition involve the following emotion indexes: (1) emotional behavior, namely, facial expression recognition, speech emotion recognition, and posture recognition (see Sections 2.1–2.3); (2) physiological pattern, which means objective emotional index after measuring PNS and CNS physiological signals (see Section 2.5); and (3) psychological measures and multimodal emotion signals, such as textual information and multimodal emotion information (see Sections 2.3 and 2.6).

2.1 Facial expression recognition

Faces may be one of the most important methods for visual communication of emotion. Though started from the 1970s, facial expression recognition is the most studied field in natural emotions machine recognition, especially in the USA and Japan, wherein studies on facial expression recognition have grown to be a hotspot of AI emotion recognition. In 1971, American psychologists Ekman and Friesen categorized facial expression into six types: anger, disgust, happiness, fear, surprise, and sadness. They also established the Facial Action Coding System (FACS) in 1978 [7], which is the earliest research of facial expression recognition. Facial expressions were deemed as observable indicators of internal emotional states, which make emotion differentiation possible.

Currently, the most-used facial expression databases included Ekman's FACS and its updated version, automated facial image analysis (AFIA) developed by Carnegie Mellon University, Japanese female expression database JAFFE and its expansion set in Japan ATR Media Information Science Laboratory, Cohn-Kanade expression database, CK+ expression database, and Rafd facial expression database established by CMU Robotics Research Institute, USA. Common facial expression picture libraries in China include the USTC-NVIE image library [8], the CFAPS facial emotion stimulating materials [9], and the Chinese facial expression intensity grading picture library [10].

The facial expression recognition included the following steps: (1) facial image acquisition, (2) image preprocessing, (3) feature extraction, and (4) emotion classification (**Table 1**).

Apart from Ekman's discrete emotion model, facial expression recognition was also conducted under the other emotional models (such as dimensional model). Ballano et al. proposed a method for continuous facial affect recognition from videos based on evaluation-activation 2D model proposed by Whissell [11].

Processes	Sub-processes and related work
Facial image acquisition	Facial images are obtained from images and videos, including static expressions and dynamic expressions
Image preprocessing	Face detection and positioning, face adjustment, editing, scale normalization, histogram equalization, dimming, light compensation, homomorphic filtering, graying, Gaussian smoothing
Feature extraction	(a) Static image. Gabor wavelet transformation, local binary patterns (LBP), scale-invariant feature transformation (SIFT), discrete cosine transformation (DCT), regional covariance matrix. (b) Dynamic image. Optical flow method, difference image method, feature point tracking, model-based method, elastic graph matching.
Emotion classification	Canonical correlation analysis, sparse representation classification, expert rule-based method[a]

[a]An expert rule-based method classifies the emotion according to a set of "if-then" statements based on expert experience or sampling with rule acquisition algorithm.

Table 1.
Facial expression recognition process.

The evaluation dimension defines the valence of emotion, while the activation dimension defines the action tendencies (e.g., active versus passive) under the emotional state. Their model extended the emotion information to continuous emotional trajectory.

Micro-expressions are quick, unconscious, and spontaneous facial movements that occur when people experience strong emotions. The duration of micro-expression is about 1/25 to 1/2 s. The fleeting micro-expression has small movement and does not appear in the upper face and the lower face at the same time, so it is quite difficult to observe and recognize correctly. Therefore, the collection and selection of micro-expression data sets are very important. Micro-expression recognition requires (1) the image acquisition and preprocessing of face image, (2) the detection of micro-expressions from the face and the extraction of its features, and (3) classifying and recognizing the categories of the micro-emoticon. Different research teams have developed different automatic micro-expression recognition systems and established databases.

Polikovsky et al. [12] explored the 3D gradient histogram method for feature extraction of facial micro-expressions in video sequences based on the Polikovsky expression library. They proposed a new approach to capture micro-expression using 200fps high-speed camera. Shreve et al. [13] established the USF-HD database and applied the optical flow method for automatic micro-expression recognition research. They developed a method of automatically spotting continuously changing facial expressions in long videos. The University of Oulu in Finland developed the spontaneous micro-expression corpus (SMIC) and SMIC2. Yan et al. [14] improved the micro-expression elicitation paradigm and developed the Chinese micro-expression database CASME. Later on they further expanded the sample number, improved the frame rate and image quality of CASME, and created CASMEII. They differentiated full suppression of facial movements from self-perceived suppression of facial movements. The micro-expressions were elicited in a well-controlled laboratory context and had high temporal resolution (200 frames/s). The best performance is 63.41% for 5-class classification.

2.2 Speech emotion recognition

As the easiest, most basic, and direct way of information communication, speech contains rich emotional information. Speech could not only convey semantic information but also reveal speaker's emotional state, for instance, a person may have a voice with high volume, heavy tones, and accelerated speed when getting angry, but sullen intonation and slow speed when feeling sad. Therefore, in order to make the computer understand people's emotions better and interact more naturally with people, it is necessary to study speech emotions. Speech emotion recognition is widely applied in man-machine interaction, such as automatic customer service system, which can transfer emotional users to manual service [15]; it monitors the driver's emotional fluctuations based upon his speech speed and volume to remind him of staying calm, thus preventing him from a car accident [16]; it helps the disabled to speak [17]; and it detects emotional state of patients with mental disorders based upon context analysis [18].

Most of the studies use prosodic features as characteristic parameters of speech emotion recognition. For example, Gharavian et al. [19] extracted parameters such as fundamental frequency, resonance peak, and Mel coefficient and then analyzed the correlation among them. The obtained 25-dimensional vectors were classified by FAMNN classification algorithm to gain a more credible emotion recognition result. Devi et al. [20] summarized speech signal preprocessing techniques, common short-term energy, MFCC features, and their applications in speech emotion recognition. Zhang et al. [21] use a multilayer deep belief network (DBN) to automatically extract the emotional features in speech signals, piece together consecutive multi-frame speeches to form an abstract high-dimensional feature, use features trained by the deep belief network as the input end of the extreme learning machine (ELM) classifier, and ultimately establish a speech emotion recognition system. Zhu et al. [22] propose a track-based space-time spectral signature speech emotion recognition method and obtain relatively accurate results. Liu and Qin [23] study the application of speech emotion recognition in manned space flight, establish a stress emotion corpus, and build speech emotion recognition model and software through feature extraction and Gaussian mixture model (GMM) to verify the accuracy of speech emotion recognition.

The emotional speech features extracted in the abovementioned study are mostly targeted at personalized speech emotion recognition, while the feature extraction for non-personalized speech emotion recognition is still a challenge. Recent efforts have been made toward development of large corpus [24]. The current speech emotion recognition study is limited by lack of unified, public and standard mandarin emotion corpus, as well as an authoritative and unified standard for building emotion corpus. Many researches are conducted based on self-recorded databases which vary in terms of age, gender, number of participants, text information, and the scale of the final corpus, making it difficult to compare between different research results. Furthermore, most of the studies are conducted based on discrete emotions, taking into consideration limited emotional dimension corpus.

2.3 Posture emotion recognition

Posture refers to the expressional actions of other parts of human body than face. It can coordinate or supplement speech content and effectively convey emotional information. Postures can be divided into body expression and gestures. Body expression is one of the ways to express emotions. People would have different postures under different emotional state, such as belly laugh when happy, arched shoulders when scared, and being fidgeted when nervous. Postures such as raising hands and akimbo can express individual emotions. People may have different postures at different emotional state and level, hence it is possible to analyze and predict emotional state by observing different expressions and intensity of the expression. Researchers have pointed out at early times that posture and movements can only reflect intensity of emotion, but not the essence and type of the emotions. Later, some put forward that posture is conducive to the expression of emotional intensity although it cannot reflect accurately emotional state. Some scholars have studied the ability of subjects to understand six basic postures, the subjects were expressionless throughout the test, and the result showed that posture can be used to identify certain emotional state, such as sorrow and fear.

Generally, there are two posture recognition methods: (1) recognizing affective content of daily behavior through analysis and (2) using the temporal and spatial characteristics of gestures (such as the rhythm, amplitude, and strength of the motion) to analyze the affective content. For example, Castellano et al. [25] proposed a method for recognizing emotions based on human motion indicators (such as amplitude, velocity, and mobility) and establishing emotional models with image sequences and motion test indicators; Bernhardt and Robinson [26] used segmentation techniques to quantify high-dimensional motion into a set of simple motion data, extract motion features, and pair them with corresponding emotions; Liu et al. [27] classified the body movement and combined motion and velocity parameters for weighting function calculation to identify the emotion expressed by certain movement. Shao and Wang [28] extracted two 3D texture features by processing the image sequences of body movement and used this as a basis for emotion classification. The recognition rate can reach 77.0% in experiment which tests seven common natural emotions in the FABO database.

The posture recognition process mainly includes four steps: motion data acquisition, preprocessing, motion feature extraction, and emotion classification. *Firstly*, motion data collection. Generally, there are two types of motion data collection methods: (1) contact type which is a wearable device embedded with various sensors, such as electronic gloves and data shoe covers, and (2) noncontact type, which generally obtains image information through the camera. The contact recognition technology has high equipment cost, uncomfortable user experience, and goes against the objective of natural man–machine interaction. *Secondly*, data preprocessing. This generally includes human body detection, image denoising, image segmentation, image binarization processing, time window, filtering processing, and others. Among them, human body detection mainly includes basic image segmentation, background difference method, interframe difference method, optical flow method, and energy minimization method. *Thirdly*, motion feature extraction. Generally speaking, motion features can be divided into four categories: (1) static features which include size, color, outline, shape, and depth; (2) dynamic features which include speed, optical flow, direction, and trajectory; (3) spatiotemporal features which include spatiotemporal context, spatiotemporal shape, and spatiotemporal interest points; and (4) descriptive features which include scenes, attributes, objects, and poses. There are three types of most-used methods for motion feature extraction, namely, time domain analysis, frequency domain analysis, and time-frequency domain analysis. *Fourthly*, emotional classification. Other classifiers than the commonly used ones are dynamic time warping, dynamic programming, potential Dirichlet distribution, probabilistic latent semantic analysis, context-free grammar, finite state machines, conditional random fields, and others.

2.4 Textual emotion recognition

Emotions are not exactly linguistic constructs. However the most convenient to emotion is through language. With the advent of social media, social media platforms are becoming a rich source of multimodal affective information, including text, videos, images, and audios. One of them is textual analysis. Affect recognition from text analysis is often used for a public opinion mining. The process of text recognition contains four steps: material collection, text preprocessing, feature extraction, and emotion classification. (1) The first step is material collection. Web crawlers are commonly used to collect materials from blogs, e-commerce sites, and news sites. (2) The second step is text preprocessing, which includes word segmentation, part-of-speech tagging, tag filtering, affix trimming, simplification and replacement, and so on. (3) The third step is feature extraction. Main text features involve words, phrases, n-gram, concepts, and others. Words containing general features can be automatically extracted, while others need to be identified by human efforts before creating emotional glossary. Other methods used are frequent pattern mining techniques and associated rule mining techniques. (4) The fourth step is emotion classification. In addition to some commonly used classifiers, it also includes central vector classification, maximum entropy, emotion-based words labeling, and word frequency-weighted statistics.

Domestic researches on text recognition mainly center around emotion recognition of social platforms such as microblog. For example, Hao et al. [29] proposed a microblog emotion recognition method based on wording features of microblogs and verified its validity. Hao et al. [30] proposed a classification method based on supervised learning for the classification and prediction of emotional polarity in microblogs, and the accuracy of the experimental analysis reached 79.9%. Huang et al. [31] proposed a multifeature fusion-based microblog theme and emotion mining model TMMMF and verified its validity; Zhang et al. [32] proposed a joint model of microblog emotion recognition and emotion incentive extraction based on neural network. The experiment shows that the F value of the model in the emotion incentive extraction task is 82.70% and the F value in the emotion recognition task is 74.74%.

2.5 Physiological model recognition

William James [33] proposed that emotions derive from peripheral physiological responses. Kreibig [34] examined the patterns of autonomic nervous system activity under different emotions, showing the specificities in different physiological responses. For example, fear would cause accelerated heart rate and respiratory rhythm and strengthened galvanic skin response. The theory confirms the role of autonomous physiological activities in emotional expression but ignores the role of the brain center in emotions. In 1929, Cannon questioned James's theory and came up with the Cannon-Bard theory (also known as the thalamus theory) with Bard. According to this theory, emotions and their corresponding physiological changes occur simultaneously, both of which are controlled by the thalamus, and the central brain determines the nature of emotions, which affirms the central nervous system's role in regulating and controlling emotions. In conclusion, the occurrence of emotions is accompanied by certain degree of physiological activation of the central and peripheral nervous system. This provides a theoretical basis for studying emotion recognition in different physiological patterns.

Early studies mainly focused on the PNS physiological signals such as skin temperature, blood pressure, electrocardiogram, electromyography, respiratory action, galvanic skin response, and blood volume fluctuation for emotion recognition. Picard et al. [35] collected four physiological signals of galvanic skin response, blood volume fluctuation, electromyographic signal, and respiratory action under different emotional states and reached 81% in terms of recognition accuracy for eight emotions. Kim and Andre [36] developed a short-term monitoring emotion recognition system based on physiological signals of multiple users. They used support vector machine (SVM) to classify and identify four emotions including sadness, depression, surprise, and anger, achieving a classification rate at 95%. Yan et al. [37] collected a variety of physiological signals through multipurpose polygraph MP150: used Fisher, k-NN, and other intelligent algorithms for feature extraction and analysis; and identified six basic emotional states with recognition rate being at 60–90%. Li et al. [38] proposed emotion recognition based on recursive quantitative analysis of physiological signals. They extracted 10 sets of nonlinear features from the recursive graphs of skin conductance signals, myoelectric signals, and respiratory signals and achieved higher emotion recognition rate. Jin et al. [39] used the updated LSTSVM for emotion recognition based on the physiological signals of electroencephalography, skin conductance, myoelectricity, and respiration and obtained higher recognition accuracy.

In recent years, with the development of neurophysiology and the rise of brain imaging technology, CNS brain signals have attracted the attention of researchers and been used in emotion recognition because of their high temporal resolution and strong functional specificity. In the early stage of the study, the most common measurement index was electroencephalogram (EEG). Some scholars pointed out that the frontal brain asymmetry is closely related to emotional valence. Studies have shown that high-frequency parts of EEG can reflect people's emotional and cognitive states and the γ and β bands can better tell the change of emotional state than the low-frequency band [40]. Jie et al. [41] realized the recognition of high and low arousal and high and low pleasure through nonlinear feature sample entropy. Duan et al. [42] used differential entropy in machine classification learning for emotion recognition, and the classification accuracy rate was up to 84.22%. It is shown that as a nonlinear EEG feature, differential entropy shows higher classification efficiency. Later, some scholars combined spontaneous physiological signals with EEG and used comprehensive information to improve the recognition rate [43, 44].

However, the EEG acquisition process is relatively complicated and often has the interference with external noise and electromyography. The cerebral blood oxygen parameter measurement method based on functional near-infrared spectroscopy (NIRS) is gaining greater popularity in emotion recognition because of its high portability, insensitivity to noise and motion, and high possibility for long-term continuous measurement. Tai and Chau [45] extracted the time domain features of prefrontal signals during affective states to identify positive and negative emotions elicited by emotional pictures. The recognition rate of 13 subjects was within the range of 75.0–96.67%.

The most critical steps in emotion recognition based on physiological signals are signal preprocessing, feature extraction and optimization, and classification identification.

1. **Emotion signal preprocessing**. This step mainly retains valid data segments during emotion induction process at its highest level and then removes noise and artifacts from the signal. The artifact removal methods mainly include filtering, normalization, independent component analysis, and so on. (a) Filters with different frequency band parameters, such as adaptive filters and Butterworth filters, are commonly used for denoising physiological signals, such as smoothing filtering of the galvanic skin to remove high-frequency glitch. (b) Normalization could reduce the adverse effects of baseline individual differences on emotion recognition [46]. (c) Independent component analysis or principal component analysis may remove electro-oculogram and artifacts [47].

2. **Feature extraction**. There are four main types of features: time domain, frequency domain, time-frequency, and nonlinear features.

    a. **Time domain**. Time domain feature extraction is found first and relatively simple. It obtains information in amplitude, mean value, standard deviation, partiality, and kurtosis by analyzing the time domain waveform of signal. In this processing, less information is lost. Common time domain analysis methods include zero-crossing analysis, histogram analysis, analysis of variance, correlation analysis, peak detection, waveform parameter analysis, and waveform recognition. Emotion recognition studies using cerebral blood oxygen parameters more often involve time domain feature analysis and extraction.

    b. **Frequency domain**. Frequency domain feature extraction is based on power spectrum analysis and widely used in analysis of ECG, respiration, EEG, and other signals, such as power spectrum ratio, power spectrum energy, and sub-band power spectral density in different frequency bands.

c. **Time-frequency feature**. The time-frequency feature extraction considers joint distribution information in terms of time domain and frequency domain. This method describes the changing relationship between signal frequencies and time and contains more comprehensive contents. Commonly used analysis methods are wavelet transform, short-time Fourier transform, Hilbert-Huang transform, and others. Wavelet transform has multiresolution, adjustable sliding time window, has good resolution in both time domain and frequency domain, and has become an effective tool for analyzing nonstationary signals, such as EEG, ECG, EMG, and other signals underlying emotion processes.

d. **Nonlinear feature**. EEG signals are created in complex limbic system with noticeable nonlinearity and chaos characteristic, so the extraction of EEG features is more complex and diverse than other physiological signals. In recent years, the analysis of nonlinear features such as entropy, correlation dimension, and fractal dimension has gradually increased in the study of emotional EEG recognition. Konstantinidis et al. [48] calculated the correlation dimension of emotional EEG for online recognition research; Liu et al. [49] extracted the nonlinear features such as the fractal dimension of EEG to obtain the ideal recognition effect and built an online application.

2.6 Multimodal emotion recognition

Most recent researches have focused on multimodal emotion recognition using visual and aural information. Human expression of emotion is mostly multimodal, including visual, audio, and textual modalities for effective communication [3]. Furthermore, physiological signals can reveal emotional state objectively, even if the subject conceals his/her expression of emotion due to complex reasons. Hence emotion recognition integrating multiple modalities has gained increasing attention, and research hotspot has shifted from single modality to multimodal emotion recognition in practical applications. D'Mello and Kory [50] used statistical methods to compare the accuracy of single modality and multimodal on different databases. Multimodal expression recognition was superior to single modality performance in the experiments. The McGurk [51] phenomenon reveals that in the process of brain perception, different senses are automatically combined unconsciously to process the information, and any lack or inaccuracy of sensory information will lead to deviations in the brain's understanding of external information. Therefore, multimodal feature fusion recognition technology has become a research hotspot in the past few years.

The widely used multimodal emotion databases are HUMAINE database [52], the Belfast database [53], the large-scale audiovisual database SEMAINE [54], the IEMOCAP emotional database [55], the audiovisual database eNTERFACE [56], the Acted Facial Expression in the Wild database (AFEW) [57] composed of audio and video clips from English movies and TV programs, and the Chinese multimodal emotional data set CHEAVD [58].

Multichannel information fusion levels can be divided into three categories: data layer, feature layer, and decision layer: (1) Data layer fusion refers to the fusion of collected raw data and then extracting feature vector from the fused data, finally classifying the emotion; (2) feature layer fusion refers to conducting preprocessing and feature extraction of the collected data of each channel first, then obtaining the feature vector by fusing extracted emotion features, and then finally classifying the emotion; and (3) decision layer fusion refers to making separate emotion classification decision for collected data of each channel and then fusing the single modality recognition result to obtain the final classification result. The commonly used information fusion methods are D-S evidence theory, artificial neural network, fuzzy set theory, Bayesian inference, cluster analysis, expert system method, and others.

Current studies on postures mainly concentrate on bimodal emotion recognition of facial expressions and postures. Castellano et al. [25] conducted a comparative study of the processing of body language and facial expression and found that body language and facial expression have similar visual processing mechanisms. The two are highly similar in terms of event-related potential (ERP) components, psychological functions, and influencing factors and are partially overlapping or adjacent to each other in potential neural bases. Gunes and Piccardi [59, 60] conducted long-term research on bimodal emotion recognition of facial expressions and postures and established the Bi-modal Face and Body Gesture Database for Automatic Analysis of Human Nonverbal Affective Behavior (FABO). Yan et al. [61] studied video-based bimodal emotion recognition of facial expression and postures and proposed an emotion recognition method based on bilateral sparse partial least squares which has low computational complexity but low recognition rate. In order to tell human emotions through video data, Wang and Shao [62] extracted emotional features of facial expression and body movements from the FABO database, used a fusion algorithm based on canonical correlation analysis (CCA) to fuse two features, and then used nearest neighbor classifier and support vector machine for emotion recognition. After using updated sparsity preserving CCA (SPCCA), they combined emotion features of facial expressions and body movements, achieving an emotion recognition rate at 90.48%. Wang et al. [63] focused on the problem of high computational complexity in video emotion recognition and proposed a bimodal emotion recognition method based on temporal-spatial local binary pattern moment (TSLBPM) which has been proven effective. Jiang et al. [64] proposed a spatiotemporal local ternary orientational pattern (SLTOP) feature description method and cloud-weighted decision fusion classification method for bimodal emotion recognition of facial expressions and postures in video sequences, achieving better recognition result than other classification recognition methods in the comparative experiments.

3. Application of emotion recognition in depressive disorder

Depressive disorder is characteristic of negative mood and anhedonia, which are two core symptoms for diagnosis of the disease. Traditionally, the clinical diagnosis for depression requires the clinicians to assess the severity of depressive symptoms according to verbal statements of patients as well as nonverbal indicators such as voices (pitch, speaking speed, and volumes) and facial expressions. Additionally, structured questionnaires (such as Beck Depression Inventory, Hamilton Depression Rating Scale) have been developed and validated in clinical populations to assess the severity of depressive symptoms. However, the physiological biomarkers of depression are still unclear. Since the 1950s the consensus has emerged that psychiatric diagnoses could be defined according to relevant biological characteristics. However, the empirical diagnostic categories such as depressive disorder failed to be reified and objectified by valid biological measures [65]. The Research Domain Criteria (RDoC) initiative attempted to link physiologic mechanisms (esp. circuit level) to dimensional constructs (e.g., positive/negative valence) rather than diagnostic categories (e.g., MDD), with the potential for alternative diagnostic processes [66].

3.1 Physiological emotion recognition

Ample evidence showed that specific brain regions including the PFC, amygdala, anterior cingulate, and insula play a major role in the neuropathological basis of affective disorders. Recent meta-analyses found evidence which is against the locationist account of emotion and suggested that brain regions corresponding to basic psychological operations are involved in emotion processing across emotional categories and are not specifically localized to discrete brain networks [67]. With its advantages in superior soft tissue contrast, high spatial resolution, and noninvasive detection, magnetic resonance imaging (MRI) has become a promising tool for detection of neurological alterations in mental disorders such as depression.

Using an experimental therapeutics approach coupled with machine learning, Liu et al. investigated the effect of a pharmacological challenge aiming to enhance dopaminergic signaling on whole-brain's response to reward-related stimuli in MDD. Artificial intelligence technology combined with MRI technology was used to find the objective biological markers of depression. The brain regions with diagnostic value included anterior cuneate lobe, cingulate gyrus, inferior marginal angular gyrus, insular, thalamus, and hippocampus. The brain regions with preventive value included the precuneus, postcentral gyrus, dorsolateral prefrontal lobe, orbitofrontal lobe, and middle temporal gyrus. The brain regions with predictive therapeutic response included the precuneus, cingulate gyrus, inferior marginal angular gyrus, middle frontal gyrus, middle occipital gyrus, inferior occipital gyrus, and lingual gyrus [68].

Studies have shown that machine learning and deep learning techniques have been widely used in the diagnosis, prevention, and treatment of depression and other neuropsychiatric diseases in recent years. Abnormal brain regions may be used as predictors of diagnostic and therapeutic responses. Research hotspot mainly focused on cortical areas rather than the midbrain limbic system or dopamine system. Collectively, the literature review suggested that the cingulate gyrus and precuneus may be the most important candidate brain regions among the objective biological markers of depression. Due to complex pathophysiological changes and etiological heterogeneity of depression, combining imaging biomarkers with other indicators (e.g., biochemical, genetic) is necessary to achieve more objective assessment of course and prognosis of depression [69].

3.2 Textual emotion recognition

With the growing amount of emotional information from social media, including text, photos, and videos, emotion recognition through multimodal information using machine learning technique is becoming a trend. Absolutist thinking represents a form of cognitive distortion typical of anxiety and depression. Al-Mosaiwi and Johnstone conducted a text analysis of 63 Internet forums (over 6400 members) using the Linguistic Inquiry and Word Count software to examine absolutist thinking. The results suggested that absolutist words, rather than negative emotion words, tracked the severity of affective disorder forums. They found elevated levels of absolutist words in depression recovery forums. This suggests that absolutist thinking may be a vulnerability factor for relapse of affective disorder [70].

The project of Proactive Suicide Prevention Online (PSPO) identified suicide-prone individuals to provide further crisis management. A microblog group was identified as a high-risk population, who commented around a Sina microblogger who committed suicide. They were assessed for suicidal thought and behavior. The frequency of death-oriented words significantly decreased after the intervention, while the frequency of future-oriented words significantly increased. This model may help people with suicidal thoughts and behaviors but with a low motivation to seek help [71].

The modeling of textual and visual features from Instagram photos successfully identified individuals diagnosed with depression. The results showed that depressed people are more likely to upload photos that are bluer, grayer, and darker. The human rating of photo attributes (happiness, sadness, interestingness, and likability) is a weak predictor of depression [72]. These findings suggest new avenues for early screening and detection of mental illness.

3.3 Facial expression and speech recognition

The physiological approaches using specific sensors for emotion signals have the advantage of being more precise, but are generally more costly and need more effort in clinical context. Facial and speech information is more applicable in these natural environments. Chronic stress, anxiety, and depressive states are three intertwined processes which constitute the vicious circle in common affective disorders such as depression. Chronic stress may induce autonomic responses concurrent with anxiety states, and anxiety may lead to depressive states when stress continues and coping strategies are ineffective. Gavrilescu and Vizireanu for the first time proposed a neural network-based architecture for predicting levels of stress, anxiety, and depression based on FACS in a nonintrusive and real-time manner. Their method allows the experts to monitor the three emotional states in real time. Additionally, 93% accuracy was achieved discriminating between healthy individuals and those with major depressive disorder (MDD) or post-traumatic stress disorder (PTSD) [73]. This method is an attractive alternative to traditional self-report measurements based on questionnaires.

A new approach to predict the depressive symptoms with Beck Depression Inventory II (BDI-II) scores from video data is proposed based on the deep convolutional neutral networks (DCNN). The proposed framework is designed to capture both the facial appearance and dynamics in the video data by integrating two deep networks into one. The method could predict with over 80% accuracy depressive behavior, achieving a comparable performance to most methods combing video and audio data [74]. Thus their method provided a more efficient and convenient way of prediction than multimodal methods.

Harati et al. used several metrics of variability to extract unsupervised features from video recordings of patients before and after deep brain stimulation (DBS) treatment for major depressive disorder (MDD). Their goal was to quantify the treatment effects on emotion indicated with facial expression. Their preliminary results indicate that unsupervised features learned from these video recordings using dynamic latent variable model (DLVM) based on multiscale entropy (MSE) of pixel intensities can distinguish different phases of depression and recovery [75]. Therefore, their methods may provide more precise markers of treatment response.

As a relatively objective and easily available variable, speech has potential value in the diagnosis of depression. The acoustic analysis of patients with mental illness showed that there is greater than moderate correlation between speech-related variables and symptom indicators [76, 77]. Pan et al. build a speech-based depression recognition model with logical regression (LR) classification methods. The results show that the speech recognition accuracy reached 82.9% [78].

They found that four voice features (PC1, PC6, PC17, PC24, $P < 0.05$, corrected) made significant contribution to depression and that the contribution effect of the voice features alone reached 35.65%. These results demonstrate that voice features have great potential in applications such as clinical diagnosis and prediction.

3.4 Multimodal emotion recognition

Facial, video, and textual information are the most available affective information in clinical context. Therefore, recent studies explored multimodal emotion recognition methods to improve the accuracies and specificities when the multimodal emotion information was input as predictors. Haque et al. present a machine learning method for measuring the severity of depressive symptoms. Their multimodal method uses 3D facial expressions and spoken language, commonly available from modern cell phones. It demonstrates an average error of 3.67 points (15.3% relative) on the clinically validated Patient Health Questionnaire (PHQ) scale. For detecting major depressive disorder, their model demonstrates 83.3% sensitivity and 82.6% specificity [79]. Yang et al. proposed new text and video features and hybridizes deep and shallow models for depression estimation and classification from audio, video, and text descriptors. They demonstrated that the proposed hybrid framework effectively improves the accuracies of both depression estimation and depression classification [80]. SimSensei Kiosk was a virtual human interviewer which aims to automatically assess the verbal and nonverbal behaviors indicative of depression, anxiety, or post-traumatic stress disorder (PSTD). A multimodal real-time sensing system was used to simultaneously capture different modalities (e.g., smile intensity, 3D head position and orientation, intensity or lack of facial expressions like anger, disgust, and joy) to model the relation between mental states and human behavior [81].

4. Conclusions

This chapter summarized the recognition of human affect based on internal and external signals of emotion, which has gained intensive attention in research fields such as artificial intelligence, psychology, cognitive neuroscience, and physiology. The reviewed empirical researches rarely deal with "social emotions" such as guilt, shame, and embarrassment. Instead of the more traditional cognitive and biological perspectives of emotion, the sociological perspective focused on functions of emotions to control social interactions and sustain the social order. Future studies need to deal with its extension to social emotions and the relevant theoretical foundations.

Emotion recognition is based on discrete and dimensional views of emotion, with underlying CNS and PNS dynamics. Single modal as well as multimodal emotion recognition rely on facial, speech, posture, physiological, and textual emotional information, which could function separately or concurrently. Integrating multimodal emotion information for emotion recognition remains challenging, and much research is needed about the way they relate to human affect.

Furthermore, the application of emotion recognition in depressive disorder may pave an avenue for more precise diagnosis of the syndrome and prediction of its disease course. Identifying specific physiological substrates of depressive disorder, combined with emotion classification technique such as machine learning, may help identify the dimensional constructs of RDoC, which are implicit in the clinical phenomena of depressive disorder.

Conflict of interest

The authors declare no conflict of interest.

Author details

Xiaotong Cheng[1†], Xiaoxia Wang[2*†], Tante Ouyang[1] and Zhengzhi Feng[1]

1 College of Psychology, Army Medical University, Chongqing, China

2 Department of Basic Psychology, College of Psychology, Army Medical University, Chongqing, China

*Address all correspondence to: lemonowang@gmail.com

† Cheng and Wang contributed equally to this article and should be considered co-first authors.

References

[1] Minsky M. The Society of Mind. New York, NY: Simon & Schuster Imprint; 1985

[2] Picard RW. Affective Computing. Cambridge, MA: The MIT Press; 1997

[3] Poria S, Cambria E, Bajpai R, Hussain A. A review of affective computing: From unimodal analysis to multimodal fusion. Information Fusion. 2017;**37**:98-125. DOI: 10.1016/j.inffus.2017.02.003

[4] Ekman P, Levenson RW, Friesen WV. Autonomic nervous system activity distinguishes among emotions. Science. 1983;**221**(4616):1208-1210. DOI: 10.1126/science.6612338

[5] Singh D. Human emotion recognition system. International Journal of Image, Graphics and Signal Processing. 2012; **4**(8):50-56. DOI: 10.5815/ijigsp.2012.08.07

[6] Quigley KS, Barrett LF. Is there consistency and specificity of autonomic changes during emotional episodes? Guidance from the conceptual act theory and psychophysiology. Biological Psychology. 2014;**98**:82-94. DOI: 10.1016/j.biopsycho.2013.12.013

[7] Ekman P, Friesen WV. Facial Action Coding System: A Technique for the Measurement of Facial Movement. Palo Alto, CA: Consulting Psychologists Press; 1978

[8] Yang C, Li H. Validity study on facereader's images recognition from Chinese facial expression database. Ergonomics. 2015;**21**:38-41. DOI: 10.13837/j.issn.1006-8309.2015.01.0008

[9] Gong X et al. Revision of the Chinese facial affective picture system. Chinese Journal of Mental Health. 2011;**250**: 40-46. DOI: 10.3969/j.issn.1000-6729.2011.01.011

[10] Liu J et al. Establishment of the Chinese facial emotion images database with intensity classification. Chinese Journal of Mental Health. 2019;**33**: 120-125. DOI: 10.3969/j.issn.1000-6729.2019.02.009

[11] Ballano S, Hupont I, Cerezo E, Baldassarri S. Recognizing Emotions from Video in a Continuous 2D Space. Berlin, Heidelberg: Springer Berlin Heidelberg; 2011. pp. 600-603

[12] Polikovsky S, Kameda Y, Ohta Y. Facial micro-expressions recognition using high speed camera and 3D-gradient descriptor. In: Proceedings of the 3rd International Conference on Crime Detection and Prevention; 3 December 2009; London. London, UK: IEEE; 2009. pp. 1-6. DOI: 10.1049/ic.2009.0244

[13] Shreve M, Godavarthy S, Manohar V, Goldgof D, Sarkar S. Towards macro- and micro-expression spotting in video using strain patterns. In: Proceedings of the IEEE Workshop on Applications of Computer Vision; 2009/12; 7-8 December 2009; Snowbird, UT. Snowbird, UT: IEEE; 2009. pp. 1-6

[14] Yan W-J, Li X, Wang S-J, Zhao G, Liu Y-J, Chen Y-H, et al. CASME II: An improved spontaneous micro-expression database and the baseline evaluation. PLoS One. 2014;**9**:e86041. DOI: 10.1371/journal.pone.0086041

[15] Lee CM, Narayanan SS. Toward detecting emotions in spoken dialogs. IEEE Transactions on Speech and Audio Processing. 2005;**13**:293-303. DOI: 10.1109/tsa.2004.838534

[16] Schuller B, Rigoll G, Lang M. Speech emotion recognition combining acoustic features and linguistic information in a hybrid support vector machine-belief network architecture. In: Proceedings of the 2004 IEEE International Conference

on Acoustics, Speech, and Signal Processing; 17-21 May 2004; Montreal. Montreal, Quebec: IEEE; 2004. pp. I-577

[17] Ververidis D, Kotropoulos C. Emotional speech recognition: Resources, features, and methods. Speech Communication. 2006;**48**: 1162-1181. DOI: 10.1016/j.specom.2006.04.003

[18] Rickheit G, Strohner H. Handbook of Communication Competence. Germany: Mouton de Gruyter; 2008

[19] Gharavian D, Sheikhan M, Nazerieh A, Garoucy S. Speech emotion recognition using FCBF feature selection method and GA-optimized fuzzy ARTMAP neural network. Neural Computing and Applications. 2012;**21**: 2115-2126. DOI: 10.1007/s00521-011-0643-1

[20] Devi JS, Yarramalle S, Prasad NS. Speaker emotion recognition based on speech features and classification techniques. International Journal of Image, Graphics and Signal Processing. 2014;**6**:61-77. DOI: 10.5815/ijigsp.2014.07.08

[21] Zhang L et al. Speech emotion recognition based on deep belief network. Journal of Taiyuan University of Technology. 2019;**50**:101-107. DOI: 10.16355/j.cnki.isn1007-9432tyut.2019.01.016

[22] Zhu Y, Bodong S, Lichen Z. Temporal and spatial spectral feature speech emotion recognition algorithm based on trajectory. Computer System Application. 2019;**28**:146-151. DOI: 10.15888/j.cnki.csa.006794

[23] Liu Y, Qin H. The application of speech emotion recognition technology in the field of manned space. In: People's Forum Academic Frontiers. 2018. pp. 69-73. DOI: 10.16619/j.cnki.rmltxsqy.2018.17.008

[24] Tao J, Tan T. Affective Computing: A Review. Berlin, Heidelberg: Springer Berlin Heidelberg; 2005

[25] Castellano G, Villalba SD, Camurri A. Recognising human emotions from body movement and gesture dynamics. In: Paiva ACR, Prada R, Picard RW, editors. Affective Computing and Intelligent Interaction. ACII 2007. Lecture Notes in Computer Science. Berlin, Heidelberg: Springer; 2007. pp. 71-82

[26] Bernhardt D, Robinson P. Detecting Emotions from Everyday Body Movements [EB/OL]. 2007. Available from: https://www.cl.cam.ac.uk/

[27] Liu Y, Liu D, Han Z. Research on emotion extraction method based on motion recognition. Computer Engineering. 2015;**41**:300-305

[28] Shao J, Wang W. Emotion recognition based on three-dimensional texture features of body movement sequences. Journal of Computer Applications. 2018;**35**:3497-3499. DOI: 10.3969 /j.issn.1001-3695.2018.11.071

[29] Hao Y et al. Method of microblog emotion recognition based on word fusion features. Computer Science. 2018;**45**:105-109. DOI: 10.11896/j.issn.1002-137X.2018.11A.018

[30] Hao M et al. Emotion classification and prediction algorithm based on Chinese microblog. Computer Application. 2018;**38**:89-96

[31] Huang F-L et al. Weibo themed emotion mining based on multi-feature fusion. Chinese Journal of Computers. 2017;**40**:872-888. DOI: 10.11897/SP.J.1016.2017.00872

[32] Zhang C, Qian T, Ji D. A joint model of microblogging emotion recognition and incentive extraction based on neural network. Computer Application. 2018;

38:2464-2468+2476. DOI: 10.11772/j.issn.1001-9081.2018020481

[33] James W. The physical basis of emotion. Psychological Review. 1994; **101**(2): 205-210. DOI: 10.1037/0033-295X.101.2.205

[34] Kreibig SD. Autonomic nervous system activity in emotion: A review. Biological Psychology. 2010;**84**: 394-421. DOI: 10.1016/j.biopsycho.2010.03.010

[35] Picard RW, Vyzas E, Healey J. Toward machine emotional intelligence: Analysis of affective physiological state. IEEE Transactions on Pattern Analysis and Machine Intelligence. 2001;**23**: 1175-1191. DOI: 10.1109/34.954607

[36] Kim J, Andre E. Emotion recognition based on physiological changes in music listening. IEEE Transactions on Pattern Analysis and Machine Intelligence. 2008;**30**: 2067-2083. DOI: 10.1109/tpami.2008.26

[37] Yan F, Liu GY, Lai XW. The research on material selection algorithm design with improved OWA in affective regulation system based on human-computer interaction. Journal of Information and Computational Science. 2013;**10**: 4477-4486. DOI: 10.12733/jics20102223

[38] Li C-L, Ye N, Huang H-P, Wang R-C. Physiological signal emotion recognition based on recursive quantitative analysis. Computer Technology and Development. 2018;**28**: 94-98. +102

[39] Jin C, Chen G. Multi-modal physiological signal emotion recognition based on optimized LSTSVM. Application of Electronic Technology. 2018;**44**:112-116. DOI: 10.16157/j.issn.0258-7998.171839

[40] Yong P, Jia-Yi Z, Wei-Long Z, Bao-Liang L. EEG-based emotion recognition with manifold regularized extreme learning machine. In: Proceedings of the 2014 36th Annual International Conference of the IEEE Engineering in Medicine and Biology Society; 26-30 August 2014; Chicago. Chicago, IL: IEEE; 2014. pp. 974-977

[41] Jie X, Cao R, Li L. Emotion recognition based on the sample entropy of EEG. Bio-Medical Materials and Engineering. 2014;**24**:1185-1192. DOI: 10.3233/bme-130919

[42] Duan R-N, Zhu J-Y, Lu B-L. Differential entropy feature for EEG-based emotion classification. In: Proceedings of the 2013 6th International IEEE/EMBS Conference on Neural Engineering (NER); November 2013; San Diego. San Diego, CA: IEEE; 2013. pp. 81-84

[43] Soleymani M, Lichtenauer J, Pun T, Pantic M. A multimodal database for affect recognition and implicit tagging. IEEE Transactions on Affective Computing. 2012;**3**:42-55. DOI: 10.1109/t-affc.2011.25

[44] Koelstra S, Muhl C, Soleymani M, Jong-Seok L, Yazdani A, Ebrahimi T, et al. Deap: A database for emotion analysis using physiological signals. IEEE Transactions on Affective Computing. 2012;**3**:18-31. DOI: 10.1109/t-affc.2011.15

[45] Tai K, Chau T. Single-trial classification of NIRS signals during emotional induction tasks: Towards a corporeal machine interface. Journal of NeuroEngineering and Rehabilitation. 2009;**6**:1-14. DOI: 10.1186/1743-0003-6-39

[46] Mandryk RL, Atkins MS. A fuzzy physiological approach for continuously modeling emotion during interaction with play technologies. International Journal of Human-Computer Studies. 2007;**65**:329-347. DOI: 10.1016/j.ijhcs.2006.11.011

[47] Zhang D, Wan B, Ming D. Research progress on emotion recognition based on physiological signals. Journal of Biomedical Engineering. 2015;**32**: 229-234

[48] Konstantinidis EI, Frantzidis CA, Pappas C, Bamidis PD. Real time emotion aware applications: A case study employing emotion evocative pictures and neuro-physiological sensing enhanced by graphic processor units. Computer Methods and Programs in Biomedicine. 2012;**107**:16-27. DOI: 10.1016/j.cmpb.2012.03.008

[49] Liu Y, Sourina O, Nguyen MK. Real-time EEG-based emotion recognition and its applications. Transactions on Computational Science XII. 2011;**6670**: 256-277. DOI: 10.1007/978-3-642-22336-5_13

[50] D'Mello SK, Kory J. A review and meta-analysis of multimodal affect detection systems. ACM Computing Surveys. 2015;**47**:1-36. DOI: 10.1145/2682899

[51] McGurk H, Macdonald J. Hearing lips and seeing voices. Nature. 1976;**264**: 746-748. DOI: 10.1038/264746a0

[52] Douglas-Cowie E, Cowie R, Sneddon I, Cox C, Lowry O, McRorie M, et al. The HUMAINE data-base: Addressing the collection and annotation of naturalistic and induced emotional data. In: Proceedings of the 2nd International Conference on Affective Computing and Intelligent Interaction. Berlin: Springer Berlin Heidelberg; 2007. pp. 488-500

[53] Douglas-Cowie E, Cowie R, Campbell N. A new emotion database: Considerations, sources and scope. In: Proceedings of the ISCA Workshop on Speech and Emotion; April 2003. Belfast: Textflow; 2000. pp. 39-44

[54] McKeown G, Valstar M, Cowie R, Pantic M, Schroder M. The SEMAINE database: Annotated multimodal records of emotionally colored conversations between a person and a limited agent. IEEE Transactions on Affective Computing. 2012;**3**:5-17. DOI: 10.1109/t-affc.2011.20

[55] Busso C, Bulut M, Lee C-C, Kazemzadeh A, Mower E, Kim S, et al. IEMOCAP: Interactive emotional dyadic motion capture database. Language Resources and Evaluation. 2008;**42**: 335-359. DOI: 10.1007/s10579-008-9076-6

[56] Martin O, Kotsia I, Macq B, Pitas I. The eNTERFACE 05 audio-visual emotion database. In: Proceedings of the 22nd International Conference on Data Engineering Workshops (ICDEW'06); 3-7 April 2006; Atlanta. Atlanta, GA, USA: IEEE; 2006. p. 8

[57] Dhall A, Goecke R, Joshi J, Hoey J, EmotiW GT. Video and group-level emotion recognition challenges. In: Proceedings of the 18th ACM International Conference on Multimodal Interaction—ICMI 2016. ACM Press; 2016. pp. 427-432

[58] Li Y, Tao J, Schuller B, Shan S, Jiang D, MEC JJ. The multimodal emotion recognition challenge of CCPR 2016. In: Tan T, Li X, Chen X, Zhou J, Yang J, Cheng H, editors. Pattern Recognition. CCPR 2016. Communications in Computer and Information Science. Vol. 2016. Singapore: Springer; 2016. pp. 667-678

[59] Gunes H, Piccardi M. A bimodal face and body gesture database for automatic analysis of human nonverbal affective behavior. In: Proceedings of the 18th International Conference on Pattern Recognition (ICPR'06); 20-24 August 2006. Hong Kong: IEEE; 2006. pp. 1148-1153

[60] Gunes H, Piccardi M. Bi-modal emotion recognition from expressive face and body gestures. Journal of

Network and Computer Applications. 2007;**30**:1334-1345. DOI: 10.1016/j.jnca.2006.09.007

[61] Yan J, Zheng W, Xin M, Qiu W. Bimodal emotion recognition based on body gesture and facial expression. Journal of Image and Graphics. 2013;**18**: 1101-1106

[62] Wang W, Shao J. Emotion recognition combining facial expressions and body movement characteristics. Television Technology. 2018;**42**:73-76.+83. DOI: 10.16280/j.videoe.2018.01:014

[63] Wang X, Hou D, Hu M, Ren F. Bimodal emotion recognition of composite spatiotemporal features. Journal of Image and Graphics. 2017;**22**: 39-48. DOI: 10.11834/jig.20170105

[64] Jiang M et al. Bimodal emotion recognition of expressions and postures in video sequences. Progress in Laser and Optoelectronics. 2018;**55**:167-174. DOI: 10.3788/LOP55.071004

[65] Yee CM, Javitt DC, Miller GA. Replacing DSM categorical analyses with dimensional analyses in psychiatry research: The research domain criteria initiative. JAMA Psychiatry. 2015: 1159-1160. DOI: 10.1001/jamapsychiatry.2015.1900

[66] Kraemer HC. Research domain criteria (RDoC) and the DSM-two methodological approaches to mental health diagnosis. JAMA Psychiatry. 2015:1163-1164. DOI: 10.1001/jamapsychiatry.2015.2134

[67] Lindquist KA, Wager TD, Kober H, Bliss-Moreau E, Barrett LF. The brain basis of emotion: A meta-analytic review. The Behavioral and Brain Sciences. 2012;**35**(3):121-143. DOI: 10.1017/S0140525X11000446

[68] Liu Y, Admon R, Belleau EL, Kaiser RH, Clegg R, Beltzer M, et al. Machine learning identifies large-scale reward-related activity modulated by dopaminergic enhancement in major depression. Biological Psychiatry: Cognitive Neuroscience and Neuroimaging. 2020;**5**(2):163-172. DOI: 10.1016/j.bpsc.2019.10.002

[69] Sun YT, Chen T, He D, Dong Z, Cheng B, Wang S, et al. Research progress of biological markers for depression based on psychoradiology and artificial intelligence. Progress in Biochemistry and Biophysics. 2019;**46**: 879-899

[70] Al-Mosaiwi M, Johnstone T. In an absolute state: Elevated use of absolutist words is a marker specific to anxiety, depression, and suicidal ideation. Clinical Psychological Science. 2019;7: 636-637. DOI: 10.1177/216770261 9843297

[71] Liu X, Liu X, Sun J, Yu NX, Sun B, Li Q, et al. Proactive suicide prevention online (PSPO): Machine identification and crisis management for Chinese social media users with suicidal thoughts and behaviors. Journal of Medical Internet Research. 2019;**21**: e11705. DOI: 10.2196/11705

[72] Reece AG, Danforth CM. Instagram photos reveal predictive markers of depression. EPJ Data Science. 2017;**6**:15. DOI: 10.1140/epjds/s13688-017-0118-4

[73] Gavrilescu M, Vizireanu N. Predicting depression, anxiety, and stress levels from videos using the facial action coding system. Sensors (Basel). 2019;**19**(17). DOI: 10.3390/s19173693

[74] Zhu Y, Shang Y, Shao Z, Guo G. Automated depression diagnosis based on deep networks to encode facial appearance and dynamics. IEEE Transactions on Affective Computing. 2018;**9**(4):578-584. DOI: 10.1109/TAFFC.2017.2650899

[75] Harati S, Crowell A, Mayberg H, Kong J, Nemati S. Discriminating

clinical phases of recovery from major depressive disorder using the dynamics of facial expression. In: 38th Annual International Conference of the IEEE Engineering in Medicine and Biology Society (EMBC); January 01, 2016; United States: IEEE. 2016

[76] Cohen AS, Najolia GM, Kim Y, Dinzeo TJ. On the boundaries of blunt affect/alogia across severe mental illness: Implications for research domain criteria. Schizophrenia Research. 2012; **140**(1–3):41-45. DOI: 10.1016/j.schres.2012.07.001

[77] Covington MA, Lunden SLA, Cristofaro SL, Wan CR, Bailey CT, Broussard B, et al. Phonetic measures of reduced tongue movement correlate with negative symptom severity in hospitalized patients with first-episode schizophrenia-spectrum disorders. Schizophrenia Research. 2012;**142**(1): 93-95. DOI: 10.1016/j.schres.2012.10.005

[78] Pan W, Flint J, Shenhav L, Liu T, Liu M, Hu B, et al. Re-examining the robustness of voice features in predicting depression: Compared with baseline of confounders. PLoS One. 2019;**14**:e0218172. DOI: 10.1371/journal.pone.0218172

[79] Haque A, Guo M, Miner AS, Fei-Fei L. Measuring depression symptom severity from spoken language and 3D facial expressions. Sound. 2018;**2**:1-7

[80] Yang L, Jiang D, Sahli H. Integrating deep and shallow models for multi-modal depression analysis—Hybrid architectures. IEEE Transactions on Affective Computing. 2018;**1**:1-16. DOI: 10.1109/TAFFC.2018.2870398

[81] David DeVault RAGB, Georgila K, Gratch J, Hartholt A, Lhommet M, Lucas G, et al. SimSensei kiosk: A virtual human interviewer for healthcare decision support. In: Proceedings of the 13th International Conference on Autonomous Agents and Multiagent Systems (AAMAS 2014). 2014

Chapter 9

Reimagining Attachment Traumas: Perspectives on Using Image-Making in Psychoeducation for People with Borderline Personality Disorder

Dominik Havsteen-Franklin, Maria Patsou, Greta Somaini and Jorge Camarena Altamirano

Abstract

Integrating arts-based practice within psychological interventions has been widely used to increase accessibility and cultural sensitivity and to enable emotional communication and expression. However, using arts within psychoeducation for people with a diagnosis of borderline personality disorder (BPD) where attachment trauma has led to interpersonal difficulties has been less well-documented. This chapter intends to illustrate the experience of patients and facilitators in a mentalization-based psychoeducational programme being delivered in adult mental health services. We will look at the relevance of how images are used to embody relational struggles and how they are used to work through themes of anticipated attachment trauma. We then describe narratives of a 12-week arts-based psychoeducational programme from both the patient and professional perspectives. We conclude that arts-based mentalization focused psychoeducation is a valuable resource for preparing patients with a diagnosis of BPD for further treatment where attachment injury is central to the presenting issues.

Keywords: attachment trauma, borderline personality disorder, art psychotherapy, psychoeducation

1. Introduction

Integrating arts-based practice within psychological interventions has been widely used to increase accessibility and cultural sensitivity and to enable emotional communication and expression. However, using arts within psychoeducation for people with a diagnosis of borderline personality disorder where traumatic events have led to interpersonal difficulties has been less well-documented. This chapter intends to illustrate the experience of patients and facilitators engaging in a mentalization-based psychoeducational programme being delivered in adult mental health services. We will look at the relevance of how images are used to embody relational struggles and how they are used to work through themes of anticipated interpersonal trauma. We then describe narratives of a 12-week arts-based psychoeducational programme from both the patient and professional perspectives.

We present an overview of the rationale of introducing arts-based psychoeducation into a mental health programme for people with a diagnosis of borderline personality disorder (BPD) followed by a description of the structure and a brief vignette of the programme. Finally, we will explore patient perceptions of the programme. All patients are anonymised and have given consent for this material to be published, including any images produced during the sessions. The authors are experienced clinician-researchers and have substantial experience of working within mental health services and related contexts.

1.1 Background

We now know that understanding the relationship between attachment, trauma and affect regulation is central to treating patients with a diagnosis of BPD. Evidence suggests that symptoms of BPD have a multifactorial psychobiological aetiology and include attachment trauma reactions to a range of harmful events, including childhood physical and sexual abuse [1–5], early neglect [6, 7] and invalidation [8]. Attachment traumas in this context refer to an intergenerational disorganised condition of relationship that results in disassociation, high affect arousal 'stemming from fright without solution' [9]. In conditions of affect dysregulation due to experiencing attachment traumas, it is hard for the person to make sense of causal factors, including traumatic events and triggers that may produce reactive high arousal states. Stawarczyk et al. [10] proposed that thought suppression is a key survival mechanism developed to mitigate the effects of predictive processing, particularly in relation to interpersonal events. Given the propensity to evade direct linking between affect arousal and events preceding the arousal, acting out emotional experience within an interpersonal context where attachment traumas are perceived to occur is a core part of the work in the restoration of a capacity to mentalize. Here we are referring to mentalizing as having the capacity to imagine intentional states of mind that influence behaviours, for example, desires, beliefs, feelings and thoughts. This is highly relevant to working with patients with a diagnosis of BPD where there is marked reduction in mentalizing [11] due to high affect arousal [12] and attachment trauma triggers within interpersonal contexts [13]. A mentalization-based verbal group model has been developed with this theoretical premise in mind [14]. Mentalizing begins in early infancy through the mirroring actions of parental care that offers a capacity to sensitise to emotional experiences and develop symbolic representations of self-and other as well as narrativisation and restoration of affective homeostasis [12]. The actions of mentalizing another, that is the attuned awareness of internal states influencing behaviours, enable a secure attachment [15]. Where unsuccessful parental mentalizing happens, for example, misattunements, insensitivity, neglect or abuse, the psychobiological vulnerability of the infant is likewise managed with non-mentalizing behaviours. As the pre-requisite for secure attachment is a capacity to mentalize this can cause transgenerational patterns of insecure attachment and attachment traumas, potentially advancing to conditions of severe avoidance of abandonment, identity disturbance, impulsivity and self-harm. These are symptomatic of severe conditions of non- mentalizing and together are considered to be primary symptoms of borderline personality disorder [16]. Most treatments for borderline personality disorder focus on the restoration of mentalizing and enabling a second-order representational system to become established [11, 17, 18]. Second to this, the development of 'positive thinking' to replace anticipated catastrophe is also considered to be helpful, particularly for impulsive behaviours [19]. Most treatments are medium to long-term and psychoeducation, as a brief intervention is still in the early stages of development for this clinical group. Given that mentalizing involves imagining mental states and developing representations of self and others, the use of image-making as a reflexive tool is proposed as being a helpful addition to the models of BPD treatment. That said, in order to mobilise the process, framing the problem, understanding the aetiology and reflecting on relational patterns of behaviour are a fundamental first step towards engaging with treatment. Whilst the authors are not intending to describe the effectiveness of the process of using art in psychoeducation for this population, the development of a trauma focused model or the long term benefits, the authors are intending to understand what happens when art is used as a focal point within a psychoeducation programme and how it effects people's experiences, self-understanding and the participant's preparedness for psychological treatment.

Psychoeducation is widely used in mental health contexts to help patients to understand living with a diagnosis of borderline BPD [20, 21], how and when presenting issues arise and to consider attachment trauma in the context of interpersonal relationships [22], identity and affect arousal [21]. Further to this, psychoeducation has been used to help impulsivity and suicidality often occurring in relation to attachment traumas [23]. In psychoeducation, participants usually engage between one and 2 hours on a weekly basis for 6–20 weeks. There is some evidence to suggest psychoeducation improves relationships, reducing attachment traumas [22] however the evidence of its effectiveness is limited to feasibility and pilot studies [20–24]. However, the true extent of the use of psychoeducation is not accounted for given that psychoeducation is often part of a psychotherapeutic intervention for borderline personality disorder [25]. Within the context of art psychotherapy this was also clear in a survey conducted by the British Association of Art Therapists [26]; it was evident that 50% of the art therapists that responded used psychoeducation as either a stand-alone intervention or as being integrated within their treatment. Springham and Whittaker [26] reflect on the survey outcomes and conclude that psychoeducation could be a 'crucial unique feature of the practice of art therapy with BPD'. This is also clear in the emerging literature in this field where art psychotherapy methods of practice within a psychoeducational framework are often used alongside conventional methods of treatment [27–31]. For example, Sweig [30] uses a model of arts in psychoeducation and 'the role of art therapy in clarifying issues and mobilizing creative energies in service of personal growth.' Likewise Thorne [32] has published a specific model of using art within a psychoeducational framework for patients diagnosed with BPD similar to the one that we employed, that offers a structured and theme-based approach to engaging in understanding and reflecting upon self- and other-experience. Thorne [23] asserts that the image-making process adds to a psychoeducation model for BPD through enabling emotions and experiences to be more richly expressed and contained.

The theoretical assumption guiding the evaluation was that the use of arts in psychoeducation encourages the patient to view the perceived attachment trauma trigger from a 'distance'. An intolerable, affectively charged trauma can be made more tolerable through seeing it as a human pattern of relating that all people may experience, and hence offering some normalisation according to human functioning [33, 34]. The nature of requesting the participant to see their experience through the lens of human patterns of relating and attachment trauma reactions helps the patient to consider potential aetiological factors. This requires the patient to relate to the subject but also to see the problem as an observer of themselves [35]. Psychoeducation uses a teaching-based model that encourages distance from the trauma and desensitisation to the predicated interpersonal response. We hypothesised that in the proposed model of psychoeducation there is a core mechanism that increases the capacity to reflect on the expected attachment trauma. The second key feature of taking a more distanced view of the attachment trauma, relates to the generalisability of the presenting difficulty. Arts psychotherapies engage the person in thinking about what they are expressing, how it is expressed and how the expression might be received. We propose that introducing arts to a psychoeducation model supports the process of imaginative reflexivity in psychoeducation as a method that enhances the person's capacity to regulate affect and improve relating to the other [36–39]. These features of developing imaginative flexibility are also described as a core mechanism in the capacity to mentalize attachment traumas [34] and therefore we deemed this as a helpful addition to the verbal methods of intervention.

Mentalization-based art psychotherapy is becoming an established method of treatment due to the accessibility, cultural sensitivity and scope for emotional communication and reflection [40, 41]. Mentalization based treatment draws on relational theory from attachment theory [42] and restoring mentalizing in the context of attachment trauma as a key part of the work [43]. The concept of mentalization also has its roots in early dynamic theory and cognitive science [44] and refers to a person's capacity to reflect on self and others' intentional states of mind [45].

2. Arts-based psychoeducation within a mentalization based programme in psychiatry

2.1 Overview of the psychoeducation programme

Arts-based mentalization focused psychoeducation is a 12-week programme developed within a secondary care mental health context as both a standalone intervention and as a preparation for an 18-month arts-based mentalization treatment programme. Patients were offered up to four sessions to assess for presenting issues relating to attachment trauma such as self-harm, identity disturbance and affect dysregulation as well as the patient's motivation for receiving therapy. To understand other stressors, a holistic view to the person's life including family, finance, social factors and a risk assessment were assessed in relation to their potential treatment and was shared with patients as an assessment formulation report co-written with the patient. The facilitators regularly reviewed the formulation with the members throughout the programme. Following this process, the facilitators offered a place on the arts-based psychoeducation programme. The sessions included arts and ran for 1 hour and 30 minutes over 12 weeks. The themes for each week were modelled on the programme designed by Karterud and Bateman [46] that described preparatory sessions for mentalization-based treatment (MBT) [47]:

Week 1: Mentalization and mentalizing stance
Week 2: What does it mean to have problems with mentalizing?
Week 3: Why do we have emotions and what are the core emotions?
Week 4: How do we register and regulate emotions?
Week 5: The significance of attachment relationships
Week 6: Attachment and mentalization
Week 7: What is borderline personality disorder?
Week 8: Mentalization-based arts therapies - Part 1
Week 9: Mentalization-based arts therapies - Part 2
Week 10: Anxiety, attachment and mentalizing
Week 11: Depression, attachment and mentalizing
Week 12: Summary and conclusion, feedback

The facilitators informed participants that the focus of the group would be on how we see ourselves and the way we relate to others and how these perceptions link to early attachment patterns and traumas to those attachments. Group rules, boundaries, confidentiality, respect for others and punctuality were discussed and agreed. Using alcohol, drugs and violence was prohibited in addition to contact between the members of the group, outside of the group. The format of the group included attendance and a refresher of the previous session, presentation and development of the theme of the current session and discussion, image making, feedback and preparation for the next session.

Each session had the purpose of clarifying the concept of mentalization and the point where it can fail, particularly in relation to anticipating attachment traumas and regulating the associated intense affect. The intention of the group was to work with recent attachment traumas, which group members had identified as being emotionally difficult. At the end of the psychoeducation group, there was a collaborative decision made whether further treatment was required.

2.2 Psychoeducation, group work and the clinical process: the art psychotherapists' perspective

The arts were introduced by the fourth author of this chapter and a co-facilitator (both art psychotherapists) to be used in an improvised and explorative way. Materials such as chalks, pens and paints were available to help the patient explore their experience of being in the group in relation to the weekly themes. The narrative uses pseudonyms for the patient names. All members of the group had a primary diagnosis of BPD which had been confirmed through the assessment process. George was a 61 year old, white British man, Henry was a 65 year old white British man, and Dalmar was a 27 year old British Somalian lady.

The artworks were treated as an important part of their personal and group experience and were kept until the end of the 12th session. Over the weeks, the patients' engagement with the arts appeared to develop in emotional complexity, competency and confidence which was reflected in the way they used the arts media. With the presence of anticipated attachment traumas, the arts were also offered as a way of regulating feelings through making doodles or experimental marks when it felt too difficult to reflect on or explore themes. As sessions passed an increasing engagement with the arts was encouraged and there was clear intent to produce figurative drawings with a narrative that related to attachment trauma and how mentalizing could be restored in relation to the themes discussed.

A way of developing initial cohesion in the group was clear in Week 3, in response to the theme of 'Why do we have emotions and what are the core emotions?', George described how his image making on the first week was driven by the curiosity of using the pencil colours that were available, as it gave him an opportunity to 'get a feel for being in a group'. In Week 3, his initial anxieties were reformulated to form rhythmically drawn patterns in distinct shades on the right top corner of the paper (**Figure 1**). The early stage of the work in the group and how the forms co-existed became a strong motif for his experience, where the spaces between people, the nuances of emotions and feelings remained compact and connected in a controlled space. We felt that the patient was using the arts materials to regulate his emotional response to feeling cornered, hemmed into a group where he was uncertain about how people could interact and function without disagreement and the resulting personal trauma and potential disassociation. His marks represented a tapestry like presence where form and colour could coexist in a similar way as his emergent feelings in the group's context.

Similarly, in the same session, Dalmar described her artwork (**Figure 2**) she said that her relationships were like these stone structures that had 'collapsed', 'heavy and helpless', 'immovable' and 'stuck'. These terms are typical of the disorganised attachment state where there is no solution or relational flexibility and ultimately there is a

Figure 1.
'Myself in the group'.

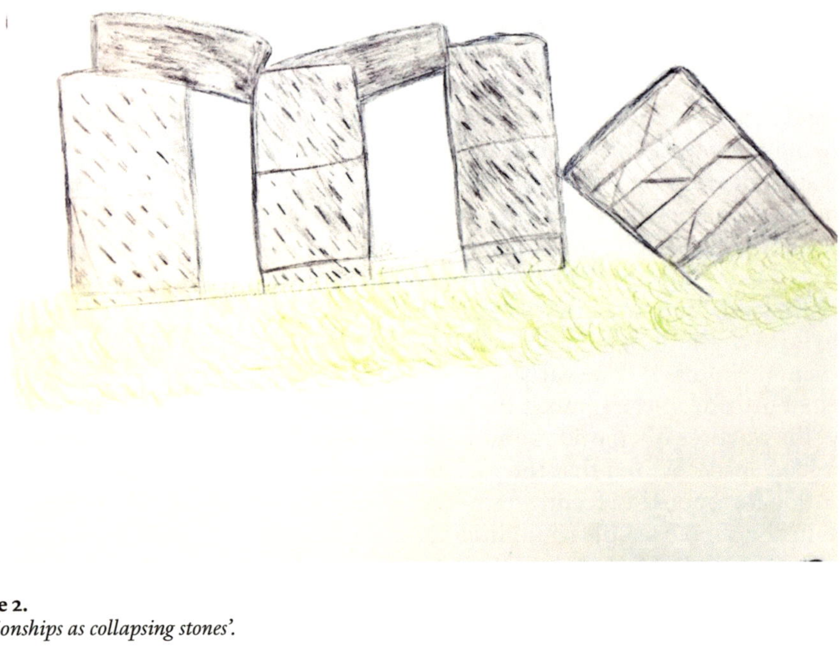

Figure 2.
'Relationships as collapsing stones'.

sense of unresponsive or misattuned neglect. These early images showed a capacity to use image making as a tool for embodying complex emotional narratives that anticipated attachment traumas in ways that could be communicated within a group context.

By Week 3 some group members mentioned how the use of the arts seemed to enable a capacity to be more aware and talk about their mental and emotional processes within an interpersonal context. In **Figures 1** and **2**, the artwork allowed the opportunity to expressively articulate thoughts and emotions that had remained unspoken. In Week 4, 'How do we register and regulate emotions?' One group member (Henry) described his image as the traffic light in the middle of his drawing (**Figure 3**). He used the image to help the group reflect on his anxieties of being out of control, again in a disorganised state where he felt helpless and unwanted. He described the predominant affect as fear, represented by the sunset as a loss of light and something blinding. He described his wish to be like the lamp on the left of the page which he commented on as having a more 'pleasant and balanced quality'. Again, key themes about the rupture to attachments as losing the sun and associated high 'fight or flight' arousal of feeling afraid were at the core of the work.

Using themes to structure sessions helped to enable experiences to be shared. For example, another group member (George) (**Figure 4**) described being 'like the hectic river which was crossing and dividing the urban and green space'. In these early sessions, we focused the content on identifying emotional states and understanding how interpersonal contexts stimulate attachment anxieties about anticipated attachment traumas. In **Figure 4**, George described the urban environment as populated with fragile homes with empty windows, and a mass of green fluidity is sharply divided by an insertion of blue. The powerful disruption also described an intense experience of disconnection that he felt was difficult to bridge due to the uncertainties contained in the green grass of the hill and the disappearing, empty-looking town again drawing on the felt experience of the unavailable and unresponsive others.

The cause of these intolerable conditions of loss of control and disorganised attachment was shared in the group. Dalmar stated that if her family understood her, they would not behave the way they do. Firmly stating, 'It's them that's the problem.' (**Figure 5**).

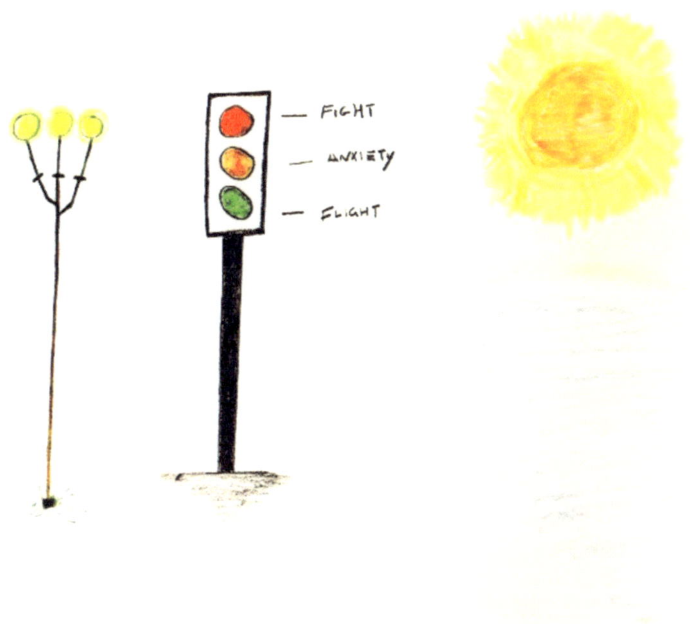

Figure 3.
'Loss of control'.

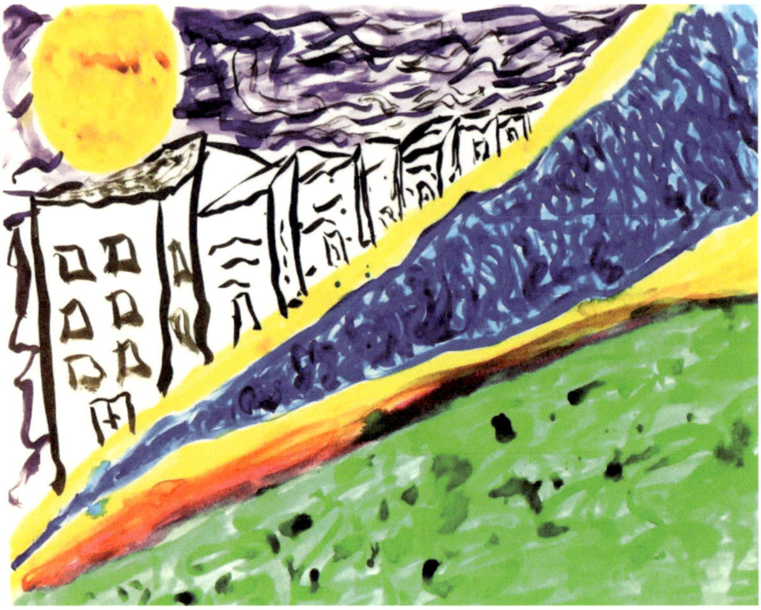

Figure 4.
'I live in the space In-between'.

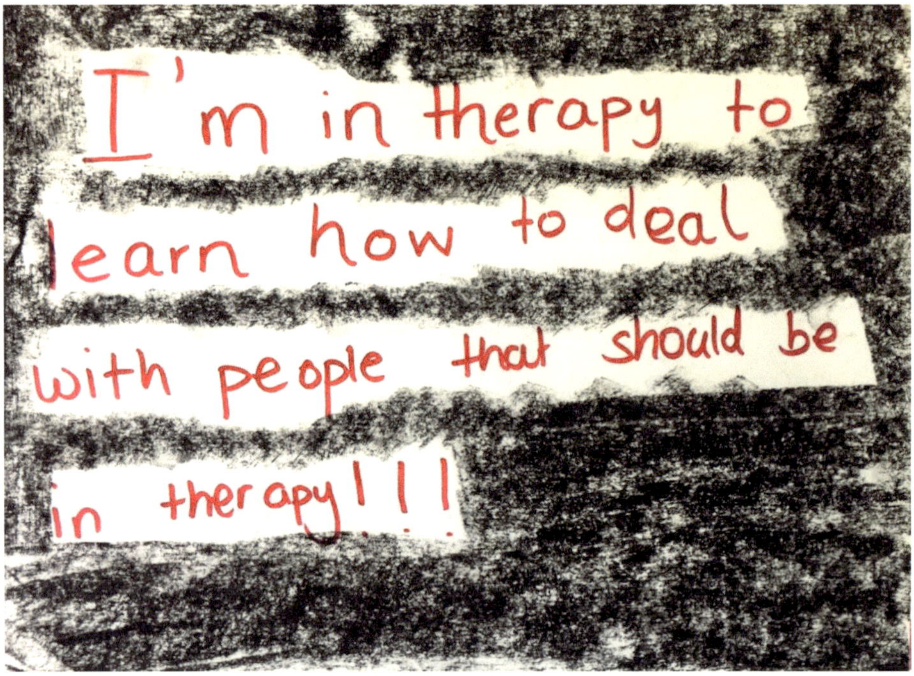

Figure 5.
'It's them that's the problem'.

The same member, later in the work during the session titled, 'Anxiety Attachment and Mentalizing', responded by describing how she manages those states of helplessness and abandonment rather than describing what causes them. She managed painful feelings by harming herself or attempting to overdose on her medication, depicting a blue and white pill in a smudged, surrounded by

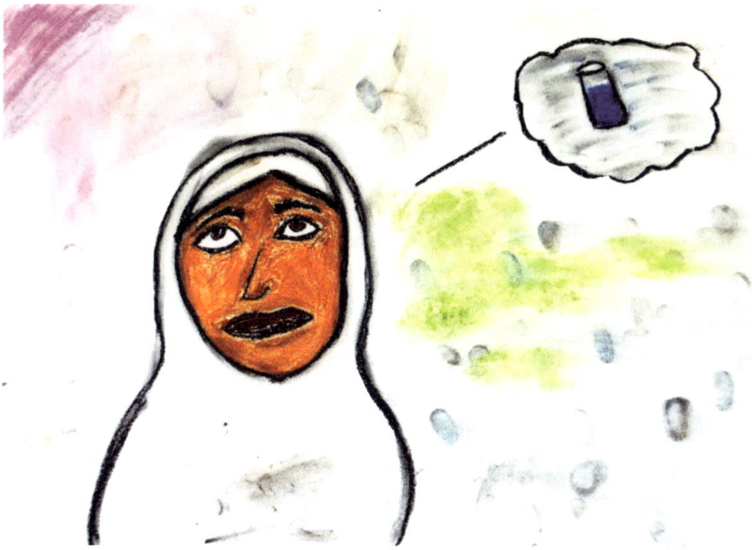

Figure 6.
'When I feel abandoned I can only think about dying'.

fingerprint smudges (**Figure 6**). The theme resonated with the group experience. Several people in the group said that this was the first time that they felt that they were being heard. The sense of having a shared experience within the group session contributed positively to the sense of being held in mind by another and developing a capacity to mentalize the other in the context of anticipated social rupture.

By the end of the 12 weeks, participants were asked to conclude the sessions through sharing thoughts about how they engaged with the use of the arts as a medium to foster reflective thinking about thoughts, emotions, beliefs, and their personal stories.

2.3 Experiences of image-making, affect and relationships: the patient perspective

Following the psychoeducation, all members were invited to give feedback about their experience for the purposes of evaluating the group and for the results to be published. Three members came forward and gave consent for their interview to be published (George, Henry and Dalmar). The interviews were conducted by honorary researchers (authors 2 and 3) who were independent from the programme and who were supervised as part of an early career research initiative [48, 49] founded with the NHS by the first author. Each interview lasted about 1 hour and was semi-structures. Key extracts that appeared to be prevalent or represent the larger themes were extracted and are contextualised within the narrative below.

The first sessions appeared to have a heightened sense of vulnerability and members were tentatively engaging. For example, one member (George.) described drawing an image of a baby without a mother in response to the theme of what it means to have problems with secure attachment, describing the image as having a re-traumatising quality. The image making was originally seen as tentative, bearing no genuine relationship to the psychoeducation, and sometimes felt uncomfortable. Members also expressed cautious engagement through feeling self-conscious and unskilled when using the art media, which they felt expressed a sense of vulnerability and the feeling that using the art media was exposing a sense of vulnerability, feeling like they would fail or not be good enough. For example, one member stuttered and looked embarrassed when she was asked about the use of the art materials.

> *'I did feel slightly embarrassed, but or not embarrassed, but...conscious and conscious that I couldn't draw really that well in that short time.'*

The unexpected effect of the image was often experienced as both offering helpful insight and emotional disturbance. George described how a sense of profound attachment re-traumatisation was immediately evoked,

> *'When [the image], features round something that impacted you like, so bad, so much...When it, when you could see what happened, bulging in front of your eyes... it brought back terrible memories.'*

Henry also expressed an experience of re-traumatisation from being in the presence of others during the group experience whilst attempting to avoid group conflicts. He described an avoidance of unmanageable disorganised attachment arousal in the group that could be provoked by group conflicts to try to keep his stability.

> *'It's just that it might have brought up memories that I didn't want to think about... I'm sort of outside the conflicts... ... [Relationships] can be rocky, chaotic, so again it's a bit like me, I'm stable now but I feel it's a bit fragile...'*

However, in this early stage, there was a sense that the structure could contain and guide, often helped to reduce anxieties through a sense of being in a group with a direction which felt supportive; being held by the frame of the task. Henry stated,

> *'And so to have that...back-up... of other people. Though they, you're not talking... you're, more or less, you know, it's more structured'. Henry said that she had begun to gain a sense of clarity regarding past relationships '[past attachment trauma] is not bothering me so much...cause the only person it's destroying it's me'.*

However, through having a practical task, the sense of accomplishment of improvising was felt to be useful and could express a state of attachment trauma rather than acting out interpersonally. George said that he used the image as a retreat when one he 'could not get a word in'. As the work progressed, members said the image making became more comfortable and automatic, perhaps less pre-meditated, but often members said that the relational tension meant that it was hard to be playful or to improvise. As the work progressed, members began to monitor themselves, restore a capacity to mentalize, using the psychoeducation to make sense of their experience. For example, using images helped Dalmar to reflect on the experience of attachment trauma, exploring what felt like part of an illness and what was felt like a 'normal' response to relationships,

> *'....in relation to like my personality disorder erm ...there is a lot of up and down and stuff... but it's unhealthy but I was just thinking how a lot of it is just normal...'*

As the group progressed, what seems to accompany the image making and inform the process were several key areas directly related to the aims of the group. Members said that image-making was used to reflect on feeling states relating to attachment traumas that had otherwise been considered as overwhelming and this marked the beginning of feeling more trusting of others.

> *'..yeah, my confidence has come back… I think I can trust them, but it's, I…, I don't know, I just don't know.'*

Members also described an experience of image-making as a way of processing over-thinking and an opportunity to make sense of the salient teaching points provided by the facilitator.

> *'I was just feeling reflective like…erm thinking about myself and thinking about what other people were saying I was just sort of processing it in my head and this is how it came out on paper.'*

During the latter sessions they described a growing sense of stability and confidence in themselves and their own agency, which enabled a capacity to be more reflective about other people's states of mind. However, this appeared to be less so with the experience of what motivated other people's actions, which often produced feelings of anxiety or distrust. Two of the participants described having a more structured interpersonal experience where they were trying to unravel their problems and consider ways of reflecting on their experience. For example, one participant stated,

> *'the psychoeducation group has helped me to step back and think about what is happening'.*

Towards the end, members suggested an experience of hope that was linked with an educational 'structure' that enabled people to be together and learn about how they might experience one another and what might cause a perceived attachment trauma. There was also an experience of being together and appreciating each other's struggles, in effect beginning to mentalize the others' experience.

> *'That other people around you, makes you feel comfortable. Make you feel… they're suffering and all. You know, others are in the same predicament as you are.' (George)*

The ending marked a hard transition and whilst the psychoeducation was successful in helping members of the group to reflect on their experience and form tentative relationships, there was also a sense that they were left with uncertainties given the brief period of the group. Members described the first steps towards alternative ways of relating, but they seemed to be left with a fragile footing.

> *'… well, I'm more positive, I'm more positive in myself. I could lose that stability any moment…'*

This brief narrative echoes some similar anxieties as the therapist's account of the session, and overall, the quality and stories of the members felt like a brief but important encounter that opened up the emotionality and contextual issues in relation to their presenting issues. Following the psychoeducation, most members agreed to continue the work of understanding mentalizing in a non-directive mentalization art psychotherapy group.

3. Conclusion

The arts-based psychoeducation offered a structured experiential approach to understanding attachment traumas and mentalizing relationships. The image making seemed to offer powerful access to feelings and experiences that sometimes, and especially at the beginning of the psychoeducation, could be uncomfortable and even 're-traumatising'. The art psychotherapists' perspective of the work provides a comprehensive narrative, highlighting the small but significant positive changes. In the follow-up evaluation we see the patient's autonomy emerging, also describing a tentative grasp of the concepts and emergent alternative forms of relating. We believe that the image-making process facilitated an affective experience of relationships, often revealing vulnerability in safe ways that could be reflected on.

The images offered a powerful account of this process, and particularly the anxieties and uncertainties about developing a secure attachment. The images also revealed anticipated attachment traumas and an invalidating environment, for example in the stuck, rigid invalidating stones; being surrounded by a family that 'should be in therapy'; the constant traffic light 'fight or flight' dance or being stuck in a turbulent place between haunting empty houses and the green grass. Whilst we believe that the use of arts is a valuable tool for communicating, engaging with and reflecting on feeling states; careful, structured and sensitive facilitation is required to maintain safe and effective practice especially where the focus is on how therapists facilitate brief educational work focusing on attachment trauma.

This study revealed that the psychoeducation can expose deep relational vulnerabilities, where the principal focus for members had often been to manage pain in isolation. Perhaps most importantly, the emergent capacity for group members to recover from attachment trauma and to restore mentalizing indicated that there was the conceptual and reflective infrastructure that formed the foundations for further work and would enable members to engage with explorative forms of psychotherapy.

Acknowledgements

The authors would like to thank the following people for their dedication to the development of the programme as honorary researchers: Charlotte Barker, Kirstin Leyton-Boyce, Dr. Jennifer Townell and the participants for their commitment to the project.

Conflict of interest

The authors declare no conflict of interest.

Author details

Dominik Havsteen-Franklin[1]*, Maria Patsou[2], Greta Somaini[2] and Jorge Camarena Altamirano[2]

1 CNWL NHS Foundation Trust, Brunel University, London, UK

2 CNWL NHS Foundation Trust, London, UK

*Address all correspondence to: dominik.havsteen-franklin@nhs.net

References

[1] Bailey JM, Shriver A. Does childhood sexual abuse cause borderline personality disorder? Journal of Sex & Marital Therapy. 1999;**25**(1):45-57

[2] Bornovalova MA, Huibregtse BM, Hicks BM, Keyes M, McGue M, Iacono W. Tests of a direct effect of childhood abuse on adult borderline personality disorder traits: A longitudinal discordant twin design. Journal of Abnormal Psychology. 2013;**122**(1):180

[3] Fossati A, Madeddu F, Maffei C. Borderline personality disorder and childhood sexual abuse: A meta-analytic study. Journal of Personality Disorders. 1999;**13**(3):268-280

[4] Howell EF. Back to the "states" victim and abuser states in borderline personality disorder. Psychoanalytic Dialogues. 2002;**12**(6):921-957

[5] Trull TJ. Structural relations between borderline personality disorder features and putative etiological correlates. Journal of Abnormal Psychology. 2001;**110**(3):471-481. DOI: 10.1037/0021-843X.110.3.471

[6] Widom CS, Czaja SJ, Paris J. A prospective investigation of borderline personality disorder in abused and neglected children followed up into adulthood. Journal of Personality Disorders. 2009;**23**(5):433-446

[7] Wildschut M, Swart S, Langeland W, Smit JH, Draijer N. An emotional neglect–personality disorder approach: Quantifying a dimensional transdiagnostic model of trauma-related and personality disorders. Journal of Personality Disorders. 2020;**34**(2):250-261

[8] Rosenthal MZ, Cheavens JS, Lejuez CW, Lynch TR. Thought suppression mediates the relationship between negative affect and borderline personality disorder symptoms. Behaviour Research and Therapy. 2005;**43**(9):1173-1185

[9] Allen JG. Restoring Mentalizing in Attachment Relationships: Treating Trauma with Plain Old Therapy. Washington DC, US & London, UK: American Psychiatric Publishing; 2012

[10] Stawarczyk D, Bezdek MA, Zacks JM. Event representations and predictive processing: The role of the midline default network core. Topics in Cognitive Science; 2019. Wiley Online Library. Available from: https://onlinelibrary.wiley.com/doi/abs/10.1111/tops.12450 [Accessed: 07 August 2020]

[11] Bateman A, Fonagy P. Mentalization based treatment for borderline personality disorder. World Psychiatry. 2010;**9**(1):11-15

[12] Fossati A, Feeney J, Maffei C, Borroni S. Thinking about feelings: Affective state mentalization, attachment styles, and borderline personality disorder features among Italian nonclinical adolescents. Psychoanalytic Psychology. 2014;**31**:41-67

[13] Fonagy P, Target M, Gergely G, Allen JG, Bateman AW. The developmental roots of borderline personality disorder in early attachment relationships: A theory and some evidence. Psychoanalytic Inquiry. 2003;**23**(3):412-459

[14] Karterud S. Mentalization-Based Group Therapy (MBT-G): A Theoretical, Clinical, and Research Manual. Oxford: OUP; 2015. Available from: https://books.google.co.uk/books?hl=en&lr=&id=lUpoCgAAQBAJ&oi=fnd&pg=PP1&dq=karterud+group+MBT&ots=025IZcQFW5&sig=5B-V_Bl0kROHFoN7GrP41nkC42E [Accessed: 02 August 2017]

[15] Kelly K, Slade A, Grienenberger JF. Maternal reflective functioning, mother–infant affective communication, and infant attachment: Exploring the link between mental states and observed caregiving behavior in the intergenerational transmission of attachment. Attachment & Human Development. 2005;**7**(3):299-311

[16] Grant BF, Chou SP, Goldstein RB, Huang B, Stinson FS, Saha TD, et al. Prevalence, correlates, disability, and comorbidity of DSM-IV borderline personality disorder: results from the Wave 2 National Epidemiologic Survey on Alcohol and Related Conditions. The Journal of Clinical Psychiatry. 2008;**69**(4):533

[17] Holmes J. Mentalizing from a psychoanalytic perspective: What's new. In: Handbook of Mentalization-Based Treatment; 2006. pp. 31-49

[18] UK NCC for MH. Borderline Personality Disorder: Treatment and Management. British Psychological Society; 2009. Available from: https://www.ncbi.nlm.nih.gov/pubmed/21796831 [Accessed: 04 July 2017]

[19] Swales HLH. Linehan's dialectical behaviour therapy (DBT) for borderline personality disorder: Overview and adaptation. Journal of Mental Health. 2000;**9**(1):7-23

[20] Allen JG, Kelly KA, Glodich A. A psychoeducational program for patients with trauma-related disorders. Bulletin of the Menninger Clinic. 1997;**61**(2):222

[21] Banerjee P, Duggan C, Huband N, Watson N. Brief psychoeducation for people with personality disorder: A pilot study. Psychology and Psychotherapy: Theory, Research and Practice. 2006;**79**(3):385-394

[22] Groat M, Allen JG. Promoting mentalizing in experiential psychoeducational groups: From agency and authority to authorship. Bulletin of the Menninger Clinic. 2011;**75**(4):315-343

[23] Bergmans Y, Links PS. A description of a psychosocial/psychoeducational intervention for persons with recurrent suicide attempts. Crisis: The Journal of Crisis Intervention and Suicide Prevention. 2002;**23**(4):156

[24] Cavanaugh MM. An Exploration of the Feasibility and Utility of the Dialectical Psychoeducational Workshop (DPEW) as a Preventative Intervention for Males at Potential Risk of Intimate Partner Violence. Pennsylvania, US: University of Pennsylvania; 2007

[25] Gunderson JG. Handbook of Good Psychiatric Management for Borderline Personality Disorder. Washington DC, US: American Psychiatric Publishing; 2014

[26] Springham N, Whitaker R. How do art therapists structure their approach to borderline personality disorder? The Arts in Psychotherapy. 2015;**43**:31-39

[27] Silverman MJ. The effect of single-session psychoeducational music therapy on verbalizations and perceptions in psychiatric patients. Journal of Music Therapy. 2009;**46**(2):105-131

[28] Silverman MJ. Psychiatric patients' perception of music therapy and other psychoeducational programming. Journal of Music Therapy. 2006;**43**(2):111-122

[29] Summer D, Soble L, Scott-Moncrieff S, Senroy P, Senroy S, Hodermarska M, et al. Healing the Inner City Child: Creative Arts Therapies with At-Risk Youth. London and Philadelphia: Jessica Kingsley Publishers; 2007

[30] Sweig TL. Women healing women: Time-limited, psychoeducational

group therapy for childhood sexual abuse survivors. Art Therapy. 2000;**17**(4):255-264

[31] Weinberg DJ. The potential of rehabilitative computer art therapy for the quadriplegic, cerebral vascular accident and brain trauma patient. Art Therapy. 1985;**2**(2):66-72

[32] Thorne D. Portrait of self and other. In: Hughes R, editor. Time-Limited Art Psychotherapy: Developments in Theory and Practice. London and New York: Routledge; 2016. pp. 92-118

[33] Morton S, Hohman M. "That's the weight of knowing": Practitioner skills and impact when delivering psychoeducational group work for women who have experienced IPV. Social Work with Groups. 2016;**39**(4):277-291

[34] Rivera ET, Fernández IT, Hendricks WA. Psychoeducational and counseling groups with Latinos. In: DeLucia-Waack J, Kalodner C, Riva M, editors. Handbook of Group Counseling and Psychotherapy. Thousand Oaks, CA, US: SAGE Publications; 2004. pp. 213-223

[35] Khalil GE. Understanding the User Experience and Emotional Involvement during eHealth Interventions: A Randomized Controlled Trial of ASPIRE. New York, US: State University of New York at Buffalo; 2015. Available from: https://search.proquest.com/openview/e9fd0bdd8e4cc5f91bc62c47c69c8fd1/1?pq-origsite=gscholar&cbl=18750&diss=y [Accessed: 07 August 2020]

[36] Collet P. Reflexivity and agency: A study of women's careers in the visual arts as a basis for reflection in art education. Australian Art Education. 1998;**21**(2):20

[37] McCaffrey R, Frock TL, Garguilo H. Understanding chronic pain and the mind-body connection. Holistic Nursing Practice. 2003;**17**(6):281-289

[38] McCaffrey T, Edwards J. Meeting art with art: Arts-based methods enhance researcher reflexivity in research with mental health service users. Journal of Music Therapy. 2015;**52**(4):515-532

[39] Weber S, Mitchell C. Art for accessibility: Art as activism; art for reflexivity; arts informed. 2004;**3**(2):7-19

[40] Havsteen-Franklin D. Mentalization-based art psychotherapy. In: Rubin J, editor. Approaches to Art Therapy Theory and Techniques. New York: Brunner/Mazel; 2016. pp. 144-164

[41] Havsteen-Franklin D. Creative arts therapies. In: Bateman AW, Fonagy P, editors. Handbook of Mentalizing in Mental Health Practice. 2nd ed. Washington, DC, US: American Psychiatric Publishing; 2019. pp. 181-197

[42] Bowlby J. Attachment theory and psychotherapy research. The Journal of Psychotherapy Practice and Research. 2001;**10**(2):133

[43] Allen JG, Fonagy P, Bateman A. The role of mentalizing in treating attachment trauma. In: Vermetten E, Lanius RA, editors. The Hidden Epidemic: The Impact of Early Life Trauma on Health and Disease. New York: Cambridge University Press; 2010. pp. 247-256

[44] Fonagy P, Luyten P, Bateman A, Gergely G, Strathearn L, Target M, et al. Attachment and personality pathology. In: Psychodynamic Psychotherapy for Personality Disorders: A Clinical Handbook. Washington DC and London: American Psychiatric Publishing; 2010. pp. 37-88

[45] Fonagy P. The mentalization-focused approach to social development. In: Busch FN, editor. Mentalization. New York, US and Hove, UK: The Analytic Press and Taylor & Francis Group; 2006. pp. 3-56

[46] Karterud S, Bateman A. Manual for Mentalization Based Psychoeducational Group Therapy (MBT-I). Oslo: Gyldendal akademisk; 2011

[47] Bateman A, Fonagy P. Mentalization-based treatment. Psychoanalytic Inquiry. 2013;**33**:595-613

[48] Havsteen-Franklin D, Maratos A, Usiskin M, Heagney M. Examining arts psychotherapies practice elements: Early findings from the Horizons Project. Approaches. 2016;**8**. Available from: http://approaches.gr/havsteen-franklin-a20160324/ [Accessed: 04 November 2016]

[49] The Horizons Project – Honorary Arts Psychotherapies Clinical Research Posts - CNWL [Internet]. Available from: http://www.cnwl.nhs.uk/health-professionals/icapt/the-horizons-project/ [Accessed: 12 September 2014]

Section 3

Social Aspects

Chapter 10

Amnesia among Indigenous Australians

Alison Husain

Abstract

Looking at the incidence of amnesia in Australian indigenous people who have experienced a legacy of intergenerational trauma and psycho-social traumas in childhood such as psychological, sexual and physical abuse, domestic violence, substance abuse, out-of-home care, and over-policing, this chapter will consider the impact of trauma-based amnesia from the perspective of social neuroscience in relation to the frequency of incidence derived from data on reported mood and neurotic group disorders to draw insights into the epidemiology of psychogenic amnesia among indigenous Australians. This chapter will also consider cultural implications as health is not just a physiological or mental status of an individual but encompasses social, emotional, and cultural connectedness which amnesia disrupts. This research seeks to create better understanding as to the causal attributes of more prevalent levels of suffering among indigenous Australians as compared to non-indigenous Australians.

Keywords: amnesia, psycho-social trauma, intergenerational trauma, indigenous Australians, mental health, epidemiology, dissociative and psychogenic amnesia

1. Introduction

While much research has been undertaken on the neural mechanisms and effect of trauma-induced amnesia, it is suggested that much less attention has been applied to the more covert and pervasive types of trauma and long-term effects of psychogenic amnesia among indigenous Australians. This chapter is essentially a study in the application of social neuroscience in the psycho-social trauma frequently associated with childhood. The objective of this social neuroscience research is to understand the epidemiology of amnesia and related neurophysiological systems that underpin the traumatic social background of indigenous Australians, and is intended to further understanding.

This article analyses themes underlying the causes of childhood trauma, considers the impact leading to amnesia, available diagnosis and mitigation. The material was informed by a review of epidemiological literature on psycho-social trauma present in indigenous Australians with consideration given to international literature to determine the elements of collective and mass trauma studies which correlate to indigenous communities in Australia. Psychogenic amnesia as a specific mental disorder has not been recorded in the data history of indigenous and non-indigenous hospitalizations. Consideration has therefore been given to the group of mood and neurotic disorders within which psychogenic amnesia lies in particular arising from stress levels. This article will contemplate memory disorders by considering memory disturbances, relationships to functionality and frequency, before turning to aspects of therapeutic interventions and culturally safe approaches.

The use of social neuroscience in exploring the incidence of amnesia caused by emotional and psychological trauma among indigenous Australians will provide broader consideration of the causal attributes of more prevalent levels of suffering among indigenous Australians as compared to non-indigenous Australians [1]. Social neuroscience perspectives on childhood trauma unite the concept that the brain responds to stress and abuse, as social behaviors stem from brain development [2]. Consideration may then be given to development of best therapeutic practices to promote healing and recovery from the damage caused to brain development by adverse experiences.

1.1 Background

It cannot be emphasized enough that the colonialist practices of dispossession, child removal, suppression of indigenous social practices, stolen heritages and oppressive government policies, resulted in long-term intergenerational trauma that is still experienced today [3]. Ongoing social inequalities are particularly apparent across health outcomes [4, 5].

Current statistics indicate there are approximately 800,000 indigenous Australians, equating to 2.8% of the Australian population [6] (**Figure 1**).

The health and welfare outcomes are significantly disproportionate as indigenous Australians experience disease at a far higher rate than non-indigenous Australians. Of these diseases, the group of mental health disorders has one of the highest disparity ratio. This group represents disorders relating to stress, anxiety, depression, alcohol and drug use, and the autism spectrum [5]. To understand the impact of trauma, the issues raised above may be viewed through Historical Trauma theory. This conceptual theory is based on the premise that where a particular population has been historically subjected to long periods of mass trauma

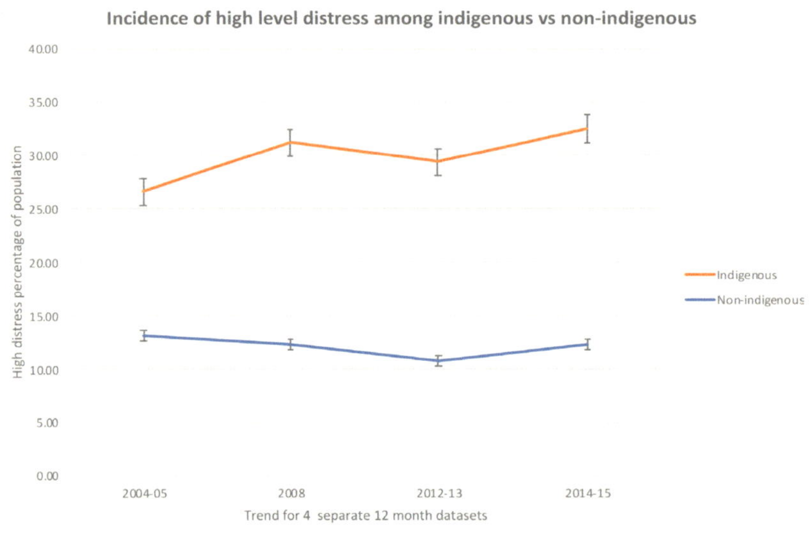

Figure 1.
Incidence of higher levels of distress among indigenous Australians compared to non-indigenous population. For indigenous Australians, the comparative distress levels are not only higher for all the four reported time periods but also show a trend of increasing levels of disparity for each consecutive period. Data for this chart were derived from Australian government report: Overcoming indigenous disadvantage 2016 [7].

(such as colonialism, genocide, slavery, and abuse) then higher incidents of poor health outcomes remain present for many generations to follow [8]. In Australia, this is evidenced by the health disparities currently present [9, 10]. Once primary trauma occurs, the intergenerational effect is amplified by the risks associated with increased vulnerability to secondary trauma identified above. As a result, a pattern of trauma is often established in family and community groups which can be viewed through the current statistics that evidence Australian indigenous children end up in out-of-home care at a greater rate than non-indigenous children and disproportionately high rates of fatal self-harm [11, 12].

1.2 Methodology

For this review, research papers were retrieved from the following databases and search engines: the Centre for Independent Studies (CIS), ProQuest, PubMed, ScienceDirect, Scopus, and Springer Link. The following: "trauma," "childhood trauma," "intergenerational trauma," "indigenous," "aboriginal," "retrograde amnesia of psychogenic origins," "dissociative and psychogenic amnesia," "mental health," "indigenous connection to country" together with "quantitative," "statistical" and "social neuroscience" were used as keywords to filter results. Other keywords to filter results were "over policing," "detention," and "close the gap." Search areas were restricted to clinical neurological science and sociology reporting on amnesia across indigenous Australians with results analyzed on the basis of the last two decades, geographical location, and types of intervention. Statistical evidence was sought from the Australian Bureau of Statistics (ABS) National Health Survey, 2014–2015, National Aboriginal and Torres Strait Islander Social Survey, 2014–2015 and Australian Institute of Health and Welfare (AIHW). Criteria for inclusion in this review were studies from the last two decades to capture political and social changes and were written in the English language. When the effect of mass trauma was analyzed for indigenous Australians on the basis of population and global geographical location, it was observed that New Zealand studies were most relevant to this review.

The exclusion criteria were reviews outside recent neurological memory loss and general indigenous research not relevant to Australian indigenous issues and papers not written in English. Research papers were also limited based on health specific records, identification of indigenous people, diagnosis mixed with other preexisting conditions. Also excluded, were reviews relating to memory loss as a result of accidents, sports, and direct physical damage to the brain, as the scope of this article focusses upon retrograde amnesia of psychogenic origins.

Data used in this article has been derived from Australian Government sources with the figures extrapolated from mental health statistics, in particular mood and neurotic disorders in which dissociative and psychogenic amnesia appears to draw conclusions.

1.3 Results

Indigenous Australians have a higher incidence of distress indicative of social and psychological trauma than non-indigenous Australians. The legacy of trauma continues to exist in indigenous life with lived experience of psychological, sexual and physical abuse (including domestic violence), alcohol and substance abuse, over-policing, dissociation from family due to out-of-home care, continuing discrimination and racism, perpetuating the cycle. The effects are hard to quantify as directly supporting statistical evidence is limited [9, 10]. The greater incidence of distress trauma present in indigenous communities correlates to a higher incidence of amnesia compared to non-indigenous counterparts.

2. Key concepts in memory and related losses: amnesia

To better understand the nature of memory and how memory loss occurs in various types of amnesia, existing knowledge about human memory and a description of the various types of amnesia relevant to this article are set out below.

2.1 Memory

All memory types have two dimensions, time and content. Considering the time dimension, memory is categorized into a further four categories based on its content. Firstly, the shortest term memory type, which lasts a second or less, described as sensory memory, here sensory receptors capture the sensation momentarily to be filed into a longer-term memory section [13]. There are five sensory receptors which provide input to sensory memory: iconic or visual, echoic or auditory, haptic or touch-based, olfactory or smell related, and a taste receptor. Secondly, there is working memory, also referred to as primary or active memory which last less than a minute. Thirdly, there is the long-term memory, the loss of which is essentially the primary subject of this article [13]. The contents of long-term memory are categorized into two main types; one is explicit or conscious memory, sometimes also referred to as declarative memory, and implicit or unconscious memory, also known as procedural memory. The explicit or conscious memory is generally subtyped into episodic memory where events and experience are recorded; and semantic memory where general facts and concepts are recorded. Episodic memory is referred to episodic autobiographical memory (EAM), if the episode recorded relates to personal experiences [14, 15].

Other memory types such as prospective memory relate to processing future tasks and have little to do with recollection of past events. Autonoetic consciousness, however, is regarded as an anchor, or sense of self, in that all past experiences or exposures over a person's lifetime are able to be retrieved and reflected upon [14, 16]. Conversely, semantic memory refers to the process of collecting general knowledge, allowing for recall of rudimentary facts and common knowledge, learned during the course of an individual's existence, not drawn from personal experiences but is interconnected with culture [14].

Independent case studies have demonstrated that both episodic and semantic memories may be lost and, given the right time and circumstances, these memories may be recovered at a later date [14]. In one case it was observed that a patient experiencing retrograde amnesia caused by a mild head trauma exacerbated by work stressors was unable to access episodic and semantic memories. Over a period of several months, the patient was observed to be able to recall some semantics until full access to his blocked memories was established. In this case, to determine full recovery the patient was required to demonstrate competency in three faculties; ability to sense time, be aware of subjective autonoetic chronology and be aware of the presence of his own self through that chronology [14]. Neuroscience research relating to the experience, absorption, and memory of various episodes in life has found little evidence of early infantile episodic memory and given the development of the brain, early episodic and autobiographical memory during infancy does not happen. It is generally agreed that these memories occur after the age of 3 years [15].

For indigenous Australians, associations with family, community, land and wellbeing are crucial; individual land ownership is not an indigenous concept. Memories are formed through "storytelling" as a form of continuous oral tradition of recording and preserving history and importance of connection to land and country [17]. Intimate knowledge of country forms a strong connection that is inherent to indigenous identity and sustains wellbeing across spiritual, physical, social and cultural perspectives. Caring for country means participating in interrelated activities which aim to promote ecological, spiritual and human health and wellbeing. Loss of autonoetic consciousness interrupts such connection to country and as such, impacts upon health and wellbeing, not just for an individual but often for a community [1, 18]. The impact of amnesia results in lost inheritance for future generations.

2.2 Amnesia

Whilst it is acknowledged that memory loss may occur as a result of accidents, sports, and direct physical damage to the brain, the scope of this article is centered upon retrograde amnesia of psychogenic origins. Retrograde amnesia is the inability to recall long-term memory, mainly episodic and autobiographical, and is caused by extreme psychological trauma typified by that experienced by indigenous Australians [19]. In severe cases, anterograde amnesia may occur preventing the formation of any further memories after the experience of an episode of severe psychogenic trauma and, although atypical, may also be accompanied by loss of semantic and factual memories [19]. Dissociative amnesia, a subtype of psychogenic amnesia, is usually triggered by a traumatic event and is illustrated by retrospective memory gaps, the inability to recall personal information, often of a traumatic or stressful nature and is too explicit to be ascribed to forgetfulness or fatigue [20]. This article will also specifically consider indigenous childhood trauma of psychogenic origins that causes the removal of painful memories from parts of the brain that are responsible for memory function. The removal of such painful memories is considered a defense mechanism to extreme emotional and psychological stress. Dissociative amnesia may also have accompanying indications of depression and anxiety, with associated displays of impulsive aggressive behaviour, self-mutilation and suicidal ideation [21, 22].

2.2.1 History of amnesia

Historically, incidents of amnesia associated with memory lapses and forgetfulness have been linked to physical, emotional, and spiritual welfare and often hypothesized through a philosophical lens [23]. Historically, memory loss was attributed to neurological disorders and physical head injuries, metabolic dysregulation, substance abuse, other acute or chronic brain illnesses. Following much debate, amnesia was identified as a memory disorder with further specificity distinguishing retrograde and anterograde categories [23]. Amnesia as a clinical feature was critical to the development of notions of dissociation of conscious from subconscious recall, and differentiation of neurogenically-based from psychogenic-based amnesia became central to understanding post-traumatic states [21].

2.2.2 Neurological observations of stress-related amnesia

Memory functionality has been found to improve when events recorded by the brain are emotionally arousing. These events tend to enable the human brain to absorb and recall events more effectively, over a longer period of time. The use of corticosteroids or cortisol, the main form of long-term stress hormones, has been considered to enhance or increase the brain's memory capacity [24]. Conversely, persistently high levels of the stress hormone cortisol, common among indigenous people can be detrimental to long-term health, mental health and, wellbeing of the individual and community [25, 26]. Episodic memory appears to be affected when the Hypothalamus-pituitary-adrenal (HPA) axis records higher amounts of glucocorticoids, released from the adrenal cortex, when stress is experienced which impacts the regions inside the brain. Central to the above is that episodic memory is not just impaired, but more specifically its access and retrieval is temporarily blocked [27].

2.2.3 Beneficial effects of amnesia

The repression of memory, whether consciously practiced or chemically induced, is considered to be a suitable coping mechanism for trauma-related or acute stress and has been observed to be good practice for sufferers of myocardial infarction [28]. The benefits of memory repression were realized whilst researching prevention, delayed onset, or reduction in the severity of post-traumatic stress disorders (PTSD) [29]. Although trauma-induced amnesia does not increase a person's functionality, intellect or powers of execution, it has been found to reduce stress disorders. The defense mechanism in the brain that induces amnesia after a severe episode of trauma has the protective effect of reducing the likelihood of PTSD, autism spectrum disorder and other associated side effects [29].

2.2.4 Treatments of psychogenic and dissociative amnesia

No agreed treatment is available for psychogenic dissociative amnesia nor any methodology in place that may lead to rehabilitation. It is suggested that this is one area where complimentary intensive research in neurophysiology may improve understanding of the disorder and produce a feasible solution to improve the quality of life for those afflicted [30]. The inherent danger in dissociative amnesia is that it statistically points to increased risk of self-harm, suicide, and life-long loss of cognitive functionality. The detection and prevalence of dissociative amnesia varies broadly nationally and internationally, making it harder to define and detect let alone attempt to mitigate its effects [30].

Consequently, this article will correlate neurophysiological research with social and demographic research pertaining to indigenous Australians to detect the presence and epidemiology of psychogenic amnesiacs. The platform of social neuroscience, where such convergence occurs, is considered a suitable area of study as outlined further below.

3. Social neuroscience and its relevance

Humans are social in nature and create evolving social structures based on an individual social grouping and the creation and evolution of accompanying cultures. These social structures have influenced the evolution of human neurobiological systems and accompanying effects on genes, cells, neural networks, and hormones. Social neuroscience is a study of the connection of the two systems as they coexist and co-influence [31]. Human neurobiological makeup has assisted in the various social constructs humans have built around themselves, which have then influenced and mutated human biology [31]. Social neuroscience is a relatively new area of academic inquiry which allows for greater understanding into the co-dependency and confluence of biological and social sciences. Insights into the cause and effect of psychological events on human neurophysiology validate the need for further research into social neuroscience [32].

Neuroscience research provides evidence that traumatic psychogenic amnesia, not directly associated with physical brain damage, impacts upon brain functions following the use of a neuroimaging technique called positron emission tomography (PET) [33]. It has been observed that a psychogenic amnesiac has different parts of the brain activated compared to non-amnesiacs in that the amygdala and other regions of the brain showed increased activity [19]. This leads to the suggestion that limbic functions and limbic cortical functions are affected by psychogenic amnesia and in case studies, patients recorded as having experienced traumatic psychogenic amnesia, also demonstrate cognitive impairments in attention, execution and intellectual capabilities [34].

4. Social, community and belief considerations

Research into trauma related amnesia in relation to indigenous people can be a sensitive issue. Much has been written about indigenous health with criticism around the research methodology, theoretical perspectives, and evaluations of programs. It is clear the "closing the gap" strategy is struggling to have a major impact on the ambitious targets set by the Australian Government [35]. Reflective practices between cultures often present different philosophical and theoretical perspectives and discrete communication and language add complexity to the problems faced. The interpretation of incidence of amnesia among indigenous Australians can aggravate the segregation of the two cultures [36]. Interventions should be in the context of the use of traditional learning processes to view health and wellbeing from traditional healing perspectives with sound solutions for the future [36]. Comparative New Zealand research into therapeutic interventions for indigenous mental health, demonstrated that treatment based on the premise that a holistic view of wellbeing which is congruent with culture, customs and values integrating aspects of spirituality, provides a greater individual sense of self and place, and should be considered in any treatment plan [37].

Within the last decade, there appears to have been a shift in the narrative around acknowledging that not all aspects of indigenous culture is positive. Recent discourse by prominent female indigenous leaders has provided a sincere snapshot into some of the continuing health issues [38]. It is conceded that indigenous communities are often desensitized to a culture of violence, with many assaults going unreported, and violence deemed the norm [39]. It is also felt that the very nature of the traditional culture continues to maintain the dominant rights for men to control women [38]. These adverse aspects of culture are regarded as detrimental to finding solutions to better health outcomes.

There is an urgent need for better evaluation of indigenous policies and programs nationally to assess outcomes. There is a lack of reliable national data reporting on how health and wellbeing measures are based. Evidence shows that when programs are well researched, supported by effective community targeting and engagement, then outcomes are positive [39]. One example of this is in relation to petrol sniffing and the implementation of OPAL fuel (a low aromatic fuel) substitution for petrol. This program resulted in a dramatic reduction in ailments arising from petrol sniffing [40]. Improved data collection around patient consultation, diagnosis, referrals to specialists, and outcome of referrals is required to better understand the impact of amnesia [41].

The concept of culture plays an important part in both the social and biological sciences as culture enables a community to make sense of their world and impacts treatment outcomes. Research provides that the biogenetic, environmental and cultural influences impact collectively on cognitive development affecting behaviour [42]. It cannot be emphasized enough that through culture, people are able to place themselves and self-identify, as such traditional healing methods should form part of health strategies and be framed through cultural messaging [43]. It has been suggested that two fields of research practice have dominated debates around health and wellbeing, one view suggests that factors such as income, socioeconomic hierarchy, and social status provide indicators of risk of disease, the second view, held by health psychologists, anthropologists and sociologists, is that risk of disease is associated with stressors and the ability of an individual or community to cope with such stressors [32]. Therefore health and wellbeing are impacted by historical legacies and politics; and the passage of time directly affects how culture shapes health trends in relation to indigenous people.

5. Incidence, detection, and impact of amnesia

Testing for amnesia is often unreliable as it is frequently associated with cognitive dysfunction identified through impairment of learning and executive functions [44]. Cognitive dysfunction is also ubiquitous with high rates of poor health, diseases, substance abuse, domestic violence, psychological stress, and trauma, as reported widely among indigenous Australians. Tests are also often based on Western premise and not tuned for cultural nuances [45]. Alcohol and substance abuse, in general, is one of the most reported concerns among indigenous Australians with misuse often resulting in impairment and toxic harm to organs and tissues, with premature aging and death. Being in a state of intoxication diminishes coordination, cognition, perception and promotes dependency [46]. It has been established that alcohol abuse alters the structure of the brain through degeneration of the cerebral cortex, and causes changes to the hypothalamus and cerebellum [47]. These changes directly impact cognitive processes associated with learning, memory, attention, rational thinking, and impulse control [48, 49]. The abuse of alcohol may cause complications giving rise to neuropsychological disorders, cancer, cardiovascular, diabetes and infectious diseases, injuries whilst intoxicated, and fetal disorders [44, 47]. Poverty and economic stress arising from poor educational outcomes, and unemployment can cause additional psychogenic trauma impacting mental health causing anxiety and depression [41]. As previously outlined, stress triggers hormonal action on the nervous system to produce a biological uninhibited reaction which often translates into violence or abuse. Continuously high stress levels lead to heightened states of hypersensitivity undermining positive health leading to mood disorders such as depression, anxiety and aggression, diabetes and high blood pressure and potentially resultant amnesia [50].

6. Neurophysiological research

Recent research into dissociative identity disorders supports the finding that highly stressful events during childhood development produce a neurological response to intolerable stress which results in the deconstruction of self-identity [51]. Stress-induced trauma may arise from physical and emotional abuse or neglect, disturbed attachment, and boundary violations with the resultant effect amplified as a result of familial, societal and cultural factors [52]. As a biopsychosocial concept, dissociative identity disorder has been validated as a chronic psychiatric disorder arising from intolerable stress and trauma grounded on interpersonal non-assimilation, cognitive and neurobiological responses and as such warrants further comparative research [51].

Research has provided insights into how stress interacts with long-term potentiation (LTP), long-term depression (LTD), stress, and memory on the hippocampus, amygdala and prefrontal cortex [53]. These three regions of the brain are impacted in time from stress-related, trauma-inducing events so that immediate impact is temporarily followed by a medium-term, then a longer term effect [54]. In relation to the hippocampus, the LTP is engaged and activated for a short period of time. After this early period lasting no more than a few minutes, LTP activity is blocked and a period of memory consolidation occurs for up to half an hour [54, 55]. During this period of consolidation new memories are suppressed and LTP is disengaged. In the amygdala region, LTP is engaged for a longer-period and emergency decision making is enabled and action is taken [54]. The prefrontal cortex reacts differently compared to the hippocampus and amygdala in that LTP is temporarily impaired, attention is divided and multitasking is enabled. After a period lasting a few minutes to an hour normal LTP induction is restored. These concurrent effects on the three parts of the brain induced by traumatic events not only show how strong psychological and emotional events induce high levels of stress, resulting in short-, medium- and long-term effects but also result in longer-term phenotype changes in their physiological structure [54]. Further evidence of the impact of trauma on neurophysiological structures is provided by PET data, which illustrates that the right hemisphere of the brain is affected by these events and visual areas of the brain are activated, directly related to the extent of trauma [19, 33, 34].

7. Epidemiology of psychogenic amnesia

In severe cases of trauma-related stress, both retrograde and anterograde memories are affected along with overall impairment of mental and physical health [26, 55]. Studies relating to the frequency of dissociative and psychogenic amnesia have been carried out in 16 countries with rates of prevalence in different countries varying from 0.2 to 7.3% [56]. This large variation in the epidemiology may partly be explained by a lack of standard testing. Therefore, combining social research with neuroimaging data and neurobiological studies of this disorder is suggested to improve understanding of the debilitating impact on its sufferers, and indigenous Australian communities in general [56].

Access to appropriate treatment is problematic given the lack of accurate testing, diagnosis and reporting. Frequently, the correlation between a patient's symptoms and traumatic experiences are not explored in depth as existing diagnostic tools are used to analyze and problem-solve which may only result in partial treatments [44]. Often trauma is treated by prescribing medicines for insomnia, anxiety and depression without understanding the etiology of the trauma condition [12, 51, 52]. There is also an increase in interventions from agencies in relation to emotional abuse, neglect and exposure to domestic violence and the need to mitigate risk to children. Again, although the paramount protection of children is the overriding concern, interventions do not address underlying issues associated with trauma and to a certain extent, perpetuate the effects [50].

According to the 2012–2013 Australian Aboriginal and Torres Strait Islander Health Survey (AATSIHS) 30% of people over 18 years old reported high or very high levels of psychological distress. Indigenous people were approximately three times likely to have experienced very high levels of psychological distress across age groups [57]. As previously mentioned, stress can impact on cognitive function and produce mental health issues. Cognitive processes affected in mood disorders include impairment of working memory, abstract reasoning, sustained attention, visuomotor skills and verbal memory [45, 53, 58]. **Figure 2** below demonstrates

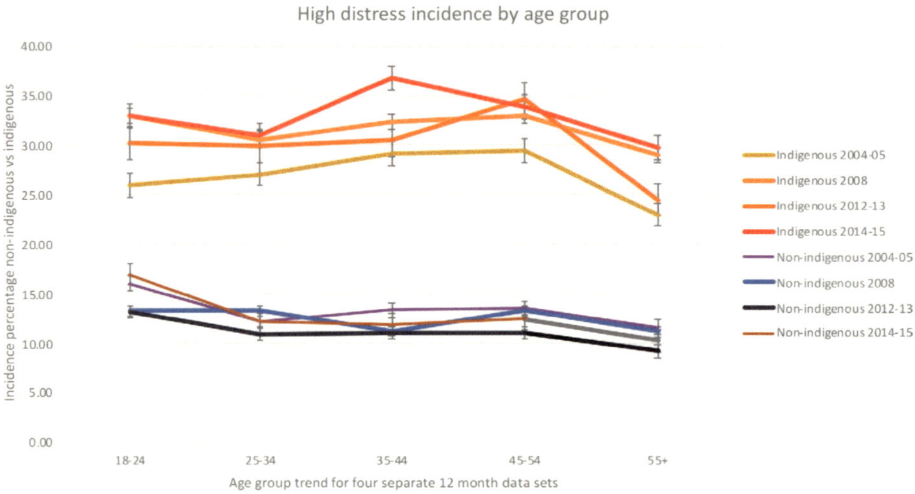

Figure 2.
Levels of distress in indigenous versus non-indigenous Australians across time and age-groups. Indigenous Australians aged 35–44 years record the highest levels of distress and non-indigenous Australians aged 55+ years record the lowest levels of distress. As time passes, stress levels appear to be increasing in all age groups in indigenous Australians and decreasing or stable in non-indigenous. Data for this chart were derived from Australian government report: Overcoming indigenous disadvantage 2016 [7].

varying levels of high distress experienced by various age groups among indigenous and non-indigenous Australians, exemplifying the huge mental health disparity between the two communities.

8. Incidence of psycho-social trauma

Childhood psychogenic trauma can be experienced in a multitude of ways. Although many indigenous children grow up in stable and loving homes, those exposed to secondary trauma, develop coping mechanisms [59]. Long-term stress arising from direct forms of psychogenic trauma and indirect transgenerational trauma gives rise to a continuous stream of cortisol. These high levels of cortisol result in the body disabling the cortisol receptors in an attempt to disengage itself from painful events. When high levels of cortisol are present in childhood, it results in children feeling withdrawn and inactive with an associated lack of stimulation [25]. Conversely, responding to the similar circumstances of high stress and unabated levels of cortisol, some children may display highly sensitive and alert behavior which eventually takes a toll on their long-term health [25]. In either case, recurring levels of stress produce psychiatric damage that continues into adulthood. The impact is then perpetuated at community levels displaying across their mental and physical health. Further, sensory emotional and physical flashbacks of repeated traumatic experiences including diagnosed post-traumatic stress disorders produce further disordered memory function. Flashbacks are more likely to occur when a person is upset, stressed or aroused by any association with the traumatic event [52].

Within indigenous Australian culture, traditional values still control communities and maintain the dominant rights of indigenous males over females. Negative aspects of this culture are associated with the intersection of customs and law whereby customary law allows for the sexual assault of under-age girls who are "promised wives" to men and suffer an early cessation of childhood [60]. Family violence also has a significant impact on the health and welfare of individuals,

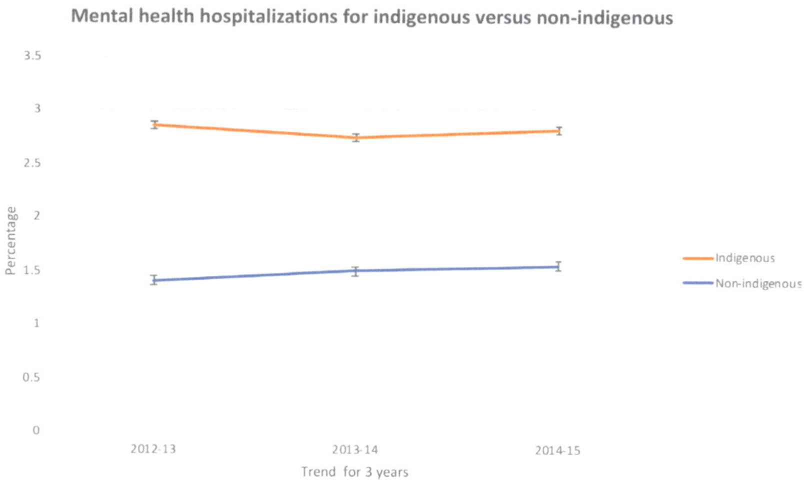

Figure 3.
All mental health hospitalizations for indigenous versus non-indigenous Australians over time indicating significant variation in population. Data for this chart were derived from Australian government report: Overcoming indigenous disadvantage 2016 [7].

families, and communities [38, 61]. In some Australian jurisdictions, police records indicate indigenous women were physically assaulted up to 11.4 times more frequently than non-Indigenous women with reports of domestic and family violence by a current partner also considerably higher than for non-indigenous women [7]. Hospitalizations for indigenous women for non-fatal family violence-related assaults were also significantly higher at 32 times the rate of non-Indigenous females [7]. Hospitalizations among indigenous population due to mental health disorders are twice as high as non-indigenous Australians as shown in **Figure 3** below.

In understanding the ongoing legacy related to trauma, consideration needs to be given to the number of children in kinship care. Kinship carers are often in an older age group, are economically poorer, with reduced health, and lower levels of education than foster carers and may appear to perpetuate the pattern of disadvantage [62]. The number of indigenous children in kinship care has grown at more than twice the rate of children in foster and residential care with some suggestions that this has been driven by increased demands for care, a shortage of foster carers, and reduction in costs [63].

Attention must also be placed on the enduring disproportionate rates of indigenous arrests, detention, and over-policing evident in many indigenous communities. The 1991 establishment of the Royal Commission into Aboriginal Deaths in Custody confirms that treatment of indigenous people in the criminal justice system was considered of national importance and left no doubt as to concerns about inappropriate violence perpetrated by Police [64–66]. More recent concerns raised by the New South Wales Ombudsman still suggest a disproportionate level of interaction, over-policing and use of Tasers against indigenous people [67].

9. What can be done and what has been achieved

Research has shown that often individual experiences of trauma underscore difficulties in recovery as the effects of trauma compound within a community on which an individual has depended, and the community becomes fragmented and disconnected [9]. An individual diagnosis of psychogenic amnesia may be better served if consideration is given to collective community trauma; individual treatment may result in disconnection from community and loss of self-connection [9]. Studies indicate that adopting evidence-based principles of family and community healing, developed internationally in mass communal disaster situations, may assist in conceptualizing a more informed response to the wellbeing for indigenous Australian communities [9].

It is acknowledged that treatment for trauma-induced amnesia is in early stages of development with robust data not readily available. It is evident that health practitioners working with indigenous Australians affected by trauma need to modify their programs to suit individual traumatic experiences and operate from a "trauma-informed" community perspective [59]. Culturally competent staff accept that trauma is individualized, and that therapeutic care must be customized for the individual to meet holistic and ecological needs [59]. Medical concepts in plain English or local language should replace technical specialist language within cross-cultural settings with the use of "story" central to shared understanding. As a society, we have a responsibility to ensure children have the opportunity to heal from trauma and have a responsibility to ensure all appropriate services and treatment methods are provided to achieve this [42].

In 2015, the Australian Government released the Implementation Plan for the National Aboriginal and Torres Strait Islander Health Plan 2013–2023 which outlines actions and strategies to be undertaken by the Government and other key stakeholders to execute the priorities [68]. Priorities include access to primary health care for early intervention to prevent hospitalizations and avoidable deaths and improved mental health outcomes. The Plan acknowledges that mental health has implications for incidence of domestic violence, substance abuse imprisonment and family disconnections and seeks a reduction in suicide and self-harm rates [68]. The Plan indicates that rates of family and community violence were unchanged between 2002 and 2014–2015 (around 22%), and risky long-term alcohol use in 2014–2015 was similar to 2002 [68]. Of concern, is that the proportion of adults reporting high levels of psychological distress increased from 27% in 2004–2005 to 33% in 2014–2015 (as shown in **Figure 1**),

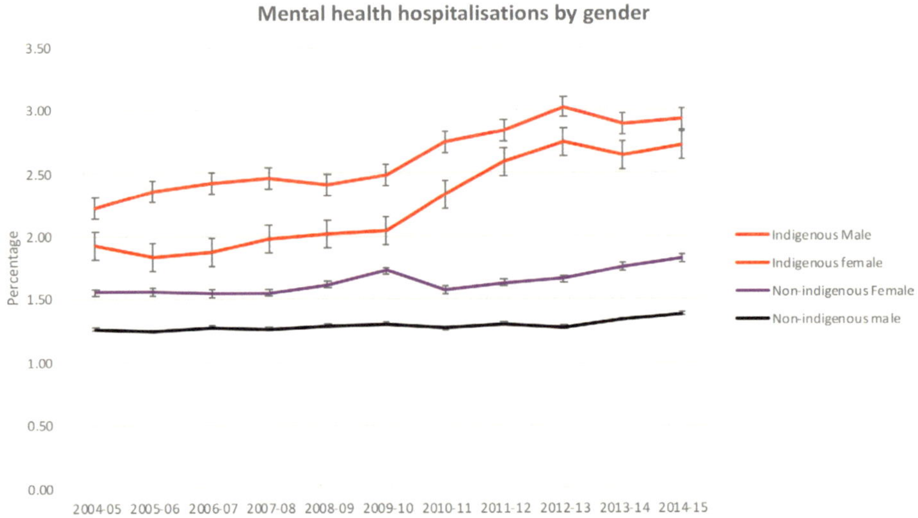

Figure 4.
Mental health hospitalizations by gender for indigenous versus non-indigenous Australians for a reported period and shows increased levels of hospitalizations for both male and female indigenous. Male indigenous hospitalizations show more than twice the level as compared to non-indigenous. Female indigenous have higher levels of hospitalizations than non-indigenous but less than male indigenous which raises possible concerns over reporting. Data for this chart were derived from Australian government report: Overcoming indigenous disadvantage 2016 [7].

and hospitalizations for self-harm increased by 56% over this period. The proportion of adults reporting substance misuse in the previous 12 months increased from 23% in 2002 to 31% in 2014–2015 [5, 68] (**Figure 4**).

It has been inspiring to see organizations implement Reconciliation Action Plans driving collective action to implement change for positive indigenous Australian health outcomes. It has been acknowledged that indigenous patient safety is inextricably linked with cultural safety and that currently, no agreed national definition of cultural safety exists [69]. Despite this some organizations have informed the view that cultural safety should be defined as the individual and institutional knowledge, skills, attitudes, and competencies needed to deliver optimal equitable health care for indigenous people [69].

The perspective of trauma-informed health care may change the lens on treatment plans for indigenous people presenting with mental illness [70, 71]. For change to occur, local indigenous communities and regional areas must be in control of determining health needs and responsible for assessing the outcome in conjunction with health professionals [72, 73]. Indigenous Australians have a "right to a good life" and past uncoordinated approaches to tackle the problems of poor health outcomes has led to a culture of low expectations [74].

10. Conclusion

This chapter has considered the psycho-social trauma and epidemiology of amnesia associated with childhood and intergenerational trauma prevalent among indigenous Australians, from the social neuroscience perspective. The legacy of destruction imposed on indigenous Australian by violence and assimilation has had severe long-term consequences contributing to the tragic health inequality present in indigenous Australian's today. The insights derived from this review indicate that the complex effects of psycho-social trauma induced amnesia should be considered in any treatment plan.

It is clear there is strong need to understand the meaning of trauma recovery in the indigenous context which differs from non-indigenous interpretations, and acknowledgment that wellbeing of indigenous people has to take into account genetic and environmental influences. Indigenous people suffering from psycho-social trauma-induced amnesia often experience additional complex factors of social disconnection. Open discussions need to address cultural dimensions that value past, present and preservation of knowledge. Taking a deeper look at the underlying causal factors of amnesia may allow consideration of a greater range of treatment options across a multitude of social neurological science disciplines may go towards informing funding for further research and training.

Conflict of interest

The author declares no conflict of interest.

Other declarations

This chapter generally uses the term "indigenous Australians" to describe Aboriginal and Torres Strait Islander Australians, as Australia's first peoples, and "non-indigenous Australians" to refer to Australians of other backgrounds, except where quoting other sources.

Author details

Alison Husain[1,2]

1 Developments in Literacy (DIL Australia), Sydney, Australia

2 New South Wales (NSW) State Government, Office of the Children's Guardian, Sydney, Australia

*Address all correspondence to: alison.husain@yahoo.com

References

[1] Kingsley J, Townsend M, Henderson-Wilson C, Bolam B, Kingsley J. Developing an exploratory framework linking Australian aboriginal peoples' connection to country and concepts of wellbeing. International Journal of Environmental Research and Public Health. 2013;**10**(2):678-698. DOI: 10.3390/ijerph10020678

[2] Twardosz S, Lutzker JR. Child maltreatment and the developing brain: A review of neuroscience perspectives. Aggression and Violent Behavior. 2010;**15**(1):59-68. DOI: 10.1016/j.avb.2009.08.003

[3] Lonne B. Re-Visioning Public Health Approaches for Protecting Children. Cham: Springer International Publishing; 2019. DOI: 10.1007/978-3-030-05858-6

[4] Australian Government Australian Institute of Health and Welfare; Aboriginal and Torres Strait Islander Health Performance Framework (HPF) Report. AIHW. 2017. Available from: https://www.aihw.gov.au/reports/indigenous-health-welfare/health-performance-framework/contents/overview [Accessed: 12 August 2019]

[5] Australian Government Australian Institute of Health and Welfare; Australian Burden of Disease Study: Impact and Causes of Illness and Death in Aboriginal and Torres Strait Islander People. AIHW. 2011. Available from https://www.aihw.gov.au/reports/burden-of-disease/australian-bod-study-2011-indigenous-australians/contents/table-of-contents [Accessed: 12 August 2019]

[6] Australian Bureau of Statistics (ABS). 3238.0.55.001 - Estimates of Aboriginal and Torres Strait Islander Australians. 2016. Available from: https://www.abs.gov.au/ausstats/abs@.nsf/mf/3238.0.55.001 [Accessed: 04 August 2019]

[7] Australia Government Steering Committee for the Review of Government Service Provision, Overcoming Indigenous Disadvantage: Key Indicators. Productivity Commission. Canberra. 2016; p. 4.61, 4.157-165, 8.2155-2158, 2444-2446, 2449-2451, 2537-2538, 2541-2542. Available from: https://www.pc.gov.au/research/ongoing/overcoming-indigenous-disadvantage/2016/report-documents/oid-2016-overcoming-indigenous-disadvantage-key-indicators-2016-report.pdf

[8] Sotero MA. Conceptual model of historical trauma: Implications for public health practice and research. Journal of Health Disparities Research and Practice. 2006;**1**(1):93-108. Available from: https://ssrn.com/abstract=1350062

[9] Krieg A. The experience of collective trauma in Australian indigenous communities. Australasian Psychiatry. 2009;**17**(1_suppl):S28-S32. DOI: 10.1080/10398560902948621

[10] Nogrady B. Trauma of Australia's indigenous 'stolen generations' is still affecting children today. Nature. 2019;**570**(7762):423-424. DOI: 10.1038/d41586-019-01948-3

[11] O'Donnell M, Nassar N, Leonard H, Jacoby P, Mathews R, Patterson Y, et al. Characteristics of non-aboriginal and aboriginal children and families with substantiated child maltreatment: A population-based study. International Journal of Epidemiology. 2010;**39**(3):921-928. DOI: 10.1093/ije/dyq005

[12] Delima J, Vimpani G. The neurobiological effects of childhood maltreatment. An often overlooked

narrative related to the long-term effects of early childhood trauma? Family Matters. 2011;**89**:42-50. Available from: https://aifs.gov.au/publications/family-matters/issue-89/neurobiological-effects-childhood-maltreatment

[13] Staniloiu A, Markowitsch HJ. The remains of the day in dissociative amnesia. Brain Sciences. MDPI AG. 2012;**2**(2):101-129. DOI: 10.3390/brainsci2020101

[14] Thomas Antérion C, Mazzola LB. Autobiographic memory: Phenomenological aspects, personal semantic knowledge, generic events and characters (one case of pure retrograde memory recovery). Neurophysiologie Clinique/Clinical Neurophysiology. Elsevier SAS; 2008;**38**(3):171-176. DOI: 10.1016/j.neucli.2008.02.006

[15] Newcombe NS, Lloyd ME, Ratliff KR. Development of episodic and autobiographical memory: A cognitive neuroscience perspective. Advances in Child Development and Behavior. 2007;**35**:37-85. DOI: 10.1016/B978-0-12-009735-7.50007-4

[16] Nyberg L, Kim A, Habib R, Levine B, Tulving E, Nyberg L. Consciousness of subjective time in the brain. Proceedings of the National Academy of Sciences, USA. 2010;**107**(51):22356-22359. DOI: 10.1073/pnas.1016823108

[17] Revealed: How Indigenous Australian storytelling accurately records sea level rises 7,000 years ago. The Guardian. 2015. Available from: https://www.theguardian.com/australia-news/2015/sep/16/indigenous-australian-storytelling-records-sea-level-rises-over-millenia [Accessed: 09 September 2019]

[18] Markowitsch HJ, Staniloiu A. 1687 – Social cognition in patients with dissociative amnesia. European Psychiatry. Elsevier SAS. 2013;**28**(1):1-1. DOI: 10.1016/S0924-9338(13)76675-6

[19] Markowitsch HJ, Staniloiu A. Neurological changes in dissociative amnesia. Journal of the Neurological Sciences. Elsevier B.V. 2015;**357**(1):e224-e224. DOI: 10.1016/j.jns.2015.08.775

[20] Leong S, Waits W, Diebold C. Dissociative amnesia and DSM-IV-TR cluster C personality traits. Psychiatry (Edgmont). 2006;**3**(1):51-55. Available from: http://search.proquest.com/docview/812134370/

[21] Papanicolaou AC, Billingsley-Marshall R. The Amnesias: A Clinical Textbook of Memory Disorders. Oxford, England, UK: Oxford University Press; 2006. pp. 214-228

[22] Markowitsch HJ. Psychogenic amnesia. NeuroImage. 2003;**20**(1):S132-S138. DOI: 10.1016/j.neuroimage.2003.09.010

[23] Bogousslavsky J, Boller F, Iwata M. A History of Neuropsychology. Basel: Karger; 2019. pp. 64-65

[24] Buchanan T, Lovallo W. Enhanced memory for emotional material following stress-level cortisol treatment in humans published in. Psychoneuroendocrinology. Elsevier Ltd; 2001;**26**(3):307-317. DOI: 10.1016/S0306-4530(00)00058-5

[25] Tracey N. Transgenerational Trauma and the Aboriginal Preschool Child: Healing Through Intervention. Lanham MD. Rowman & Littlefield. 2014. pp. 109-131

[26] Tracey N. The autistic core in aboriginal trauma: Breaking down or breaking out of the autistic defence. Psychoanalysis. Culture and Society. 2012;**17**(4):356-372. DOI: 10.1057/pcs.2012.35

[27] Wolf OT. Stress and memory in humans: Twelve years of progress. Brain Research. Elsevier B.V; 2009;**1293**:142-154. DOI: 10.1016/j.brainres.2009.04.013

[28] Cunningham J, Paradies Y. Socio-demographic factors and psychological distress in indigenous and non-indigenous Australian adults aged 18-64 years: Analysis of National Survey Data. BMC Public Health. BioMed Central. 2012;**12**(1):95. DOI: 10.1186/1471-2458-12-95

[29] Zohar J, Sonnino R, Juven-Wetzler A, Cohen H, Zohar J. Can posttraumatic stress disorder be prevented? CNS Spectrums. 2009;**14**(1 Suppl 1):44-51. Available from: http://search.proquest.com/docview/66849311/

[30] Staniloiu A, Markowitsch HJ. Dissociative amnesia. The Lancet Psychiatry. Elsevier Ltd. 2014;**1**(3): 226-241. DOI: 10.1016/S2215-0366(14)70279-2

[31] Cacioppo JT, Berntson GG, Decety J, Cacioppo JT. Social neuroscience and its relationship to social psychology. Social Cognition. 2010;**28**(6):675-685. DOI: 10.1521/soco.2010.28.6.675

[32] Kedia G, Harris L, Lelieveld GJ, van Dillen L. From the brain to the field: The applications of social neuroscience to economics, health and Law. Brain Sciences. 2017;7(8):6. DOI: 10.3390/brainsci7080094

[33] Cabeza R, Mangels J, Nyberg L, Habib R, Houle S, McIntosh AR, et al. Brain regions differentially involved in remembering what and when: A PET study. Neuron. 1997;**19**(4):863-870. DOI: 10.1016/S0896-6273(00)80967-8

[34] Yasuno F, Nishikawa T, Nakagawa Y, Ikejiri Y, Tokunaga H, Mizuta I, et al. Functional anatomical study of psychogenic amnesia. Psychiatry. 2000;**99**(1):43-57. DOI: 10.1016/S0925-4927(00)00057-3

[35] Jacobs C. Submission to the Department of Prime Minister and Cabinet – Consultation Paper: COAG Closing the Gap Refresh Indigenous Research Program. The Centre for Independent Studies CIS. 2018. pp. 2-9. Available from: https://www.cis.org.au/app/uploads/2018/05/Submission-Closing-the-Gap-Refresh-The-Centre-for-Independent-Studies.pdf

[36] Williams R. Djambatj Mala: Why warriors lie down and die: Towards an understanding of why the aboriginal people of Arnhem Land face the greatest crisis In health and education since European contact. The Australian Journal of Rural Health. 2001;**9**(5):259-261. DOI: 10.1046/j.1440-1584.2001.00392

[37] Cone E, Wilson L. A study of New Zealand occupational therapists' use of the recovery approach. New Zealand Journal of Occupational Therapy. 2012;**59**(2):30-35

[38] Price JN. Homeland truths: the unspoken epidemic of violence in indigenous communities. The Centre for Independent Studies CIS. Occasional papers 148. 2016. Available from: https://www.cis.org.au/app/uploads/2016/08/op148.pdf

[39] Price JN, Langton M, Cashman J. Ending the violence in indigenous communities, the Centre for Independent Studies CIS. Occasional Paper. 2016;**152**:1-18. Available from: https://www.cis.org.au/app/uploads/2016/12/op152.pdf

[40] Opal fuel leads to 70pc drop in petrol sniffing. Australian Broadcasting Corporation (ABC) News. 2010. Available from: https://www.abc.net.au/news/2010-06-24/opal-fuel-leads-to-70pc-drop-in-petrol-sniffing/879990 [Accessed: 09 September 2019]

[41] Hudson S. Closing the Accountability Gap: The First Step Towards Better Indigenous Health. The Centre for Independent Studies. Policy

Monograph 105. 2009. p. 4, 11. Available from: https://www.cis.org.au/app/uploads/2015/07/pm105.pdf

[42] Struik A. Treating chronically traumatised children with the sleeping dogs method: Don't let sleeping dogs lie! Children Australia. 2017;**42**(2):93-103. DOI: 10.1017/cha.2017.13

[43] Green BL. Culture is treatment. Journal of Psychosocial Nursing and Mental Health Services. 2010;**48**(7):27-34. DOI: 10.3928/02793695-20100504-04

[44] Dingwall K, Gray A, Mccarthy A, Delima J, Bowden S. Exploring the reliability and acceptability of cognitive tests for indigenous Australians: A pilot study. BMC Psychology. 2017;**5**(1):1-16. DOI: 10.1186/s40359-017-0195-y

[45] Olga Gray A. Determining acceptable and reliable cognitive testing methods in an Australian Aboriginal population [thesis]. Charles Darwin University; 2015. pp. 1-2, 58-60. Available from: http://espace.cdu.edu.au/eserv/cdu:56203/Thesis_CDU_56203_Gray_A.pdf

[46] World Health Organisation. Global Status Report on Alcohol and Health. Geneva: World Health Organization; 2018. p. 11, 73, 348, 372. Available from: https://apps.who.int/iris/bitstream/handle/10665/274603/9789241565639-eng.pdf?ua=1 [Accessed: 19 July 2019]

[47] Roussotte FF, Bramen JE, Nunez S, Christopher Q, Lorna C, Smith L, et al. Abnormal brain activation during working memory in children with prenatal exposure to drugs of abuse: The effects of methamphetamine, alcohol, and polydrug exposure. NeuroImage. 2011;**54**(4):3067-3075. DOI: 10.1016/j.neuroimage.2010.10.072

[48] Heffernan T. Time based prospective memory deficits associated with binge drinking: Evidence from the Cambridge prospective memory test (CAMPROMPT). Drug and Alcohol Dependence, Elsevier Science Ltd. 2012;**123**(1-3):207-212. DOI: 10.1016/j.drugalcdep.2011.11.014

[49] Chen Y, Yang C, Chen S, Chen Y, Su C. Everyday memory problems in alcohol abuse and dependence: Frequency, patterns and patient-proxy agreement. Psychiatry Research. Elsevier B.V. 2018;**261**:488-497. DOI: 10.1016/j.psychres.2018.01.016

[50] Higgins D. Protecting children: Evolving systems. Family Matters. Australian Institute of Family Studies. 2011 Dec;**89**:5. Available from: https://aifs.gov.au/publications/family-matters/issue-89/protecting-children

[51] Şar V, Dorahy MJ, Kruger C. Revisiting the etiological aspects of dissociative identity disorder: A biopsychosocial perspective. Psychology Research and Behavior Management. 2017:137-146. DOI: 10.2147/PRBM.S113743

[52] Benjamin R, Haliburn J, King S. Humanising Mental Health Care in Australia: A Guide to Trauma-Informed Approaches. London: Routledge; 2019. pp. 11-12

[53] Lupien SJ, Maheu F, Tu M, Fiocco A, Schramek TE. The effects of stress and stress hormones on human cognition: Implications for the field of brain and cognition. Brain and Cognition. 2007;**65**(3):209-237. DOI: 10.1016/j.bandc.2007.02.007

[54] Diamond DM, Campbell AM, Park CR, Halonen J, Zoladz PR. The temporal dynamics model of emotional memory processing: A synthesis on the neurobiological basis of stress-induced Amnesia, flashbulb and traumatic memories, and the Yerkes-Dodson Law. Neural Plasticity. 2007;**2007**(2007):60803. DOI: 10.1155/2007/60803

[55] Sanjay K, Shobini R, Biju S, Gangadhar BN. Widespread cognitive impairment in psychogenic anterograde Amnesia. Psychiatry and Clinical Neurosciences. Blackwell Publishing Asia. 2007;**61**(6):583-586. DOI: 10.1111/j.1440-1819.2007.01735.x

[56] Staniloiu A, Markowitsch HJ. Dissociative amnesia—A challenge to therapy. International Journal of Psychotherapy Practice and Research. 2018;**1**(2):34-47. DOI: 10.14302/issn.2574-612X.ijpr-18-2246

[57] Australian Bureau of Statistics (ABS). 4727.0.55.001 - Australian Aboriginal and Torres Strait Islander Health Survey: Psychological Distress 2012-2013. Available from: https://www.abs.gov.au/ausstats/abs@.nsf/Lookup/9F3C9BDE98B3C5F1CA257C2F00145721?opendocument [Accessed: 06 August 2019]

[58] Gould TJ. Addiction and cognition. Addiction Science and Clinical Practice. 2010;**5**(2):4-14. Available from: https://www.ncbi.nlm.nih.gov/pmc/articles/PMC3120118/

[59] Australian Government Australian Institute of Health and Welfare. Studies Resource Sheet no. 21 produced for the Closing the Gap Clearinghouse. Atkinson J. Trauma-Informed Services and Trauma-Specific Care for Indigenous Australian Children. 2013. pp. 4-9. Available from: https://earlytraumagrief.anu.edu.au/files/ctg-rs21.pdf

[60] Brown K. Customary Law: Sex with under-age promised wives. Alternative Law Journal. 2007;**32**(1):11-15. DOI: 10.1177/1037969X0703200105

[61] McGlade H. Justice as healing: Developing aboriginal justice models to address child sexual assault. Indigenous Law Bulletin 10. 2007;**7m**(1):10-13. Available from: http://www.austlii.edu.au/au/journals/IndigLawB/2007/59.html

[62] Sammut J. The Kinship Conundrum: The Impact of Aboriginal Self-Determination on Indigenous Child Protection. The Centre for Independent Studies. Policy Monograph 44. 2014. Available from: https://www.cis.org.au/app/uploads/2015/07/pm144.pdf

[63] Kiraly M, James J, Humphreys C. 'It's a family responsibility': Family and cultural connection for aboriginal Children in kinship care. Children Australia. 2015;**40**(1):23-32. DOI: 10.1017/cha.2014.36

[64] Cunneen C, Tauri J. Violence and Indigenous Communities. In: DeKeseredy W, Rennison C, Hall-Sanchez A. editors. The Routledge International Handbook of Violence Studies, Routledge, New York. 2019. p. 350-361. Available from: https://ssrn.com/abstract=3308924

[65] Australian Government Royal Commission into Aboriginal Deaths in Custody. RCADIC. National Report. Canberra: Australian Government Publishing Service; 1991. Available from: http://www.austlii.edu.au/au/other/IndigLRes/rciadic/

[66] Wootten H. Reflections on the 20th anniversary of the Royal Commission into aboriginal deaths in custody (Australia). Indigenous Law Bulletin, University of New South Wales, Indigenous Law Centre. 2011;**7**(27):3-8. Available from: http://www.austlii.edu.au/au/journals/AUIndigLawRw/2011/1.pdf

[67] New South Wales Ombudsman. How Are Taser Weapons Used by the NSW Police Force? Sydney: New South Wales Ombudsman; 2012. Available from: https://www.ombo.nsw.gov.au/__data/assets/pdf_file/0004/6970/How-are-Taser-weapons-used-by-NSW-Police-Force-Special-report-to-Parliament-October-2012-.pdf

[68] Australian Government Department of Health, Implementation Plan for the National Aboriginal and Torres Strait Islander Health Plan 2013-2023. Australian Government, Canberra. 2015. pp. 10-34. Available from: https://www1.health.gov.au/internet/main/publishing.nsf/Content/AC51639D3C8CD4ECCA257E8B00007AC5/$File/DOH_ImplementationPlan_v3.pdf

[69] Australian Health Practitioner Regulation Agency (AHPRA). Reconciliation Action Plan for the Australian Health Practitioner Regulation Agency. 2019. Available from: https://www.ahpra.gov.au/documents/default.aspx?record=WD18%2f25725&dbid=AP&chksum=zr4TMBVOgd2gtzNaG%2fya9w%3d%3d

[70] Lucas T. Crossing cultures: Land and encounters. The Lancet. 2015;**385**(9986):2452-2453. DOI: 10.1016/S0140-6736(15)61126-6

[71] Isobel S. Humanising mental health Care in Australia: A guide to trauma-informed approaches. Australasian Psychiatry. SAGE Publications. 2019;**27**(4):409-409. DOI: 10.1177/1039856219842642

[72] Nagel T, Hinton R, Griffin C. Yarning about indigenous mental health: Translation of a recovery paradigm to practice. Advances in Mental Health. Routledge. 2012;**10**(3):216-223. DOI: 10.5172/jamh.2012.10.3.216

[73] Lawson C, Woods D, McKenna T. Towards Indigenous Australian Knowing in Art Therapy in Australia. Leiden: Koninklijke Brill NV; 2019. DOI: 10.1163/9789004368262_002

[74] Langton M. The right to the good life: Improving educational outcomes for aboriginal and Torres Strait islander Children. The Centre for Independent Studies CIS. Occasional Paper. 2013;**133**: 2-14. Available from: https://www.cis.org.au/app/uploads/2015/07/op133.pdf

Chapter 11

Psychosocial Autopsy of Mass Suicides: Changing Patterns in Contemporary Times

Nishi Misra, Harshita Jha and Komal Tiwari

Abstract

Incidents of mass suicides have been reported since ancient times wherein a large number of people killed themselves at the same time. These suicides occur for different reasons and goals. Historical perspective has revealed the presence of religious inspiration, death pacts and cults. Out of the various methods adopted for deciphering the psychological state of a person prior to committing suicide, plus a host of emotional, social, economic and cultural reasons, psychosocial autopsy is a promising one. It helps in investigating and analyzing the relevance of these interacting factors in self-inflicted deaths and provides an answer to the family members and friends of individuals who have died this way. A look into the literature reveals that there has been a change in pattern and motive of mass suicides across generations. An understanding of the decedent's personality, behavior patterns, motives, presence or absence of mental illness helps researchers in unearthing the suicidal risk factors that mitigate or aggravate suicidal behavior in masses. The present chapter discusses the change in pattern of mass suicide with the advent of computers and social media by citing some case studies from India and abroad.

Keywords: mass suicide, psychosocial autopsy, suicidal risk factors, suicidal pattern, suicidal behavior

1. Introduction

India recently witnessed two unnerving suicide events. In 2018, 10 family members of the Chundawat family from *Burari* were found hanged, while the oldest family member, the grandmother, was strangled. The *Burari* deaths are infamously known as the "*Burari* case" or "*Burari Kand*." In another wave of suicides, in 2019, over 20 students killed themselves in a span of 1 week since Telangana Intermediate Examination results were announced. These two events, even though isolated in space and time, can be categorized under the phenomenon of mass or cluster suicides. While the major underlying cause of Telangana deaths was identified as failure of students in examination, it is the Burari case that perplexed one and all. This case was beyond the scrutiny of logic as it could not be explained by the usual causes of suicide in India, such as health concerns (mental and physical), bankruptcy and indebtedness [1]. Thus, Burari and Telangana point towards two different motives for suicide. With the help of these two examples, the authors wish to highlight the complexity and diversity prevalent in suicidal behavior.

The phenomenon of suicide can be viewed as a spectrum and the only way to arrive at any meaningful suicide prevention strategy is to first understand this psycho-social phenomenon in its different expressions. At a time when India is grappling with issues of mental health, this chapter aims to draw attention to the emerging trend of clustering and contagion in suicidal behavior, its nature as well as its manifestation, as witnessed in the contemporary Indian social cultural set-up.

1.1 From mass to cluster: Emerging trends in suicidal behavior in India

Recently, the rate of cluster suicides in India has been growing rapidly since the last decade. It is a matter of deep concern as it became a massive social problem and thus, effective interventions and solution for suicide prevention need to be developed at the earliest.

There is a shift in the predominance of the number of suicides from the elderly to the younger people all over the world. India is labeled as "Suicide Capital of South-East Asia' as it has recorded the highest number of suicides in South-East Asia in 2012, according to a WHO report [2] also in 2016 the number of suicides in India had increased to 230,314 and suicide was the most common cause of death in both the age groups of 15–29 years and 15–39 years. India has a major contribution to global suicide deaths as it increased from 25·3% in 1990 to 36·6% in 2016 among women, and from 18·7 to 24·3% among men.

There are several different types of mass suicide events that can occur, each for a different reason and for different goals. Form historical perspective the most infamous events of mass suicides are those that are related to religious groups or cults.

1.2 Suicide in ancient India

An understanding of the historical trends with respect to suicide in India takes us back to the ancient scriptures that emerged in the Indian society. After having reviewed different Indian scriptures such as the Upanishads, the Bhagvad Gita and the Brahma Sutras it was concluded that suicide is not either explicitly condemned or glorified nor is it seen as a crime in these ancient Indian texts [3]. Although suicide does find mention in the great epics of Ramayana and Mahabharata, it appears that whether such behavior was approved or disapproved depended on the intent of killing oneself, which was perhaps more important than the behavior itself. Thus, if suicide was undertaken due to selfish reasons, it was likely to be disapproved, but if it was undertaken for heroic or self-sacrificial reasons, it was seen in a more positive light. Within the Indian context, it is also debatable whether taking one's life to attain self-realization or enlightenment should be considered "suicide" or not. In such instances, a more suitable term seems to be "leaving one's body" rather than "killing oneself." Some Indian philosophical systems have emphasized on the existence of soul or atman, which is eternal and imperishable in nature, therefore death is then considered an end to the body or gross physical matter and not the soul.

In some religions such as Jainism there is provision known as "sallekhana" or "sanyasa-marana." It can be defined as the religious practice of voluntarily fasting to death by gradually reducing the intake of food. It is linked to the attainment of "moksha," the liberation from the cycle of life and death [4]. Sallekhana is sanctified morally and ethically by the Jain community, thus it is not considered an act of suicide. These observations point towards the increasing necessity of a culturally based understanding of suicide. Hinduism condemns suicide, but in specific instances accepts it as a meritorious act of self-sacrifice. It is cited in the Manusmriti that libations of water, which are usually offered to the departed souls, should not be offered to those who commit suicide.

In India's past, there have also been widespread instances of "Sati" and "Jauhar" or "Juhar." These practices were considered courageous and an act to save honor. "Jauhar" or "Juhar" was practiced by Rajput women and involved mass self-immolation, primarily to avoid capture, enslavement and rape by any foreign invader. While, "Jauhar" happens to be an example of mass suicide in India, when it comes to contemporary times the picture is different. There are growing instances of cluster suicide in India. The Burari deaths and the Telangana student suicides are examples of this growing trend.

1.3 Mass suicides in the world

History is replete with unforgettable cases of mass suicides. Mass suicide of Jonestown is perhaps one such haunting example that springs to memory. It is popularly known as "People's temple mass suicide." In the 1970s, Jim Jones, a self-styled prophet established a "socialist community" in Guyana named Jonestown. Jones was popular for his notorious image and was under the scanner for financial fraud and child abuse. Establishing an isolated community in a remote corner was perhaps one of the best ways to sustain his delusions and escape arrest. However, even after he moved to Guyana investigations against him continued. Moreover, his followers who moved with him soon discovered that the utopian world promised to them i.e. "an agricultural commune rich with food, where there were no mosquitoes or snakes and where temperatures hovered around a perfect 72° every single day" was a big lie. Instead, they were starving, living in hot and humid climate, full of mosquitoes and snakes. Naturally, his followers began looking for ways to flee. It has been reported that distressed by his followers' attempts to run away; he ordered them to consume a cyanide-laced potion, which eventually resulted in the death of over 900 people. Later analysis has revealed it as more appropriately a case of mass homicide rather than suicide, as his followers were surrounded by Jones's armed guards, thus they were left with no other option than to die. Jonestown massacre is a classic example of how one man's delusion can be contagious to a mass of people.

Similar cases of mass suicide have been reported in different areas of the world, including the Heaven's Gate Mass Suicide in California, where 39 people of the eccentric Heaven's Gate cult committed suicide. They were all dressed identically, were lying on their bunk beds with plastic bags around their heads. They were misled by their Marshall that a UFO was following the comet Hale Bopp and leaving the human world was the only way to evacuate this earth and reach a better cosmic world [5].

In Uganda, the Movement of the Restoration of ten Commandments of God (MRTCG) was a Catholic group that was convinced that the world would come to an end when the millennium calendar began. On 17 March 2000, they resorted to self-immolation and poisoning.

In all of these cases, it can be observed that the self-proclaimed cult leaders exploited the vulnerabilities of people to meet their own ends. The fabled utopian land is often based on religious foundation. These cases are also testimony to the failure of reason. People when promised of "ideal land" and "perfect future" are willing to stake everything that they have; blindly following the one "messiah" that promises them a better life or rather a better death.

1.4 Mass suicides and cluster suicides

Mass suicide can be defined as the simultaneous suicide of all the members of a social group [6]. Mancinelli has subdivided mass suicides into two categories:

Firstly, (a) hetero-induced, in which a particular population has reacted to oppression, it is typical of defeated and colonized populations forced to escape from reality that does not acknowledge their human dignity, thus people may choose to kill themselves rather than submit to their oppressors. These deaths are often looked upon as heroic and may find a place among cultural myths and legends. Secondly, (b) self-induced, in which the motivation is related to a distorted evaluation of reality, without there being either an intolerable situation or a real risk of death. The question perhaps is whether these categorizations are enough to encompass the range of suicidal behavior that occurs in the present Indian society.

Suicide cluster has been defined as "a series of three or more closely grouped deaths within three months that can be linked by space or social relationships. In the absence of transparent social connectedness, evidence of space and time linkages are required to define a candidate cluster. In the presence of a strong demonstrated social connection, only temporal significance is required" [7]. Another type of suicide cluster referred to as "mass clusters", has been commonly defined as "a temporary increase in the total frequency of suicides within an entire population relative to the period immediately before and after the cluster, with no spatial clustering" [8].

Cluster suicide can be differentiated from mass suicide as a "pocket" phenomenon. It is defined by its contextual factors. Generally, studying clusters becomes more difficult than studying masses, as both temporality and spatiality of the event takes prime importance in its understanding. Again the Burari deaths and Telangana student suicides prove to be examples of the importance of local factors that played a role in these acts.

1.5 Types of suicide cluster

There are two main types of suicide clusters: **point** and **mass** [9–11].

1. **Point cluster**- Point clusters are time space clustering close in both location and time, that occurs in small communities, and involve a temporary increase in frequency of suicides above a baseline rate observed in the community and surrounding area [9–12].

2. **Mass clusters**- occur when a large amount of people kills themselves at the same time. It involves a temporary increase in suicides across a whole population. The difference between point and mass is that it is close in time but not necessarily location. Mass clusters have been documented following suicides of high-profile celebrities or others who receive considerable media attention [10, 12].

A new concept has been introduced recently that is **Echo cluster**, the occurrence of subsequent, indigenous suicide which takes place in the same location after an initial suicide [7, 13].

Most attention has focused until recently on a greater than expected number of suicides in specific locations and time periods ("point clusters"), such as the cluster of suicides that occurred in Burari in Delhi where 11 members of a family committed suicide cumulatively.

It is observed that the mechanisms underlying suicide clusters are unclear. It has been proposed that point clusters may result from a process of "contagion," whereby one person's suicidal thoughts and behaviors are transmitted from one victim to another through social or interpersonal connections [10, 12].

1.6 Categories of suicide

In India there are several categories of suicide cluster which are related with their area of profession. Some of them are students' suicide, family suicide and farmers' suicide.

Student suicide: Now a day's education is becoming society's most critical responsibility as it is more related with social status. Students have to face many challenges that affect their life directly or indirectly like academic stress caused by the very system of education, acquisition of grades, coping up with peer pressure & parental pressure and the emotional disturbances to secure good marks and position. Poor scholastic performance, rising expectations from parents, getting involved in relationships these are the reasons which prompt a student to commit suicide.

Kota in State of Rajasthan in India is well known for its coaching of students for various admission exams after 12th standard. It has become the suicide city as the number of students committing suicide has increased drastically. By the end of the year 2018 three medical/ IIT students committed suicide within four days which brought unsettling case of students suicides. Total 19 students committed suicide in 2018.

A recent example of student suicide cluster was in Indian state of Telangana where more than 20 students killed themselves within a week after declaration of intermediate examination results. Due to the occurrence of these incidents, India's education system is criticized as a poor one in which students are under heavy pressure not just to pass examinations but to exceed expectations at all costs. The instrumental value of education in India is its potential in generating socio-economic and cultural capital through a promise of decent job opportunities in the future.

Family suicide: takes place when a whole family is unanimously agreeing to take the critical step to commit suicide together. There has been a vast increase in the family suicide cases in last 2–3 years. This phenomenon came in light after the death of 11 members of family in the mysterious Burari case'. After few days of Burari case, seven members of family committed suicide in July 2018, According to police, the family was reeling under financial hardships. In March, 2013 the same thing happened in Gangapur District of Rajasthan where eight members of a family consumed poison to committed suicide together. The family was highly religious. They also made a video before suicide.

Recently in July, 2019 three members of a family ended up their life by consuming some toxins in Punjab. According to police records, some sort of family tension within the household led to this extreme step. Again after few days three of family members were found hanging on IIT campus.

Farmer Suicide: Two thirds of India's population are dependent on agriculture for their livelihood. The earth is most generous employer in this country of a billion [14] 'It is the agricultural sector that the battle for long term economic development will be won or lost. For over a decade, famer suicides have been a serious public policy concern. More recently, this has also led to shrill outcry from the media and much politicking. The government response to the crisis of farmer suicide has mostly been simplistic and in some cases perhaps aggravating [1].

This is a particular concern for country. It is observed that huge debts, inadequate income from agriculture to repay the borrowed money, the absence of any help from outer sources, are the main cause of farmer's suicide, making them choose to end their lives. Factors contributing to the high rate of suicide in this vulnerable population include economic adversity, exclusive dependence on rainfall for agriculture, and possibly monetary compensation to the family following suicide.

1.7 Mechanisms involved in mass suicides

1.7.1 Contagion of suicidal behavior

Contagion has been defined as an underlying assumption that "suicidal behavior may facilitate the occurrence of subsequent suicidal behavior, either directly (via contact or friendship with the index suicide) or indirectly (via the media) [9].

1.7.2 Imitation

It is necessary to distinguish various types of individual suicide that might be imitated. One type of suicide relates to some symbolic or group activity which creates group pressure(s) that cause an individual to kill oneself (a form of altruistic suicide). A second type that might trigger imitative suicide involves individual's prominence in specialized occupations, e.g., a well-known artist or businessperson. It is possible that such suicides might cause suicide among individuals with similar occupational backgrounds who have experienced crisis or failure. However, this imitation is only likely to occur among a small subgroup of the population. A third category that might trigger imitative suicide is the suicide of national celebrities, i.e., individuals who are well known and recognized by name and pictorial image by the larger American public. These individuals have usually achieved prominence in an occupation subject to significant public exposure, but some social actors may become celebrities through their social connections with other prominent celebrities [15].

1.7.3 Suggestibility

Philips [16] examined U.S. and U.K. suicide rates from 1947 to 1968 and reported that suicides increased after highly publicized deaths by suicide. He proposed that news reports of suicides influenced suicide risk by means of "suggestion". He dubbed this the "Werther effect." Projective identification has been regarded as a psychoanalytical concept, which refers to feelings of empathy towards suicide. There is a blurring of self and suicide followed by a re-internalization of projection, leading to suicidal behavior.

In Priming [17], activation of one thought may trigger related pre-programmed thoughts. Media images stimulate related thoughts in the minds of audience members.

Social Integration and regulation: Where there is a lack of social ties in the community, social integration is low, leading to individualism and egoistic suicide and where interests of groups dominate those of individuals, altruistic suicides result [18].

Homophily or assortative relating [10]: The tendency of people to preferentially associate with one another and associative susceptibility, [19] where a stressful event occurring in a local community will affect several vulnerable individuals independently of each other.

Certain religious beliefs may leave people feeling guilty for things they have done and may lead them to think that they cannot be forgiven. Some believe that sacrificing themselves will earn them a reward (like going to heaven) or in countries like Japan, shame or dishonor may be a reason, like hara-kiri or seppuku.

1.8 Multidimensional nature of suicide

The multidimensional nature of suicides is reflected in the array of motives and risk factors associated with it. It has been referred to as "multidimensional, multifactorial malaise" [20]. Previous researches have mostly studied the psychosocial risk factors associated with suicides. It appears that both individual factors as well as situational factors intermingle in a complex manner to determine suicidal behavior. The demographics of suicide in India [21] reveals factors such as Age, Gender, Marital status, Education, Family structure, Urban vs. rural residence, Occupation and Precipitating event, play a role determining suicidal behavior. As per the National Crime Records Bureau 2009 data [22], the top 10 causes or correlates of suicide in 2009 were identified as family problems (23.7%), illness (21%) [including insanity/mental illness (6.7%)], unemployment (1.9%), love affairs (2.9%), drug abuse/addiction (2.3%), failure in examination (1.6%), bankruptcy or sudden change in economic status (2.5%), poverty (2.3%), and dowry dispute (2.3%). In addition, the high rates of suicide among persons with mental illness and drug abuse/addiction are of much concern. Substance abuse, problems with parents-in-law and spouses and mental illness are the risk factors that are increasingly gaining momentum in the Indian society [23].

There are vulnerable individuals with negative self-esteem, socially isolated, who tend to internalize feelings and conflicts and are over-dependent on their families. Drug and alcohol abuse, employment problems, a history of self-harm have been quoted as possible causes [24].

Mass suicides are seen as suicide pacts in couples or families rather than as part of religious cults as in western societies. Suicide pacts almost always involve people well known to each other, mostly spouses, most of them childless. However, there is an emerging trend for cyber-based internet-facilitated suicide pacts which increasingly involve two or more strangers who meet on the internet and share similar world views. Such cases have been reported in the press, but have not been studied in a scientific manner [20].

1.9 Role of mental illness in suicides

Those who are especially susceptible to suicide contagion are adolescents with suicidal thoughts and people with depression, bipolar disorder, anxiety, schizophrenia and PTSD.

Exposure to previous trauma makes a person susceptible to develop PTSD, especially in cases of physical and emotional proximity to the event and victim. Rumination followed by intrusive thinking are additional causes. In such instances long term emotional support is needed, which if found missing, has its adverse consequences. The mass trauma caused by mass suicide is likely to affect the mental health of individuals. Depression has been regarded as a key risk factor for suicide. Substance abuse, chronic pain, a family history of suicide, a prior suicide attempt and impulsiveness plays a major role in adolescent suicides.

1.10 The dual role of media

The media sometimes gives intense publicity to "suicide clusters" - a series of suicides that occur mainly among young people in a small area within a short period of time. These have a contagious effect especially when they have been glamorized, provoking imitation or "copycat suicides". This phenomenon has been observed in India on many occasions, especially after the death of a celebrity, most often a movie star or a politician. The wide exposure given to these suicides by the media has led to suicides in a similar manner. Copying methods shown in movies are also not uncommon. This is a serious problem especially in India where film stars enjoy an iconic status and wield enormous influence especially over the young who often look up to them as role models.

2. Methods of suicide study

Two prominent methods are psychological and psychosocial autopsy.

In depth study of the history of suicide prior to the suicidal act is known as psychological autopsy [25]. Psychological autopsy is a method created by Shneidman [26]. It has become widespread in the last 2–3 decades.

Psychological autopsy is a depth study of a person's mental state by analyzing medical records, interviewing friends and family and conducting research into their state of mind prior to death.

The psychological autopsy report provides detailed information about the death using various sources including the autopsy report, medical records, relevant documents and information gathered from interviews with key informants.

It was conceived as a means to help forensic pathologists clarify the nature of deaths regarded as unresolved and that could be associated with natural or accidental causes, suicide or homicide. The method was also used to investigate the reasons behind self-inflicted deaths and to provide comfort to family members of individuals who have died this way.

2.1 Psychosocial autopsy

Psychosocial autopsy is understanding of emotional, social, economic and cultural reasons and circumstances associated with suicide among individuals. The aim is to investigate and analyze the relevance of interacting variables.

Some of the key goals of the Psychological Autopsy:

Obtaining an in-depth understanding of the decedent's personality, behavior patterns, and possible motives for suicide; identify behavior patterns—reactions to stress, adaptability, changes in habits or routine Establish presence or absence of mental illness.

3. Methodological issues in studying clusters

The demographic and clinical features of suicide cluster victims have been described by researchers. Only some studies [19, 27] adopt a more methodologically robust design, such as case–control study. Only a small number of possible risk factors for suicide were examined, like gender, age-group, marital status, area of residence, method of suicide. Studies using multi-level methodology are needed to determine which individual or contextual factors contribute to clustering of suicidal behavior. Longitudinal studies on suicide clusters combined with environmental factors are needed. It is not always possible to determine retrospectively whether or not a person in a suicide cluster knew about the suicide of another cluster member [28].

4. Prevention strategies

Suicide is often related to depression, social isolation and loss of meaning in life. Some strategies at the individual level are:

1. Talk to those intimately connected first prior to media coverage, possibly one who is trained in crisis care therapy.

2. Identify vulnerable persons for mass/cluster suicides, e.g. people who had a negative interaction with the person before suicide and feel that they were

responsible for suicide, people who were in suicide pact, people who were previously suicidal.

3. Screen those at high risk, screening by trained counselors, screening for emotional and mental health problems, symptoms of depression and suicide risk.

4. Provide post-care after suicide counseling by crisis counselors available in schools and make sure students know these resources are readily available.

5. Offer case-management services at schools and universities.

6. Provide mental health screening for depression and suicide.

7. Share information about mental health with parents.

4.1 Community level

Mass suicides can be prevented at community level by designing of strategies by community leaders. All sectors of the community need to be included: public health, mental health, Education, Local government, parent groups, media, as no single agency has the requisite expertise to deal with the suicide cluster. The plans need to be adapted to the particular needs, resources and cultural characteristics of the community. Suicide prevention training needs to be provided in schools. Peer-helping needs to be encouraged. It is based on the premise that an informal helping network exists. This group teaches how to reach out adults for help. Tele-health services need to be in places which are manned by counselors, mental health clinicians, social workers and clinical psychologists. Having counselors on the sites of memorials, suicide anniversaries and other events related to suicides can also be of great help.

Addressing the environment, e.g. the internet environment and how students interact with each other on the net is also needed. Mass suicides can impact those living in the community deeply. Hence strategies at the community level have a great role to play.

4.2 Role of culture

The cultural/social resources include guidance from elders for addressing grief, informal community gatherings, where community members share stories and draw on a shared sense of spirituality and cultural history to overcome crises and impact of suicides and suicide clusters. The elders can pass on the wisdom and traditions on how to thrive through harsh conditions. The mutual care and concern for others, shared purpose. Spirituality helps to a great extent in dealing with traumas of life. Traditional culture helps to ground individuals and provide a framework to view their place in the world. Communities need to connect youth to their culture. Elders can share stories of how they used to deal with crisis situations in the past before our generation. School–based programs need to be organized on suicide signs and risk factors. Developing and promoting prosocial adult and peer mentors and role models are likely to help in a great way. Culture camps can be organized where youth (at community and school level) are exposed to their traditional life ways.

4.3 Role of media

Psychological autopsy studies have found that media can be of great help by not publishing/telecasting the method used to kill oneself, not suggesting that the death was due to a similar reason or achieved a goal such as fame or revenge and listing resources to those who are struggling.

4.4 Addressing the symptoms of mental illness

Treatment of mental illness can reduce the risk for suicide and increase the quality of life. One needs to be beware of warning signs like increased use of drugs/ alcohol, statements threatening to hurt self, looking for access to fire arms, pills etc. statements of hopelessness, helplessness etc., increased anger and rage, highly reckless behavior, paired with recent losses, including deaths, break-ups, job or financial losses.

5. Conclusions

Mass suicide in across the globe is an age-old act which was carried out by individuals and was neither condemned nor glorified nor seen as a crime. The intent of the act determined its approval or disapproval. With the change in scenario, more number of cluster suicides has been reported in the present Indian society which can be categorized into family, farmers and students. Psychosocial autopsy has revealed imitation, suggestibility, contagion, lack of social integration, priming, associative susceptibility, guilt, mental illness and a host of other causes behind this act. Preventive strategies need to be addressed at individual, community and cultural level. In future, more methodologically sound and preferably longitudinal studies are needed to gain better insight into this suicide type so that preventive strategies can be targeted appropriately.

Author details

Nishi Misra*, Harshita Jha and Komal Tiwari
Defence Institute of Psychological Research (DIPR), Delhi, India

*Address all correspondence to: nishi.nishi067@gmail.com

References

[1] Ravi S. A reality check of suicides in India. In: Brookings India IMPACT Series. New Delhi: Brookings Institution India Center; 2015. pp. 6-7

[2] WHO retrieved from http://www.searo.who.int/india/topics/suicide/en on 19 Jun 2019

[3] Nrugham L. Suicide in Indian hindu scriptures: Condemned or glorified. In: Kumar U, editor. Handbook of Suicidal Behaviour. Nature Singapore: Springer; 2017. pp. 23-37

[4] Somasundaram O, Murthy AGT, Raghavan DV. Jainism – Its relevance to psychiatric practice; with special reference to the practice of Sallekhana. Indian Journal of Psychiatry. 2016;**58**(4):471-474

[5] Zeller BE. Heaven's Gate: America's UFO Religion. NYU Press; 2014

[6] Mancinelli I, Comparelli A, Giradi P, Tatarelli R. Mass suicide: Historical and psychodynamic considerations. Suicide and Life Threatening Behaviour. 2002;**32**(1):91-100

[7] Larkin GL, Beautrais A. Geospatial Mapping of Suicide Clusters. Auckland: Te Pou o Te Whakaaro Nui, the National Centre of Mental Health Research, Information and Workforce Development; 2012

[8] Arensman E, Mc Auliffe C. Clustering and contagion of suicidal behaviour. In: Kumar U, editor. Suicidal Behaviour: Underlying Dynamics. London, UK: Routledge; 2015. pp. 110-120

[9] Haw C, Hawton K, Niedzwiedz C, Platt S. Suicide clusters: A review of risk factors and mechanisms. Suicide and Life-threatening Behavior. 2013;**43**(1):97-108

[10] Joiner JE. The clustering and contagion of suicide. Current Directions in Psychological Science (Wiley-Blackwell). 1999;**8**(3):89

[11] Rezaeian M. Suicide clusters: Introducing a novel type of categorization. Violence and Victims. 2012;**27**(1):125-132

[12] Cox G, Robinson J, Williamson M, Lockley A, Cheung Y, Pirkis J. Suicide clusters in young people: Evidence for the effectiveness of postvention strategies. Crisis. 2012;**33**(4):208-214

[13] Hanssens L. "Echo- cluster" are they a unique phenomenon of indigenous attempted and complete suicide? Aboriginal and Islander Health Worker Journal. 2010;**34**(1):17-26

[14] Gunnar M. Asian Drama. New York: Pantheon; 1968

[15] Wasserman D. Imitation and suicide: A re-examination of the Werther effect. American Sociological Review. 1984;**49**:427-436

[16] Phillips DP. The influence of suggestion on suicide: Substantive and theoretical implications of the Werther effect. American Sociological Review. 1974;**39**:340-354

[17] Berkowitz L. Some effects of thoughts on anti- and prosocial influence of media events: A cognitive neo-associationist analysis. Psychological Bulletin. 1984;**95**:410-427

[18] Durkheim E. Suicide. Translated by John a. Spaulding 1951 and George Simpson. New York: Free Press; 1897

[19] Chotai J. Suicide aggregation in relation to socio-demographic variables and the suicide method in a general population: Assortative susceptibility.

Nordic Journal of Psychiatry. 2005;**59**(5):325-330

[20] Vijayakumar L. Suicide and its prevention: The urgent need in India. Indian Journal of Psychiatry. 2007;**49**:81-84

[21] Radhakrishnan R, Andrade C. Suicide: An Indian perspective. Indian Journal of Psychiatry. 2012;**54**(4):304-319

[22] National Crime Records Bureau. 2009. Available from: data.gov.in

[23] Ponnudurai R, Jeyakar J, Saraswathy M. Attempted suicides in Madras. Indian Journal of Psychiatry. 1986;**28**:59-62

[24] Davies D, Wilkes TCR. Cluster suicide in rural Western Canada. Canadian Journal of Psychiatry. 1993;**38**:515-519

[25] Unni KE. Human self-destructive behaviour. In: Vyas JN, Ahuja N, editors. Postgraduate Psychiatry. Jaypee Brothers Medical Publishers: New Delhi; 1999. pp. 526-556

[26] Shneidman ES. Suicide thoughts and reflections, 1960-1980. Suicide Life-Threatening Behaviour. 1981;**11**:195-364

[27] Davidson, L, Suicide clusters: A critical review. Suicide and Life-threatening Behavior, 1989; 19: 17-27. GOU

[28] McKenzie N, Landau S, Kapur N, Meehan J, Robinson J, Bickley H, et al. Clustering of suicides among people with mental illness. British Journal of Psychiatry. 2005;**187**:476-480

Chapter 12

Neurocognitive Perspective of Transient Global Amnesia

Eugenia Marin-Garcia

Abstract

Transient global amnesia (TGA) is a neuropsychological syndrome that involves a sudden and temporary episode of memory loss that includes inability to create new memories. It has been shown that this disorder is related with a transitory deficit of the hippocampus function. In this chapter, the preserved and impaired memory pattern of TGA patients will be discussed considering the classical memory systems model. The analysis of this perspective leads to some contradictory or unresolved issues. In order to try to resolve these inconsistencies and considering that TGA is associated with hippocampal perturbation, new research about the hippocampus is analyzed. This new perspective focused on the hippocampal function provides a deeper understanding of the memory loss pattern associated with TGA, and it points out new questions that are not studied yet in the TGA population.

Keywords: transient global amnesia, anterograde amnesia, retrograde amnesia, hippocampus, memory systems, spatial representation, temporal representation, relational memory

1. Introduction

Transient global amnesia (TGA) is a neuropsychological syndrome, which shows a severe, sudden, and transitory loss of the ability to create new memories and, to some degree, to recover past events [1, 2]. The main goal of this chapter is to provide a neurocognitive perspective of the deficits and preserved abilities of this type of amnesia. Cognitive neuroscience is the scientific field that studies the neural bases of the cognitive processes as memory and learning [3]. As it has been shown that TGA is related with a transitory deficit of the hippocampus function, in this chapter the cognitive consequences of this deficit will be discussed. These consequences are going to be framed in a classical memory systems perspective, which considers that the hippocampus is engaged in declarative and explicit memory but not in non-declarative and implicit memory. This perspective leads to some inconsistencies and unresolved issues that will be confronted having a more precise and updated description of the function of the hippocampus.

The chapter starts with a review of basic characteristics of TGA including diagnostic criteria, etiology, and differential diagnosis. Then, the preserved and impaired memory pattern of TGA patients will be discussed considering the classical memory systems model. This includes both, the analysis of the ability of the TGA patients to recall knowledge acquired before the TGA (retrograde amnesia) and to learn new knowledge during the amnesic episode (anterograde amnesia). And finally, based on new insights from the hippocampal function research, some inconsistencies derived from the memory systems perspective will be analyzed.

IntechOpen

2. Transient global amnesia

2.1 Diagnostic criteria

In order to have a clear diagnosis of the TGA, the following diagnostic criteria [4, 5] must be fulfilled: (a) there must be clear anterograde amnesia (inability to create new memories) during the attack that it is witnessed by an observer. (b) Consciousness loss and personal identity loss must be absent, and the cognitive impairment must be limited to the amnesia. (c) The patient's neurological examination is otherwise normal. No signs of pathology should appear in the electroencephalogram (EEG) of the TGA patient, with no epileptic-form activity or postictal abnormalities [6]. (d) Epileptic features must be absent. (e) Patients with recent history of head trauma or seizures must be excluded from this diagnosis. (f) The amnesic episode must be resolved within 24 hours. (g) Mild vegetative symptoms (headache, nausea, or dizziness) might be present during the acute phase [7].

2.2 Epidemiology

Concerning TGA epidemiology, the annual TGA incidence varies between 3 and 10 per 100,000 in different studies [5, 8–11]. In population older than 50 years old, the TGA rate increases until 23–32/100,000 [9, 10], and it is very rare before 40 [5]. The second TGA episode recurrence rate varies between 6 and 15% [9, 12]; thus it is not very frequent to have another episode.

2.3 Characteristics of a TGA episode

During TGA, patients show severe anterograde amnesia, which makes them unable to create new memories and to have the sense of present. This makes them disoriented in space and specifically in time, but they do not produce confabulations (false memories which are taken by the patient as true to fill the gaps in memory) [13]. In a study with 17 TGA patients, there were no significant differences in spatial orientation with the control group, while the temporal orientation was severely affected during the amnesic episode, and it was recovered after a week [14]. This difference between spatial and temporal disorientation may be reflecting their ability to use contextual information and previous semantic knowledge to make inferences about where they are. But those inferences were not helpful enough to make them orientate in time. During amnesic episode, patients maintain their attention, and they are able to perform complex tasks as gardening or driving [15, 16]. Patients usually are aware of their disease state, but they are unable to identify the nature of their memory deficits and they overestimate their memory ability [14, 17].

Witnesses of TGA episode usually report a sudden expressive or behavioral change in the patient [18]. A characteristic feature of TGA is the repetitive comments or questions that are repeated using the same words and making the same comments to the answers that they receive [13]. The episode lasts some hours and then the memory is recovered gradually. But the memory of the period of the amnesic episode is never recovered.

2.4 TGA settings

The settings where the TGA episode usually occurs include immersion in water, temperature change, painful experiences (e.g., renal pain [19]), physical activity, emotional stress (e.g., increased work load [5, 20]), sexual intercourse [21], driving and traveling, medical procedures, Valsalva-associated maneuvers, and other activities as walks, house works, meetings, etc. [12, 17, 22–27]. In most of the settings, the patient is doing a routine or automatized activity and usually is alone or not in an active communication with others. Thus, it seems that patients are in a default functioning state. Additionally, certain personality traits have been related with the TGA as psychological or emotional instability [12] and higher occurrence of personal or family history of psychiatric disorders [28]. TGA has been associated with the intake of different substances such as sildenafil, vasodilator drug for erectile dysfunction [29, 30], or ergotic drugs to treat migraine. But in both cases, it could be a coincidence of events, drug intake and amnesia, and not a causal relationship between them [31]. It is important to consider that the percentage of TGA without a triggering factor or special setting is high, between 44% [24] and 52% [12] with more than 800 patients in each review.

2.5 Etiology

MRI data suggest that during the TGA there is a temporary perturbation of the hippocampal function, mainly in the CA1 field of the hippocampus [6, 22]. Various factors such as migraine and vascular abnormalities have been suggested to be involved in the TGA etiology, but the causal mechanisms underlying these hippocampal perturbations remain unclear.

Several studies have reported a higher incidence of migraine in patients with TGA than healthy, age-marched controls [4, 12, 23, 32–34]. But patients do not usually have migraine episodes before TGA or migrainous features during TGA episode. TGA usually occurs after 50 years old, while migraine appears through the life-span [35] and migraine is a recurrent disease, and TGA usually has only one episode [28]. Thus, migraine could be a risk factor for TGA, and its correlation could reflect a sharing mechanism [36] but probably is not a direct cause of a typical TGA.

Some studies have related TGA with ischemic deficits, but even there are cases of transient amnesia with ischemic etiology (transient ischemic amnesia (TIA)) [1, 8], they do not share many characteristic with TGA. For example, TIA is associated with stroke risk factors that are not common in TGA patients [5, 7, 12, 32, 34, 37], and TGA patients usually do not develop cerebrovascular diseases [9, 15, 33].

Another transient amnesia is transient epileptic amnesia [38], which is caused by focal seizure activity, and it can be differentiated from TGA by the briefness and high frequency of the amnesic episodes [6].

Some data suggests that the impairment of the hippocampal function during TGA may be related to the metabolic stress of the hippocampal neurons [22]. This stress-related change may trigger a hypometabolic event associated with the *cortical spreading depression*, which is described as a short-lasting depolarization wave followed by neuronal depression and regionally decreased blood flow [22, 39]. In support to this idea, decreased oxygen and cerebral blood flow in the temporal region has been reported in TGA patients [40–43]. Furthermore, CA1 region of the hippocampus shows a selective vulnerability to metabolic stress caused by different situations as neurotoxicity [44].

In the same direction, Kessler et al. [45] proposed that TGA might be related with the biochemical imbalance associated with psychological stress and anxiety through the increase of stress hormones' level. There is an overlap between the brain areas affected during TGA, as hippocampus, and regions with high density of glucocorticoid receptors, which are stress hormones [45]. In fact, a special sensitivity of the TGA patients to psychological stress [12] and high prevalence of emotional stress in these patients have been suggested [32]. Additionally, several studies have pointed out that emotional, physical, and behavioral stress situations lead to the onset of TGA in many cases [22]. And studies on the animal hippocampus have shown that emotional and behavioral stresses impair long-term potentiation and enhance long-term depression in CA1 neurons, disturbing the hippocampus-dependent memory [46].

In conclusion, the causal mechanisms underlying hippocampal perturbations of TGA remain unclear, but it seems probable that TGA is related with metabolic stress of hippocampal neurons.

3. Memory systems and TGA

Traditionally, a memory system perspective has been used to describe which processes are affected and preserved during amnesia. From this perspective, memory is considered as a not unitary entity, with relatively independent but interacting systems that process different types of information, which have different cognitive rules and that are implemented in specific cerebral networks [47]. In order to define this systems, animal and human, behavioral, clinical, neuropsychological, and neuroimaging studies have been used [48–50]. The combination of these findings has helped to classify the different memory systems.

In order to describe the complexity of memory, initially binary models were suggested. Cohen and Squire [51] proposed that long-term memory could be subdivided between declarative memory, which is representational, can be verbalized, and is severely impaired during amnesia, and procedural memory, which is expressed through action, is independent from conscious awareness, and is preserved during amnesia. On the other hand, Graf et al. [52] suggested that long-term memory is divided into implicit memory that is acquired and used unconsciously and explicit memory that is conscious and intentional.

Later, a more complex model was proposed, which is considered a classical classification model of memory systems [47, 53]. This model includes the following memory systems: episodic memory, working memory, semantic memory, priming, and procedural memory. This proposal assumes that there is a continuum between explicit/implicit and declarative/procedural dimensions through different memory systems. In the following sections, each system will be defined, and the impairments and preservation pattern associated with the TGA will be described.

3.1 Procedural memory

Procedural memory is the system that allows no-conscious acquisition, maintenance, and the use of motor and cognitive skills. It is characterized by gradual or progressive acquisition, which typically results in increased speed or accuracy with repetition. It includes heterogeneous set of subsystems: motor and cognitive abilities, habits, conditioning, and nonassociative learning. It is implicit and non-declarative, it is not hippocampal dependent, and it is spared in amnesia [53].

3.1.1 Skills acquired before the TGA

During the TGA episode, patients are able to perform complex but automatized activities learnt before the attack. For example, they are able to play the organ [54], conduct a talk [17], cook [24], drive a car [55], or conduct a concert [56]. These and similar activities, which are usually quite complex, when becoming routine procedures no longer need the involvement of the hippocampus. Thus, during the TGA procedural memories acquired before the TGA tend to be preserved [56].

3.1.2 Acquisition of new procedural skills during the TGA

In addition, the ability to learn new procedural skills remains preserved as well during TGA episode. For example, Eustache et al. [40] showed that TGA patients are able to acquire mirror-reading skill at the same learning speed as the control group.

Another example of implicit learning phenomenon is the mere exposure effect, which is defined as preference enhancement to previously exposed stimuli [57]. Mere exposure effect is preserved in TGA patients during the amnesic episode, showing enhanced preference for previously exposed faces, in spite of the severe anterograde memory loss [27].

Classical conditioning is another subtype of procedural memory that is based on associative learning. In classical conditioning, repeated pairings of a neutral conditioned stimulus (CS), such as a tone, and an unconditioned stimulus (US) such as an air-puff to the eye result in the CS alone, eliciting conditioned response (CR) such as an eyeblink [58]. Traditionally, it is considered that fear and eyeblink conditioning are unaffected in patients with hippocampal damage [59, 60]. So far, there are no studies with TGA patients assessing these types of classical conditioning, but more complex conditioning paradigms, as trace conditioning and fear conditioning, seem to be affected in TGA population. This contradictory result will be described in Section 3.

3.2 Perceptual representation system

The perceptual representation system [47] facilitates word and object identification identification based on form and structure information , but not considering meaning or associative properties. It is pre-semantic, implicit, not hippocampal dependent, and Usually it is spared in amnesia. Priming is a phenomenon dependent of this system. It implies a behavioral change that is reflected in speed or accuracy change with stimulus processed following prior exposure [61]. For example, the word "plane" will produce faster response when it is preceded by the word "rain," because both words are auditorily similar, comparing when it is preceded by the word "frog."

There is some empirical evidence that suggests that PRS remains preserved during TGA episodes. Kapur et al. [62] showed that perceptual priming was spared during TGA through a fragmented figure completion task with visually degraded drawings. And even 1 week after the amnestic episode, the patient continued to show priming effect with the figures studied during the TGA episode compared with new figures. This result has been confirmed using different learning materials as fragmented numbers [13] and verbal material with a word completion task [40].

3.3 Semantic memory

Semantic memory refers to the acquisition, retention, and use of general knowledge (facts, concepts, vocabulary, and knowledge about the world and the individuals). It is declarative, independent of contextual information, and it is usually not affected in amnesia [63].

3.3.1 Retrieval of semantic knowledge acquired before the TGA

During the TGA, language is intact. According to Caplan [17], patients show spontaneous speech and normal vocabulary, and they do not present aphasic errors.

They maintain the ability to repeat oral language, to read, and to write. They can describe not present objects, geographical details, and familiar places using their semantic knowledge. Patients with TGA are able to recognize and name objects and colors [64] and to point at drawings in response to words [65]. In addition, nonverbal semantic knowledge, assessed with a task that requires matching conceptually related figures, is also preserved [65].

Regarding verbal fluency tasks, in which participants have to produce as many words as possible from a category in a given time, there are contradictory results. While in some studies [40, 45, 66–68], TGA patients presented lower production of category examples than the control group, both with words within a semantic category (category fluency) and with words starting with a given letter (letter fluency); in other investigations [64, 65, 69, 70] no significant differences were found between TGA patients and the control group, although the former produced more perseverations.

Regarding knowledge about the world, memory for past public events and famous people is impaired during TGA [62], especially for events and people from recent decades [64]. TGA patients are able to differentiate between real events from fictional events, probably based on their implicit knowledge. But their ability to localize these events in time, primarily those from the closest decades to the amnesic episode, is impaired [71, 72]. Recognition of famous people faces seems to be preserved in some cases [64, 71], but there is some contradictory data [72], especially regarding faces linked to recent experiences.

3.3.2 Acquisition of new semantic knowledge during the TGA

It is not clear if TGA patients are able to learn new semantic memory during amnesic episode. It is important to address this question. Interestingly, there is evidence of preserved semantic priming during TGA [73, 74]. TGA patients showed semantic priming during TGA episode, and this effect persisted for 1 day [73]. But there is no data about the ability of TGA patients to acquire semantic facts. Previous research has shown that the left hippocampus is involved in successful incidental acquisition of new facts about the world [75].

Furthermore, there is evidence of patients with medial temporal lobe lesions that are impaired to learn new semantic knowledge [76]. Thus, it would be interesting to study this issue with TGA patients. Based on permanent amnesia impairment pattern, new semantic knowledge acquisition is expected to be affected during TGA.

3.4 Working memory

Short-term memory implies the conscious retention for information over a few seconds, often through active rehearsal. When the information held in short-term memory is manipulated or another task is performed, this is often referred to as working memory [77].

Based on previous research, TGA patients have preserved capacity to maintain activated a limited amount of information for a brief period of time. This has been addressed using digit span task [13, 71, 78–80], immediate memory for rhythms [81, 82], memory for spatial positions measured with the Corsi block-tapping task [45, 70, 71, 78, 80], and immediate recall for letters and objects [81]. Regarding working memory during TGA, there are no conclusive results, probably due to the diversity of required processes and the variability of complexity level through different tasks. **Table 1** summarizes the data.

Task	During TGA	References
Stroop task (inhibition to avoid reading and focus on the ink color)	Preserved	[64, 65, 68, 70]
Card sorting task (flexibility to change matching criteria)	Impaired. Only one classification criteria of the six possible	[13]
Trail making test (connect fastest possible numbers placed randomly in a paper sheet)	Preserved	[65, 68]
Backward memory span (recall stimuli in reverse order of the presentation)	Preserved	[70, 71]
	Impaired	[78, 80, 83]
Updating task (listen to auditory-presented letters, and decide if each letter that is added matches one of the previous three letters)	Preserved	[70]
Brown-Peterson's experimental paradigm (retain three consonant letters while performing a distractor task)	Deficit with 3- and 6- second delay intervals	[70]
Raven's progressive matrices (nonverbal abstract reasoning: to find a missing element to complete a pattern)	Preserved	[65]

Table 1.
Summary of studies assessing working memory in TGA patients with different tasks.

3.5 Episodic memory

Episodic memory encodes, stores, and recovers memories about past events in a spatio-temporal context. This memory allows to reexperience the past episodes as in a mental "time travel." The episodic system is declarative, explicit, hippocampus dependent, and severely damaged in amnesia [63].

3.5.1 Acquisition of new episodic information during the TGA

One of the most characteristic features of TGA is the deficit to form lasting memories of new episodic information. This impairment affects the acquisition of any kind of information: visual (figures and words), tactile, olfactory, or auditory (environmental sounds and speech) [84].

Different laboratory tests have been used to measure episodic memory. Free recall, the ability to reproduce previously presented material, is severely impaired, using visually presented words [40, 66, 67, 70, 78], auditory-presented words [27, 64, 85], semantically unrelated word pairs [72, 86], prose passages [40, 62, 72, 81, 86], or complex geometric figures [40, 64, 78, 85, 86].

Regarding cue-recall, the ability to retrieve information with a recovery cue that guides searching processes, there are no conclusive data. Some patients obtain preserved cue-recall scores, and other patients show significantly lower performance than the control group [27, 69, 70, 81]. And it seems that is not related with the type of cueing methods but with the patient, since contradictory outputs have been found using the same method. In a study with a bigger sample, there was a significant difference between TGA patients and the control group in cue-recall, being impaired for the patients [27].

Regarding recognition, the ability to recognize previously presented stimuli, is impaired in patients with TGA, both with words and drawings [41, 66, 69, 80, 85]. Recognition is usually subdivided into two component processes: recollection and familiarity, frequently measured with the "remember/know" (R/K) paradigm.

Recollection implies the retrieval of contextual details of the previous event, and familiarity is based on the feeling that the event was previously experienced but without details or context [87]. Recollection has been traditionally linked with episodic memory and hippocampal function, while familiarity is related with semantic memory and it is independent from the hippocampus [88]. Impaired R/K response pattern has been shown in TGA patients [70, 89], with usually lower recollection scores in TGA patients than in controls, while no significant difference in familiarity scores between TGA and controls [80].

3.6 Autobiographical memory

Autobiographical memory is a uniquely human system that integrates memories of past experiences into a life narrative [90], and it allows to mentally travel in time [63]. There are two components of autobiographical memory: episodic and semantic autobiographical memory. Episodic autobiographical memory refers to the memories of our personal past, and it is usually assessed with interviews that cover events from childhood until hours before the amnesic episode. Semantic autobiographical memory refers to the recollection of personal facts and general self-knowledge independent of a specific time and space [91]. This division between episodic and semantic components of autobiographical memory is based on dissociations found with amnesic patients as KC [92], which shows an episodic autobiographical memory disturbed while the semantic component is preserved.

3.6.1 Acquisition of new autobiographical information during TGA

TGA patients are not able to create autobiographical memories during the TGA episode showing a severely anterograde amnesia for this self-related information. When recovering from the TGA episode, patients show a memory gap of those hours that is never recovered.

3.6.2 Retrieval of autobiographical memories acquired before the TGA

Neuropsychological studies of TGA patients have shown that they have problems to remember their past, even though this deficit is milder than anterograde deficit. During TGA, episodic autobiographical memories from different periods of life are affected, showing deficit of details, absence of spatial and temporal context, and even sometimes confusion between memories [67, 69, 72, 89]. This retrograde amnesia usually is temporally graded [22], and it follows Ribot's Law [93], which implies deeper impairment of the closest memories compared with remote memories.

In contrast, semantic autobiographical memory is preserved. TGA patients usually recall personal information such as age, place of birth, past addresses, phone number, names of teachers, and educational and professional history [17, 94].

3.7 Conclusion about memory systems and TGA

This section has shown the memory deficit pattern of TGA based on the classical memory systems perspective, which considers that the hippocampus is engaged in declarative and explicit memory but not in non-declarative and implicit memory. This perspective leads to some inconsistencies. For example, it seems that some types of classical conditioning as trace conditioning and fear conditioning are affected in TGA patients, but based on the memory systems perspective, they should be preserved. Furthermore, working memory should be preserved as well in TGA patients, but some complex working memory tasks seem to be affected. It is also important to point out that there is not much understanding of the TGA patients' ability to acquire very complex stimuli as people's faces or complex semantic knowledge during the TGA. In the following section, in order to try to resolve these inconsistencies, new research about the hippocampus is analyzed.

4. New insights from the hippocampal function research

Since the famous case of the HM patient, the hippocampus has been considered a key structure for memory. HMs' medial temporal lobe (including hippocampi) was removed in order to try to control intractable seizures [95]. This produced him a profound amnesia specially to acquire new memories. Since that time, extensive research has been conducted in order to understand the hippocampus involvement in learning and memory and in other cognitive domains.

As it was mentioned before, there is a temporary perturbation of the hippocampal function during the TGA. Therefore, this section reviews the theories about the hippocampal function and its consequences to interpret the amnesic pattern of TGA patients. These theories are organized based on the nature of the memory processes involved and the type of information that is processed.

4.1 Memory processes

There are three main processes involved in human memory: encoding, which allows converting perceived information into a more permanent form; consolidation, which stabilizes a memory trace after its initial acquisition; and retrieval, which involves re-accessing events or information from the past [96]. There is a general agreement that episodic memories depend on the hippocampus during the encoding of new memories [95]. But the involvement of the hippocampus on retrieving remote memories is controversial.

The Standard Model of Consolidation considers that episodic and semantic memories become less dependent on the hippocampus until they are completely independent [97]. On the contrary, multi-trace theory defends that the hippocampus is crucial for acquisition of both, episodic and semantic memories. But the recollection of episodic memories remains dependent on the hippocampus in order to retrieve contextual and detailed memories, whereas semantic memories become independent from the hippocampus [98].

There is a historic debate whether the hippocampus is required to retrieve remote autobiographical memories [99]. Considering this type of memories, two patterns emerge from the literature about patients with medial temporal lobe damage: complete autobiographical memory loss across all time points, recent and remote [100, 101], and memory loss with a temporal gradient, with recent memories lost but remote memories preserved [102]. These patterns could be reflecting at least two different explanations: that autobiographical memories become less detailed and more semanticized over time and thus less dependent of the hippocampus, which could explain the apparent preservation of remote autobiographical memories in some patients [98], or that the brain damage extension is different between patients and those with widespread damage are the ones showing remote autobiographical memories impaired [103].

In fMRI studies, it has been shown that the hippocampus is associated with retrieving autobiographical memories, which are detailed and vivid, anytime that they are recalled, regardless of age of the memory [75, 104]. And studies using multivoxel pattern analysis (MVPA) has shown that more recent memories engage the anterior hippocampus but the posterior hippocampus is especially essential for remote memories [105] . This shows that there is a temporal gradient representation within the hippocampus itself. Thus, the neuropsychological loss pattern of each patient may depend on the location and extent of the damage within the hippocampus.

In TGA patients, the autobiographic memory loss has two different patterns: a continuous pattern, when memories from a limited period are affected, and an irregular pattern, when memory loss is selective without a clear time interval [78, 86, 105]. This could be related with the temporal gradient shown within the hippocampus itself [105]. But in most cases, TGA patients follow Ribot's Law [93], so that recent memories are more likely to be lost than more remote memories. This is coherent with the pattern shown in patient with permanent hippocampal damage (e.g., [102]).

4.2 Type of processed information

4.2.1 Navigation and spatial representation

Spatial information is a type of information that has been proposed to be processed by the hippocampus. Animal studies have shown that place cells in the hippocampus encode location while moving in the environment, and these cells fire when a specific place field is entered, irrespective of where the animal is looking [106]. Thus, the hippocampus provides an internal space representation or cognitive map of the environment that is allocentric (world-centered) and not egocentric (self-centered) [107]. As it seems that the hippocampus is a relevant structure for both, episodic memory and spatial representation, it has been proposed that the spatial representations of the hippocampus could support spatial context to the episodic memories [108].

fMRI studies with humans support the idea that the hippocampus is engaged when mentally or virtually navigating an environment [109]. Furthermore, studies with permanent amnesic patients show that hippocampal damage impairs the spatial learning of new environments [101], but it is not essential to navigate in familiar places. In the same direction, TGA patients are able to return to familiar places or to drive in well-learnt routes [55]. This is coherent with the diminished hippocampal activation when navigating in familiar environment [110].

However, a further question important to address is if TGA patients are able to learn to navigate in a new environment while they are under the amnesic episode. Considering the hippocampus involvement in both, acquisition of new explicit knowledge and representation of space, an impaired performance is expected.

4.2.2 Temporal representation

Another type of knowledge that is related with the hippocampus is temporal information. There are some cell ensembles in the hippocampus, especially in the CA1 area, which fire when an animal is at a particular moment in a temporally structured experience. Firing patterns of these hippocampal neurons change gradually over time representing the flow of time in an experience [111]. Literature about patients with permanent temporal lobe amnesia shows that they are able to arrange information into a sequential narrative and they seem to understand the concept of time [112]. As we mentioned before, temporal orientation is severely affected during TGA [14], and they show an absence of temporal details when trying to remember their episodic autobiographical memories [67, 69, 72, 89]. But it would be interesting to study in more detail the concept of time in TGA patients, including the representation of the duration of an event, the coding of temporal order of the elements in an episode, and the subjective sense of time [113].

4.2.3 Relational representation

The relational memory theory assumes that the hippocampus' main function is to represent associations between different elements in order to bind together multiple inputs into a single representation [114, 115]. In this sense, hippocampus may represent bindings between items (e.g., who and what) and context (e.g., where and when) [116, 117]. Furthermore, the hippocampus allows to recall these flexible relational representations and to use that information for inference in novel situations [118].

Regarding relational memory in TGA patients, two different types of contextual details have been studied: the recall of spatial information about the learning session (e.g., if words are presented on the top or bottom of the screen) and temporal information of specific items (e.g., if words belong to a first or second word list). TGA patients were very impaired remembering spatiotemporal details associated with individual items or events [67, 89].

Another insight from studies in patients with permanent hippocampal damage about relational memory is that these patients are able to recognize associations between items of the same domain (e.g., word-word), but they have problems to recognize associations between items of different kind (e.g., word-face) [119, 120]. Thus, when the task requires increased relational complexity, it is more dependent on the hippocampus and specially affected in patients with hippocampal damage. Thus, TGA patients may be impaired in across-domain association recognition as well, but this issue should be studied.

A further example of hippocampal involvement in complex processing is scene reconstruction. It has been proposed that the main function of the hippocampus is scene reconstruction [121], which may be considered as a special case of relational memory theory. Scene processing requires combining individual features across domains in a complex and coherent representation of the world. Scene components need to be integrated from modality-specific representation into a spatially coherent representation [108]. It has been shown that scene recognition is impaired in patients with medial temporal lobe damage [118, 119], and even though it has not been properly studied, it may be impaired in TGA patients as well.

There are additional examples about the hippocampal contribution when relational complexity increases, both in conditioning and in working memory. As it has been mentioned before, there is no hippocampus involvement in classical conditioning, but trace conditioning, which occurs when there is a time interval between offset of the conditioned stimulus and delivery of the unconditioned stimulus, requires hippocampal functioning [122]. Thus, the processing of a temporal contiguity delay in associative learning adds more complexity and requires the hippocampus. It would be interesting to study this type of conditioning with TGA patients. Contextual fear conditioning is another example of classical conditioning paradigm that requires complex associations and hippocampus involvement. This conditioning involves placing the animal in a novel environment, providing an aversive stimulus. When the animal is returned to the same environment, generally will recover the association between environment and the aversive stimulus and it will activate fear response (freezing response). TGA patients showed contextual fear conditioning impairment compared with the control group [123], which reflects the relationship between hippocampal functioning and relational complexity of the associations.

As it has been mentioned before, working memory has traditionally been considered as immune from hippocampal damage. But, it has been shown that when working memory task requires more complex stimuli or relational binding, then it shows to be affected when hippocampus is disturbed [108, 124]. This may partially explain the contradictory results of working memory in TGA that are considered in Section 2.

In order to account hippocampal sensitivity to complexity and precision, it has been proposed pattern separation as the underlying computational mechanism [99]. This pattern separation enables to differentiate with precision between items with overlapping features or relations [125]. It would be desirable to study this mechanism in TGA patients in order to understand deeply the deficit associated with this syndrome.

Thus, predictions from memory system model would expect that, for example, conditioning and working memory are immune to hippocampal damage and preserved during TGA. But a deeper analysis of the function of the hippocampus shows the hippocampal involvement, and its impairment in amnesia is related with the level of relational complexity of the processed information and with the computations needed in this processing.

4.2.4 Future and imagination

Traditionally, the hippocampus has been considered essential to retrieve memories from the past, but recent research suggests that it may also be related to envision and predict the future events and to imagine fictitious episodes [126]. It has been shown that the hippocampus and connected areas recombine elements of existing episodic memories to create new scenarios, and this allows creating a representation of the future and imagining new events [127]. Regarding the ability to imagine future events in patients with permanent hippocampal amnesia, usually they show problems answering questions about the future [128], and they show less richness and less integration of contextual details than the control group in imagining fictitious events or scenes [129, 130].

Research with TGA patients has shown that even though they can imagine past and future events, they provide fewer and less detailed events than the control group [131]. In another study, TGA patients showed prospective memory deficit, which involves remembering to perform an intended action at some point in the future [132], and this deficit was correlated with their retrograde impairment [68]. This probably reflects shared processes between remembering the past and projecting into the future.

In relation to future planning, mind-wandering is a form of spontaneous self-generated thinking independent from the current perceptual surrounding [133]. It has been shown that people with selective bilateral hippocampal damage are able to engage in mind-wandering as controls. However, their form and content of mind-wandering are different, showing less flexible and scene-based content and more abstract and semanticized representation [134]. An open question to be addressed is mind-wandering and creative thinking in TGA patients.

5. Conclusion

The main goal of this chapter was to present a neurocognitive perspective of the deficits and preserved abilities of TGA. In order to carry out this goal, basic characteristics of TGA were analyzed, including diagnostic criteria, etiology, and differential diagnosis. Then, the deficit pattern of TGA was presented based on the classical memory systems model. This perspective assumes that declarative and explicit memory systems, as episodic and semantic memory, are severely affected during TGA. On the contrary, procedural and implicit memory systems, as procedural memory and perceptual representation system, and also working memory are preserved, while they are not dependent on hippocampal processing. The analysis of this perspective leads to some contradictory or unresolved issues.

Afterward, in order to try to understand these inconsistencies and considering that TGA is associated with transitory perturbation of the hippocampal function, new research about the hippocampus and its cognitive mechanisms are analyzed. It seems that declarative/procedural and implicit/explicit dimensions are not decisive to be affected by hippocampus damage. Nevertheless, processes as associative or relational binding and pattern separation, which operate regardless of declarative level and conscious awareness, are especially sensitive to hippocampal impairment. Moreover, the complexity level of those processes seems to be a modulating factor that affects the impairment degree both in permanent hippocampal amnesias and in TGA.

This new perspective focused on the hippocampal function has proportioned a better understanding of inconsistent results, and it has pointed out new questions that are not studied yet with TGA population.

Acknowledgements

I am grateful to Yeray Mera for his help to prepare the References section of this chapter.

Conflict of interest

The author declares no conflict of interest.

Author details

Eugenia Marin-Garcia
University of the Basque Country (UPV/EHU), San Sebastián, Spain

*Address all correspondence to: eugenia.marin@ehu.eus

References

[1] Fisher CM, Adams R. Transient global amnesia. Acta Neurologica Scandinavica. 1964;**40**:1-83

[2] Kapur N. Memory Disorders in Clinical Practice. Hove: Lawrence Erlbaum; 1994. 289 p

[3] Gazzaniga MS, Ivry R, Mangun GR, editors. Cognitive Neuroscience: The Biology of the Mind. 2nd ed. Nueva York: W.W. Norton; 2002. 1377 p

[4] Caplan L. Transient global amnesia. In: Jam F, editor. Handbook of Clinical Neurology. Amsterdam: Elsevier Science; 1985. pp. 205-2018

[5] Hodges JR, Warlow CP. Syndromes of transient amnesia: Towards a classification. A study of 153 cases. Journal of Neurology, Neurosurgery, and Psychiatry. 1990;**53**:834-843. DOI: 10.1136/jnnp.53.10.834

[6] Bartsch T, Butler C. Transient amnesic syndromes. Nature Reviews. Neurology. 2013;**9**:86-97

[7] Hodges J. Unraveling the enigma of transient global amnesia. Annals of Neurology. 1998;**43**:151-153. DOI: 10.1002/ana.410430203

[8] Matías-Guiu J, Blanquer J, Falip R, Oltra A, Martín M. Incidence of transient global amnesia in Alcoi (Spain). Acta Neurologica Scandinavica. 1992;**86**:221. DOI: 10.1111/j.1600-0404.1992.tb05071.x

[9] Miller JW, Petersen RC, Metter EJ, Millikan CH, Yanagira T. Transient global amnesia: Clinical characteristics and prognosis. Neurology. 1987;**37**:733-737. DOI: 10.1212/WNL.37.5.733

[10] Koski KJ, Marttila RJ. Transient global amnesia: Incidence in an urban population. Acta Neurologica Scandinavica. 1990;**81**:358-360. DOI: 10.1111/j.1600-0404.1990.tb01571.x

[11] Lauria G, Gentile M, Fassetta G, Casetta I, Caneve G. Incidence of transient global amnesia in the Belluno province, Italy: 1985 through 1995. Acta Neurologica Scandinavica. 1997;**95**:303-310. DOI: 10.1111/j.1600-0404.1997.tb00215.x

[12] Quinette P, Guillery-Girard B, Dayan J, De la Sayette V, Marquis S, Viader F, et al. What does transient global amnesia really mean? Review of the literature and thorough study of 142 cases. Brain. 2006;**129**:1640-1658. DOI: 10.1093/brain/awl105

[13] Goldenberg G. Transient global amnesia. In: Baddeley AD, Wilson BA, Watts FN, editors. Handbook of Memory Disorders. Chichester: John Wiley & Sons; 1995. pp. 109-133

[14] Marin-Garcia E, Ruiz-Vargas JM. Memory and metamemory during transient global amnesia: A comparative study about long-term follow up. Revista de Neurologia. 2011;**53**(1):15-21

[15] Gass A, Gaa J, Hirsch J, Schwartz A, Hennerici MG. Lack of evidence of acute ischemic tissue change in transient global amnesia on single-shot echo-planar diffusion-weighted MRI. Stroke. 1999;**30**:2070-2072. DOI: 10.1161/01.STR.30.10.2070

[16] Zeman A, Hodges J. Transient global amnesia. British Journal of Hospital Medicine. 1997;**58**:257-260

[17] Hainselin M, Quinette P, Desgranges B, Marinaud O, de La SAyette V, Hannequin D, et al. Awareness of disease state without explicit knowledge of memory failure in transient global amnesia. Cortex. 2012;**48**(8):1079-1084. DOI: 10.1016/j.cortex.2012.02.003

[18] Caplan L. Transient global amnesia: Characteristic features

and overview. In: Markowitsch HJ, editor. Transient Global Amnesia and Related Disorders. Ashland: Hogrefe & Huber; 1990. pp. 15-27. DOI: 10.1016/0022-510X(91)90172-4

[19] Durrani M, Milas J, Parson G, Pescatore R. Temporary memory steal: Transient global amnesia secondary to nephrolithiasis. Clinical Practice and Cases in Emergency Medicine. 2018;**2**(4):334-337. DOI: 10.5811/cpcem.2018.9.39338

[20] Berlit P. Successful prophylaxis of recurrent transient global amnesia with metoprolol. Neurology. 2000;**55**:1937-1938. DOI: 10.1212/WNL.55.12.1937

[21] Maloy K, Davis JE. "Forgettable" sex: A case of transient global amnesia presenting to the emergency department. Journal of Emergency Medicine. 2011;**41**(3):257-260

[22] Bartsch T, Deuschl G. Transient global amnesia: Functional anatomy and clinical implications. The Lancet Neurology. 2010;**9**:205-214

[23] Santos S, López del Val J, Tejero C, Íñiguez C, Lalana JM, Morales F. Amnesia global transitoria: revisión de 58 casos. Revista de Neurologia. 2000;**30**:1113-1117. DOI: 10.33588/rn.3012.2000083

[24] Sander K, Sander D. New insights into transient global amnesia: Recent imaging and clinical findings. The Lancet Neurology. 2005;**4**:437-444. DOI: 10.1016/S1474-4422(05)70121-6

[25] Kushner MJ, Hauser WA. Transient global amnesia: a case-control study. Annals of Neurology. 1985;**18**(6):684-691. DOI: 10.1002/ana.410180610

[26] Alonso-Navarro H, Jiménez-Jiménez FJ. Amnesia global transitoria durante el coito. Revista de Neurologia. 2006;**42**:382-383. DOI: 10.33588/rn.4206.2005493

[27] Marin-Garcia E, Ruiz-Vargas JM, Kapur N. Mere exposure effect can be elicited in transient global amnesia. Journal of Clinical and Experimental Neuropsychology. 2013;**35**(10):1007-1014. DOI: 10.1080/13803395.2013.844774

[28] Pantoni L, Lamassa D, Inzitari D. Transient global amnesia: A review emphasizing pathogenic aspects. Acta Neurologica Scandinavica. 2000;**102**:275-283. DOI: 10.1034/j.1600-0404.2000.102005275.x

[29] Savitz SA, Caplan LR. Transient global amnesia after sildenafil (Viagra) use. Neurology. 2002;**59**:778. DOI: 10.1212/WNL.59.5.778

[30] Gandolfo C, Sugo A, Del Sette M. Sildenafil and transient global amnesia. Neurological Sciences. 2003;**24**:145-146. DOI: 10.1007/s10072-003-0102-6

[31] Marin-Garcia E, Ruiz-Vargas JM. Transient global amnesia: A review. I. Clinical aspects. Revista de Neurologia. 2008;**46**(1):53-60

[32] Melo T, Ferro J, Ferro H. Transient global amnesia: a case study. Brain. 1992;**115**:261-270. DOI: 10.1093/brain/115.1.261

[33] Piñol-Ripoll G, De la Puerta González-Moró I, Martínez L, Alberti-González O, Santos S, Pascual-Millán LF, et al. Estudio de factores de riesgo en la amnesia global transitoria y su diferenciación del accidente isquémico transitorio. Revista de Neurologia. 2005;**41**:513-516. DOI: 10.33588/rn.4109.2005315

[34] Moreno-Lugris XC, Martínez-Álvarez J, Brañas F, Martínez-Vázquez F, Cortés-Laiño JA. Amnesia global transitoria. Estudio caso-control sobre 24 casos. Revista de Neurologia. 1996;**24**:554-557. DOI: 10.33588/rn.24129.96566

[35] Evans RW, Lewis SL. Transient global amnesia and migraine. Headache The Journal of Head and Face Pain. 2005;**45**:1408-1410. DOI: 10.1111/j.1526-4610.2005.00275.x

[36] Stracciari A, Rebucci GG. Transient global amnesia and migraine: familial incidence. Journal of Neurology, Neurosurgery, and Psychiatry. 1986;**49**:716. DOI: 10.1136/jnnp.49.6.716

[37] Pantoni L, Bertini E, Lamassa M, Pracucci G, Inzitari D. Clinical features, risk factors, and prognosis in transient global amnesia: A follow-up study. European Journal of Neurology. 2005;**4**:350-356. DOI: 10.1111/j.1468-1331.2004.00982.x

[38] Kapur N. Transient epileptic amnesia: A clinical distinct form of neurological memory disorder. In: Markowitsch HJ, editor. Transient Global Amnesia and Related Disorders. Ashland: Hogrefe & Huber Publishers; 1990. pp. 140-151

[39] Jovin TG, Vitti RA, McCluskey LF. Evolution of temporal lobe hypoperfusion in transient global amnesia: A serial single photon emission computed tomography study. Journal of Neuroimaging. 2000;**10**:238-241. DOI: 10.1111/jon2000104238

[40] Eustache F, Desgrandes B, Petit-Taboué MC, De la Sayette V, Piot V, Sablé C, et al. Transient global amnesia: Implicit/explicit memory dissociation and PET assessment of brain perfusion and oxygen metabolism in the acute stage. Journal of Neurology, Neurosurgery, and Psychiatry. 1997;**63**:357-367. DOI: 10.1136/jnnp.63.3.357

[41] Stillhard G, Landis T, Schiess R, Regard M, Sialer G. Bitemporal hypoperfusion in transient global amnesia: 99m-Tc-HM-PAO SPECT and neuropsychological findings during and after an attack. Journal of Neurology, Neurosurgery, and Psychiatry. 1990;**53**:339-342. DOI: 10.1136/jnnp.53.4.339

[42] Sakashita Y, Sugimoto T, Taki S, Matsuda H. Abnormal cerebral flow following transient global amnesia. Journal of Neurology, Neurosurgery, and Psychiatry. 1993;**56**:1327-1329. DOI: 10.1136/jnnp.56.12.1327

[43] Lampl Y, Sadeh M, Lorberboym M. Transient global amnesia - not always a benign process. Acta Neurologica Scandinavica. 2004;**110**:75-79. DOI: 10.1111/j.1600-0404.2004.00275.x

[44] Kosuge Y, Imai T, Kawaguchi M, Kihara T, Ishige K, Ito Y. Subregion-specific vulnerability to endoplasmic reticulum stress-induced neurotoxicity in rat hippocampal neurons. Neurochemistry International. 2008;**52**:1204-1211

[45] Kessler J, Markowitsch HJ, Rudolf J, Heiss WD. Continuing cognitive impairment after isolated transient global amnesia. International Journal of Neuroscience. 2001;**106**:159-168. DOI: 10.3109/00207450109149746

[46] Howland JG, Wang YT. Synaptic plasticity in learning and memory: Stress effects in the hippocampus. Progress in Brain Research. 2008;**169**:145-158

[47] Schacter DL, Tulving E. What are the memory systems of 1994? In: Schacter DL, Tulving E, editors. Memory Systems. Vol. 1994. Cambridge, MA: The MIT Press; 1994. p. 424

[48] Warrington EK, Weiskrantz L. The amnesic syndrome: Consolidation or retrieval? Nature. 1970;**228**:628-630

[49] Nyberg L, Tulving E. Classifying human long-term memory: Evidence from converging dissociations. European Journal of Cognitive Psychology. 1996;**8**(2):163-183

[50] Cabeza R, Nyberg L. Imaging cognition II: An empirical review of 275 PET and fMRI studies. Journal of Cognitive Neuroscience. 2000;**12**:1-47

[51] Cohen NJ, Squire LR. Preserved learning and retention of pattern-analysing skill in amnesia: Dissociation of "knowing how" and "knowing that". Science. 1980;**210**:207-209

[52] Graf P, Schacter DL. Implicit and explicit memory for new associations in normal and amnesic subjects. Journal of Experimental Psychology. Learning, Memory, and Cognition. 1985;**11**:501-518

[53] Schacter DL, Wagner AD, Buckner RL. Memory systems of 1999. In: Tulving E, Craik F, editors. The Oxford Handbook of Memory. New York: Oxford University Press; 2000. pp. 627-643

[54] Byer JA, Crowley WJ. Musical performance during transient amnesia. Neurology. 1980;**30**:80-82. DOI: 10.1212/wnl.30.1.80

[55] Shuping R, Rollison R, Toole J. Transient global amnesia. Annals of Neurology. 1980;**7**:281-285. DOI: 10.1002/ana.410070313

[56] Evers S, Frese A, Bethke F. Conducting without memory – A case report on transient global amnesia. European Journal of Neurology. 2002;**9**:695-696. DOI: 10.1046/j.1468-1331.2002.00447_8.x

[57] Zajonc RB. Mere exposure: A gateway to the subliminal. Current Directions in Psychological Science. 2001;**10**(6):224-228

[58] Cheng DT, Disterhoft JF, Power JM, Ellis DA, Desmond JE. Neural substrates underlying human delay and trace eyeblink conditioning. Proceedings of the National Academy of Sciences of the United States of America. 2008;**105**(23):8108-8113

[59] Bechara A, Tranel D, Damasio H, Adolphs R, Rockland C, Damasio A. Double dissociation of conditioning and declarative knowledge relative to the amygdala and hippocampus in humans. Science. 1995;**269**:1115-1118

[60] Gabrieli JDE, McGlinchey-Berroth R, Carrillo MC, Gluck MA, Cermak LS, Disterhoft JF. Intact delay-eyeblink classical conditioning in amnesia. Behavioral Neuroscience. 1995;**109**:819-827

[61] Schacter DL, Dobbins IG, Schnyer DM. Specificity of priming: A cognitive neuroscience perspective. Nature Reviews. Neuroscience. 2004;**5**:853-862

[62] Kapur N, Abbott P, Footitt D, Millar J. Long-term perceptual priming in transient global amnesia. Brain and Cognition. 1996;**31**:63-74. DOI: 10.1006/brcg.1996.0025

[63] Tulving E. Episodic memory and autonoesis: Uniquely human? In: Terrace HS, Metcalfe J, editors. The Missing Link in Cognition. New York, NY: Oxford University Press; 2005. pp. 4-56

[64] Regard M, Landis T. Transient global amnesia: Neuropsychological dysfunction during attack and recovery in two 'pure' cases. Journal of Neurology, Neurosurgery, and Psychiatry. 1984;**47**:668-672. DOI: 10.1136/jnnp.47.7.668

[65] Hodges JR. Semantic memory and frontal executive function during transient global amnesia. Journal of Neurology, Neurosurgery, and Psychiatry. 1994;**57**:605-608. DOI: 10.1136/jnnp.57.5.605

[66] Eustache F, Desgrandes B, Laville P, Guillery B, Lalevée C, Schaeffer S, et al.

Episodic memory in transient global amnesia: Encoding, storage, or retrieval deficit? Journal of Neurology, Neurosurgery, and Psychiatry. 1999;**66**:148-154. DOI: 10.1136/jnnp.66.2.148

[67] Guillery B, Desgrandes B, De la Sayette V, Landeau B, Eustache F, Baron J. Transient global amnesia: Concomitant episodic memory and positron emission tomography assessment in two additional patients. Neuroscience Letters. 2002;**325**:62-66. DOI: 10.1016/S0304-3940(02)00233-1

[68] Hainselin M, Quinette P, Desgranges B, Martinaud O, Hannequin D, de La Sayette V, et al. Can we remember future actions yet forget the last two minutes? Study in transient global amnesia. Journal of Cognitive Neuroscience. 2011;**23**(12):4138-4149

[69] Guillery B, Desgrandes B, Piolino P, Laville P, De la Sayette V, Eustache F. Extensive temporally graded retrograde amnesia for personal episodic facts in transient global amnesia. Neurocase. 2000;**6**:205-210. DOI: 10.1080/13554790008402771

[70] Quinette P, Guillery B, Desgrandes B, De la Sayette V, Viader F, Eustache F. Working memory and executive functions in transient global amnesia. Brain 2003;126:1917-1934. DOI: 10.1093/brain/awg201

[71] Evans J, Wilson B, Wraight P, Hodges J. Neuropsychological and SPECT scan findings during and after transient global amnesia: Evidence for the differential impairment of remote episodic memory. Journal of Neurology, Neurosurgery, and Psychiatry. 1993;**56**:1227-1230. DOI: 10.1136/jnnp.56.11.1227

[72] Hodges JR. Transient Amnesia. Clinical and Neuropsychological Aspects. London: W.B. Saunders; 1991. p. 171

[73] Guillery B, Desgranges B, Katis S, de la Sayette V, Viader F, Eustache F. Semantic acquisition without memories: Evidence from transient global amnesia. Neuroreport. 2001;**12**(17):3865-3869

[74] Beauregard M, Weiner J, Gold D, Chertkow H. Word priming during and after transient global amnesia. Neurocase. 1997;**3**(6):451-459

[75] Maguire EA, Frith CD. Lateral asymmetry in the hippocampal response to the remoteness of autobiographical memories. The Journal of Neuroscience. 2003;**23**:5302-5307

[76] Bayley PJ, Squire LR. Failure to acquire new semantic knowledge in patients with large medial temporal lobe lesions. Hippocampus. 2005;**15**(2):273-280

[77] Baddeley AD. Working Memory. Oxford: Oxford University Press; 1986. 289 p

[78] Stracciari A, Rebucci GG, Gallassi R. Transient global amnesia: Neuropsychological study of a 'pure' case. Journal of Neurology. 1987;**234**:126-127. DOI: 10.1007/BF00314119

[79] Bucuk M, Muzur A, Willheim K, Jurjevic A, Tomic Z, Tuskan-Mohar L. Make love to forget: Two cases of transient global amnesia triggered by sexual intercourse. Collegium Antropologicum. 2004;**28**:899-905

[80] Noël A, Quinette P, Guillery-Girard B, Dayan J, Piolino P, Marquis S, et al. Psychopathological factors, memory disorders and transient global amnesia. The British Journal of Psychiatry. 2008;**193**(2):145-151. DOI: 10.1192/bjp.bp.107.045716

[81] Gordon B, Marin O. Transient global amnesia: an extensive case report. Journal of Neurology, Neurosurgery,

and Psychiatry. 1979;**42**:572-575. DOI: 10.1093/neucas/2.1.51-e

[82] Caffarra P, Moretti G, Mazzucchi A, Parma M. Neuropsychological testing during transient global amnesia episode and its follow-up. Acta Neurologica Scandinavica. 1981;**63**:44-50. DOI: 10.1111/j.1600-0404.1981.tb00747.x

[83] Hodges JR, Ward C. Observations during transient global amnesia. Brain. 1989;**112**:595-620

[84] Shuttleworth E, Wise G. Transient global amnesia due to arterial embolism. Archives of Neurology. 1973;**29**:340-342. DOI: 10.1093/neucas/2.1.51-p

[85] Goldenberg G, Podreka I, Pfaffelmeyer N, Wessely P, Deecke L. Thalamic ischemia in transient global amnesia: A SPECT study. Neurology. 1991;**41**:1748-1752. DOI: 10.1212/WNL.41.11.1748

[86] Kritchevsky M, Squire LR, Zouzounis JA. Transient global amnesia: Characterization of anterograde and retrograde amnesia. Neurology. 1988;**38**:213-219. DOI: 10.1212/WNL.38.2.213

[87] Yonelinas AP. The nature of recollection and familiarity: A review of 30 years of research. Journal of Memory and Language. 2002;**46**:441-517

[88] Gardiner JM, Richardson-Klavehn A. Remembering and knowing. In: Tulving E, Craik FIM, editors. The Oxford Handbook of Memory. New York: Oxford University Press; 2000. pp. 229-244

[89] Guillery-Girard B, Desgrandes B, Urban C, Piolino P, De la Sayette V, Eustache F. The dynamic time course of memory recovery in transient global amnesia. Journal of Neurology, Neurosurgery, and Psychiatry. 2004;**75**:1532-1540. DOI: 10.1136/jnnp.2003.024968

[90] Fivush R. The development of autobiographical memory. Annual Review of Psychology. 2011;**62**:559-582. DOI: 10.1146/annurev.psych.121208.131702

[91] Kopelman MD, Wilson B, Baddeley A. The Autobiographical Memory Interview. Thames Valley Test Company: Bury St Edmunds; 1990

[92] Tulving E, Schacter DL, McLachlan DR, Moscovitch M. Priming of semantic autobiographical knowledge: A case study of retrograde amnesia. Brain and Cognition. 1988;**8**:2-20

[93] Ribot T. Les maladies de la mémoire. Paris: Ballière; 1881. 169 p

[94] Zeman A. Episodic memory in transient global amnesia. Journal of Neurology, Neurosurgery, and Psychiatry. 1999;**66**:135

[95] Scoville WB, Milner B. Loss of recent memory after bilateral hippocampal lesions. Journal of Neurology, Neurosurgery, and Psychiatry. 1957;**20**:11-21. DOI: 10.1136/jnnp.20.1.11

[96] Tulving E. Organization of memory: Quo vadis? In: Gazzaniga MS, editor. The Cognitive Neurosciences. Cambridge, MA: The MIT Press. 1995. pp. 753-847

[97] Squire LR, Wixted JT. The cognitive neuroscience of human memory since H.M.Annual Review of Neuroscience. 2011;**34**:259-288. DOI: 10.1146/annurev-neuro-061010-113720

[98] Winocur G, Moscovitch M. Memory transformation and systems consolidation. Journal of the International Neuropsychological Society. 2011;**17**:766-780. DOI: 10.1017/S1355617711000683

[99] Moscovitch M, Cabeza R, Winocur G, Nadel L. Episodic memory

and beyond: The hippocampus and neocortex in transformation. Annual Review of Psychology. 2016;**67**:105-134

[100] Cipolotti L, Shallice T, Chan D, Fox N, Scahill R, et al. Long-term retrograde amnesia... the crucial role of the hippocampus. Neuropsychologia. 2001;**39**:151-172

[101] Maguire EA, Nannery R, Spiers HJ. Navigation around London by a taxi driver with bilateral hippocampal lesions. Brain. 2006;**129**:2894-2907. DOI: 10.1093/brain/awl286

[102] Squire LR, Zola SM. Episodic memory, semantic memory, and amnesia. Hippocampus. 1998;**8**:205-211

[103] Reed JM, Squire LR. Retrograde amnesia for facts and events: Findings from four new cases. The Journal of Neuroscience. 1998;**18**:3943-3945

[104] Gilboa A, Winocur G, Grady CL, Hevenor SJ, Moscovitch M. Remembering our past: Functional neuroanatomy of recollection of recent and very remote personal events. Cerebral Cortex. 2004;**14**:1214-1225

[105] Bonnici HM, Chadwick MJ, Lutti A, Hassabis D, Weiskopf N, Maguire EA. Detecting representations of recent and remote autobiographical memories in vmPFC and hippocampus. The Journal of Neuroscience. 2012;**32**:16982-16991

[106] O'Keefe J, Dostrovsky J. The hippocampus as a spatial map. Preliminary evidence from unit activity in the freely-moving rat. Brain Research. 1971;**34**:171-175. DOI: 10.1016/0006-8993(71)90358-1

[107] O'Keefe J, Nadel L. The Hippocampus as a Cognitive Map. Oxford: Clarendon Press; 1978. 570 p. DOI: 10.2307/1422119

[108] Clark IA, Maguire EA. Remembering preservation in hippocampal amnesia. Annual Review of Psychology. 2016;**67**:51-82. DOI: 10.1146/annurev-psych-122414-033739

[109] Spiers HJ, Maguire EA. Thoughts, behaviour, and brain dynamics during navigation in the real world. NeuroImage. 2006;**31**:1826-1840. DOI: 10.1016/j.neuroimage.2006.01.037

[110] Hirshhorn M, Grady C, Rosenbaum RS, Winocur G, Moscovitch M. The hippocampus is involved in mental navigation for a recently learned, but not a highly familiar environment: A longitudinal fMRI study. Hippocampus. 2012;**22**:842-852

[111] Eichenbaum H. Time cells in the hippocampus: A new dimension for mapping memories. Nature Reviews. Neuroscience. 2014;**15**:732-744

[112] Mullally SL, Maguire EA. Counterfactual thinking in patients with amnesia. Hippocampus. 2014;**24**:1261-1266

[113] Schacter DL, Addis DR, Hassabis D, Martin VC, Spreng RN, Szpunar KK. The future of memory: Remembering, imagining, and the brain. Neuron. 2012;**76**:677-694

[114] Cohen NJ, Eichenbaum H. Memory, Amnesia and the Hippocampal System. Cambridge: MIT Press; 1993. 326 p

[115] Eichenbaum H. Hippocampus: Cognitive processes and neural representations that underlie declarative memory. Neuron. 2004;**44**:109-120

[116] Eichenbaum H, Yonelinas AR, Ranganath C. The medial temporal lobe and recognition memory. Annual Review of Neuroscience. 2007;**30**:123-152. DOI: 10.1146/annurev.neuro.30.051606.094328

[117] Ranganath C. A unified framework for the functional organization of the medial temporal lobes and the phenomenology of episodic memory. Hippocampus. 2010;**20**:1263-1290

[118] Bird CM, Burgess N. The hippocampus supports recognition memory for familiar words but not unfamiliar faces. Current Biology. 2008;**18**:1932-1936. DOI: 10.1016/j.cub.2008.10.046

[119] Mayes AR, Holdstock JS, Isaac CL, Montaldi D, Grigor J, et al. Associative recognition in a patient with selective hippocampal lesions and relatively normal item recognition. Hippocampus. 2004;**14**:763-784

[120] Konkel A, Warren DE, Duff MC, Tranel D, Cohen NJ. Hippocampal amnesia impairs all manner of relational memory. Frontiers in Human Neuroscience. 2008;**2**:15. DOI: 10.3389/neuro.09.015.2008

[121] Hassabis D, Maguire EA. Deconstructing episodic memory with construction. Trends in Cognitive Sciences. 2007;**11**:299-306. DOI: 10.1016/j.tics.2007.05.001

[122] McGlinchey-Berroth R, Carrillo MC, Gabrieli JD, Brawn CM, Disterhoft JF. Impaired trace eyeblink conditioning in bilateral, medial-temporal lobe amnesia. Behavioral Neuroscience. 1997;**111**(5):873-882

[123] Nees F, Griebe M, Ebert A, Ruttorf M, Gerber B, Wolf OT, et al. Implicit learning in transient global amnesia and the role of stress. Frontiers in Behavioral Neuroscience. 2016;**10**:222. DOI: 10.3389/fnbeh.2016.00222

[124] Olsen RK, Moses SN, Riggs L, Ryan JD. The hippocampus supports multiple cognitive processes through relational binding and comparison. Frontiers in Human Neuroscience. 2012;**6**:146

[125] Hunsaker MR, Kesner RP. The operation of pattern separation and pattern completion processes associated with different attributes or domains of memory. Neuroscience and Biobehavioral Reviews. 2013;**37**:36-58

[126] Buckner RL. The role of the hippocampus in prediction and imagination. Annual Review of Psychology. 2010;**61**:27-48

[127] Schacter DL, Addis DR. Constructive memory: The ghosts of past and future. Nature. 2007;**445**:27. DOI: 10.1038/445027a

[128] Klein SB, Loftus J, Kihlstrom JF. Memory and temporal experience: The effects of episodic memory loss on an amnesic patient's ability to remember the past and imagine the future. Social Cognitive and Affective Neuroscience. 2002;**20**:353-379

[129] Hassabis D, Kumaran D, Vann SD, Maguire EA. Patients with hippocampal amnesia cannot imagine new experiences. Proceedings of the National Academy of Sciences of the United States of America. 2007;**104**:1726-1731

[130] Rosenbaum RS, Gilboa A, Levine B, Winocur G, Moscovitch M. Amnesia as an impairment of detail generation and binding: Evidence from personal, fictional, and semantic narratives in K.C. Neuropsychologia. 2009;**47**:2181-2187

[131] Juskenaite A, Quinette P, Desgranges B, de La Sayette V, Viader F, Eustache F. Mental simulation of future scenarios in transient global amnesia. Neuropsychologia. 2014;**63**:1-9

[132] Einstein GO, McDaniel MA, Richardson SL, Guynn MJ, Cunfer AR. Aging and prospective memory: Examining the influences of self-initiated retrieval processes. Journal of Experimental Psychology.

Learning, Memory, and Cognition. *2018*;**21**(4):996-1007. DOI: 10.1037/0278-7393.21.4.996

[133] Smallwood J, Schooler JW. The Science of Mind Wandering: Empirically Navigating the Stream of Consciousness. Annual Review of Psychology. 2015;**66**(1):487-518

[134] McCormick C, Rosenthal CR, Miller TD, Maguire EA. Mind-wandering in people with hippocampal damage. The Journal of Neuroscience. 2008;**38**(11):2745-2754. DOI: 10.1523/JNEUROSCI.1812-17.2018